Disease Free

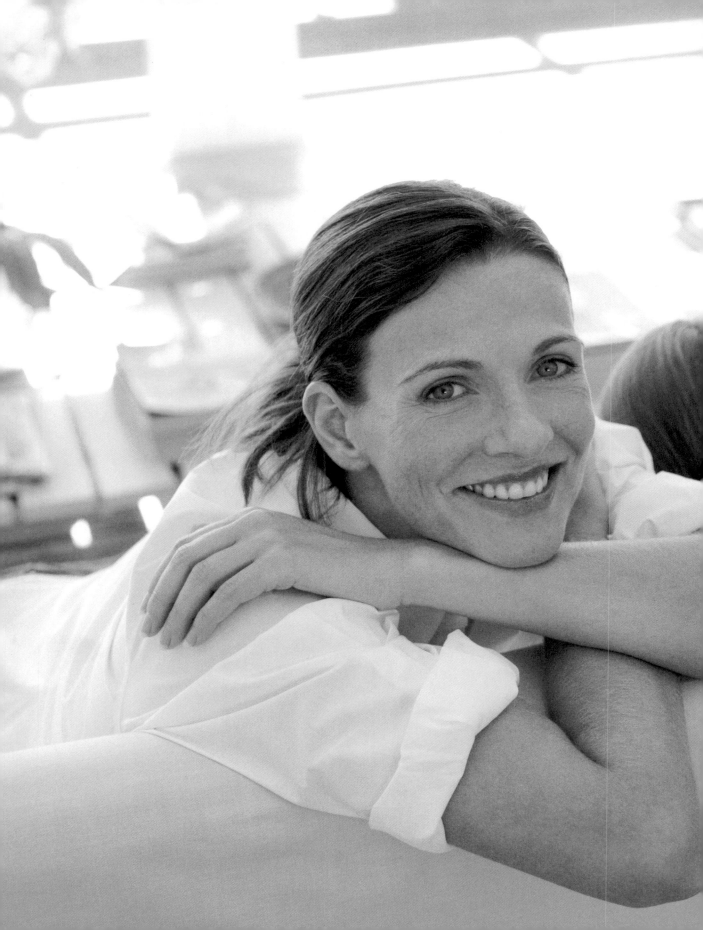

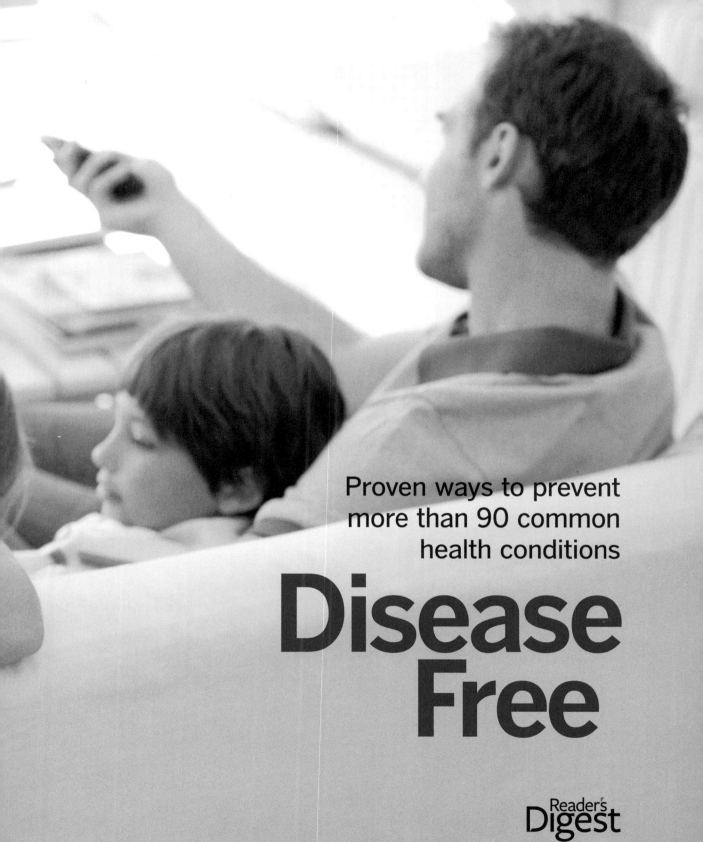

Proven ways to prevent
more than 90 common
health conditions

Disease Free

Reader's Digest

Published by The Reader's Digest Association, Inc.
London   New York   Sydney   Montreal

CONSULTANTS

Vince Forte BA (Cantab) MB BS(Lond) MRCGP MSc DA

Fiona Hunter BSc Nutrition Dip Dietetics

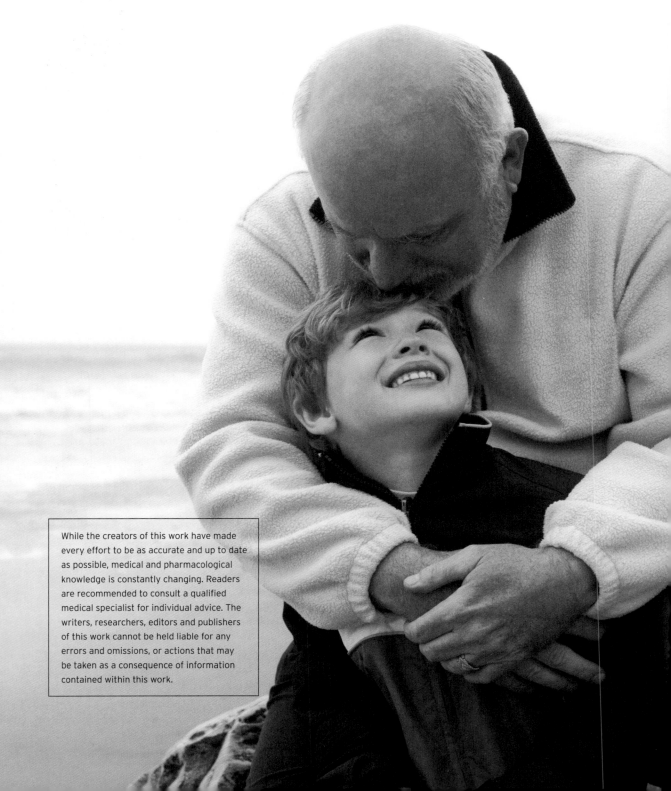

Contents

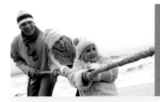

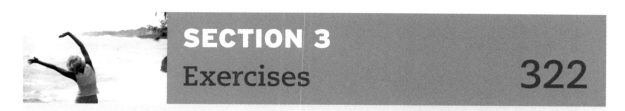

SECTION 3
Exercises
322

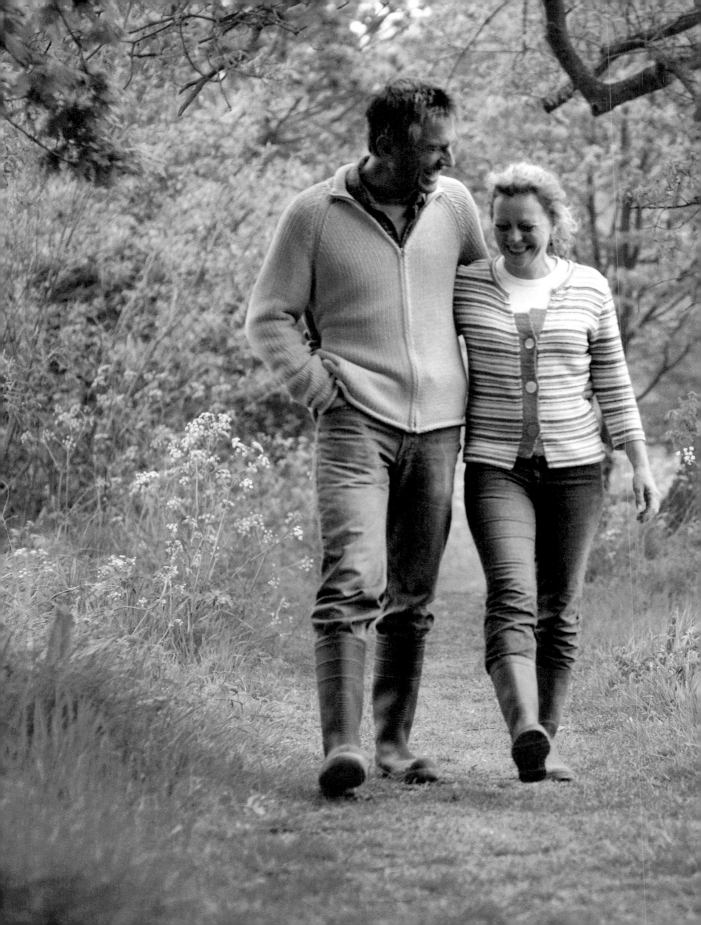

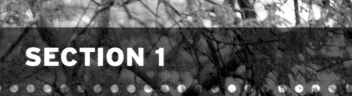

SECTION 1

Disease-free Living

Whoever said 'life is short' didn't realise just how long you can live – and how well – when you're free of illness. Many happy, healthy years is an attractive goal.

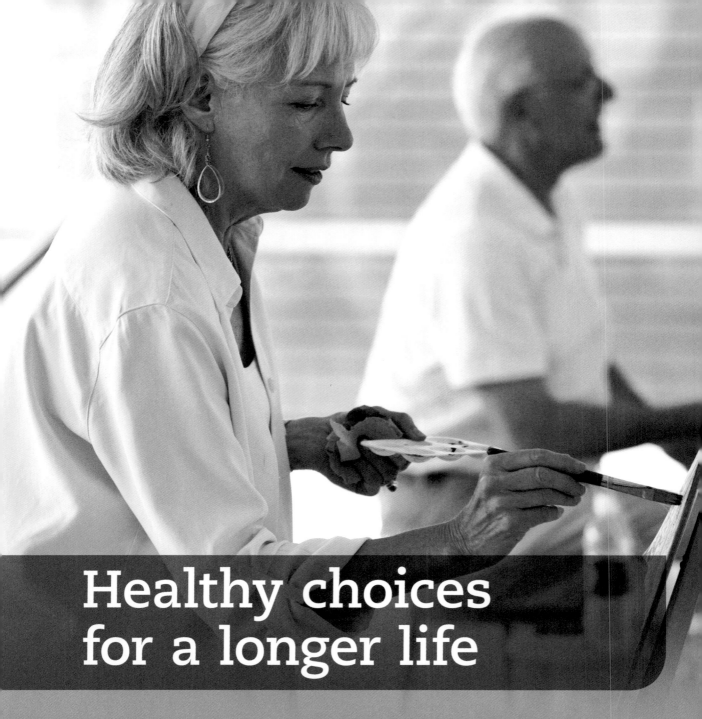

Healthy choices for a longer life

What if you were told you could live an extra decade? We're not talking about years of withering away in a nursing home but about really living. Pursuing a new hobby, playing with your great-grandchildren or fulfilling other dreams. If you stay disease free, it's not just possible – it's likely.

You hold the power

About half of all adults live with one or more chronic conditions, yet many of the diseases people face today are preventable. In creating this book, more than 100 doctors specialising in preventive medicine were surveyed by Reader's Digest in the USA, and asked a raft of questions relating to chronic diseases and how to avoid them. More than half the doctors in this survey said that at least 60 per cent of cases of chronic disease could be avoided.

The upshot of this is that the power you hold to prevent disease and live a long healthy life is nothing short of amazing. One 2008 US study of more than 2,000 men found that those who met four simple criteria – they didn't smoke, weren't overweight, exercised regularly and consumed alcohol in moderation, if at all – lived an average of 10 years longer than men who didn't fit at least one of these descriptions – and 10 years of good health at that. More than two-thirds of the men who lived to 90 rated their late-life health as either excellent or very good. And it's reasonable to surmise that the men who lived longer were also happier; you'll find out more about the connection between health and emotional wellbeing later on.

The men in the study didn't make dramatic changes to protect themselves from disease, and you don't have to either, regardless of whether you're male or female. In fact, doing just one thing – getting half an hour of exercise on most days – could dramatically turn your health around and strengthen your resistance to disease.

You may already be taking positive steps to help prevent disease. Did you have a flu jab this year? Do you have regular cervical smears? When did you last have your blood pressure checked? Study after study confirms that each of these measures saves lives. In 'Key steps to disease prevention', starting on page 60, you'll learn which ones scored highest in the survey. All of the steps outlined in that chapter can be seen as a simple 'action guide' for living a healthier life. But first, here are a few highlights of the survey and Reader's Digest's own research.

Your life, your health

Our understanding of what causes chronic disease has changed radically over the past decade. Even as researchers discover more links between genetic make-up and health, it's clearer than ever that the underlying causes of most chronic diseases are lifestyle factors most people can control.

> *Doing just **one thing** – getting half an hour of exercise on most days – could dramatically **turn your health around** and strengthen your resistance to disease.*

Say goodbye to disease

Doctors list the following diseases as those that can be virtually eliminated with lifestyle measures.

- Chronic obstructive pulmonary disease
- Type 2 diabetes
- High blood pressure
- Heart disease
- Lung cancer
- Obesity
- Stroke
- Sexually transmitted infections

For some, the initial response to that statement is: 'How can I help or prevent heart disease or diabetes when I have a strong family history of those conditions?' 'What if I come from a long line of people who had heart disease or diabetes?' 'What good will eating salads and exercising do if I was dealt a poor hand of genes at birth?'

These are fair questions, but the science is indisputable: genes may increase your risk for certain conditions, but lifestyle choices have a far greater impact on your health and longevity. Imagine the factors that determine your life span depicted in a pie chart. Studies of identical twins, who share identical genes, suggest that DNA dictates only 25 to 33 per cent of how long you live, or a quarter to a third of the pie. The rest? That depends on how you live. Unfortunately, or fortunately, depending on how you look at it, the way we live – what and how much we eat and drink, the amount of stress we're under, what we do or don't do with our leisure time – is the reason so many of us accumulate health problems as we age.

The 'new' causes of disease

In the Reader's Digest Disease Prevention Survey (see page 11), the number-one cause of chronic disease wasn't bad genes; it wasn't even high cholesterol. It was something many people assume is relatively harmless: high blood pressure, which is why it's often called the silent killer. Fortunately, it's a condition that most doctors listed as preventable. If you have untreated high blood pressure, now is the time to deal with it.

Also ranked above genes and high cholesterol in the Disease Prevention Survey was something you might find more or less right under your nose: intra-abdominal fat, the kind of fat that surrounds internal organs and contributes to everything from diabetes to heart attack. If you have a large waistline, you probably have this type of fat (see page 24 for more details).

If you're overweight, there's a pretty good chance you have another high-ranking disease risk: insulin resistance, in which the body no longer uses the hormone insulin effectively to transport blood glucose into muscle cells. The most likely explanation for the current wave of insulin resistance is our sedentary lifestyle and the foods that many of us tend to favour, including potatoes, white rice and pasta, white bread and sugary processed foods – all of which raise blood glucose quickly, and essentially begin to wear out the insulin response. It's a major leap down the path to diabetes, but insulin resistance is also turning out to contribute to heart attack, stroke and poor circulation.

High blood pressure, intra-abdominal fat and insulin resistance are all linked to chronic heart disease, the leading cause of death in the developed world. But they have something else in common: their solutions. If all of us lost excess weight, exercised more often and ate more fruit and vegetables and less saturated fat, these conditions would be drastically reduced in a relatively short amount of time.

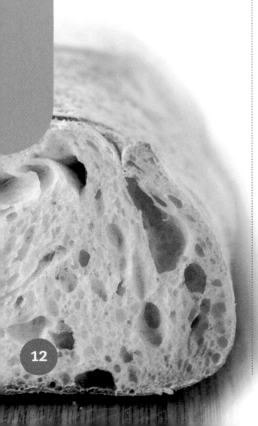

The 'new' keys to health

Although the basic messages about good health haven't changed, the survey revealed a new health message. The experts who participated made it clear that having positive relationships was intimately connected to health. In the survey, 79 per cent of the doctors polled said that being socially isolated was to the 'utmost detriment' of or 'extremely detrimental' to health. And they rated having 'happy interactions with friends and family' above 'cutting most saturated fat from your diet' as prevention strategies.

One reason why family and friends may be so important is because they help combat stress and depression. And many doctors mentioned stress as a contributing factor in major disease. They ranked it as even more dangerous than being 15kg (33lb) overweight. Depression was ranked significantly higher than high cholesterol as a condition with the greatest potential for causing chronic disease.

Simply put, what happens in your mind and heart (the figurative one this time) affects your body in profound ways. Chronic stress lowers the immune system's ability to function effectively – even making vaccines less effective. It raises levels of stress hormones, such as cortisol, and high cortisol levels can not only keep you up at night, they can also raise blood pressure, contribute to high blood glucose and increase intra-abdominal fat. There's also the more obvious effect that stress, depression and loneliness have on us every day. As one doctor put it, 'Mental stress and conflict, etc., drive the majority of bad physical habits and practices' – in other words, getting too little sleep, being too sedentary and eating too many calories.

Chronic stress also raises the risk of depression, and if you're depressed the chances are you're not going to exercise or eat well. Depression often goes hand in hand with a whole litany of diseases, from heart disease to cancer, and doctors aren't always sure which causes which. But they do know that having depression and a serious illness tends to make the symptoms of that illness worse.

Considering the known dangers of stress and depression, it's not surprising that many doctors in the survey advocated relaxation techniques such as meditation and happy daily interactions with

Surprising advice from the prevention experts

Staying healthy is not all about eating a suitable volume of fruit and vegetables, although that obviously helps. In the Disease Prevention Survey, the following advice appears to confirm that health really does originate from a life well lived.

- 'Believe in something good.'
- 'Focus on a higher sense of purpose.'
- 'Develop your unique potential.'
- 'Eat less, exercise more and have fun.'
- 'Love the ones you're with (spouse, children, extended family, neighbours, colleagues).'
- 'Achieve balance in your life.'
- 'Exercise every day, eat a well-balanced diet, maintain meaningful social interactions and relationships, and choose work that is important to you.'
- 'Find meaning in your life.'
- 'Get 8 hours or more of sleep a day.'
- 'Manage stress and enjoy your friends.'
- 'Stay positive and have a family doctor who helps you to prevent disease and improve health.'

Being **socially isolated** *was to the 'utmost detriment' of or 'extremely detrimental' to health*

13

others. It's important to find something meaningful or fulfilling to do in life, or to have a higher sense of purpose to both take our minds off our worries and to provide inspiration for daily life. Many doctors know that having this kind of focus can be just as important as medication.

It can be difficult to know the answer to the question of whether you are connected to others in a meaningful way, so ask yourself: 'Do I have people I can turn to?', 'Do I get up every day with a sense of optimism or purpose?' or 'Do I dread my to-do list or feel nothing much at all because, actually, I lost the sense of what was possible many years ago?' It's never too late to become interested in something new or to reach out and make personal connections with others.

Getting yourself to act

People who exercise and eat well tend to live a long time, often surviving others by up to a decade or more. So why don't more of us get moving? Because it can be hard to get started if exercise has never been a regular habit. The chances are that choosing just one healthy habit to adopt, or one bad habit to quit, will make you feel good both physically and emotionally – good enough to want to choose another. On pages 18-19, the quiz will help you identify your current habits.

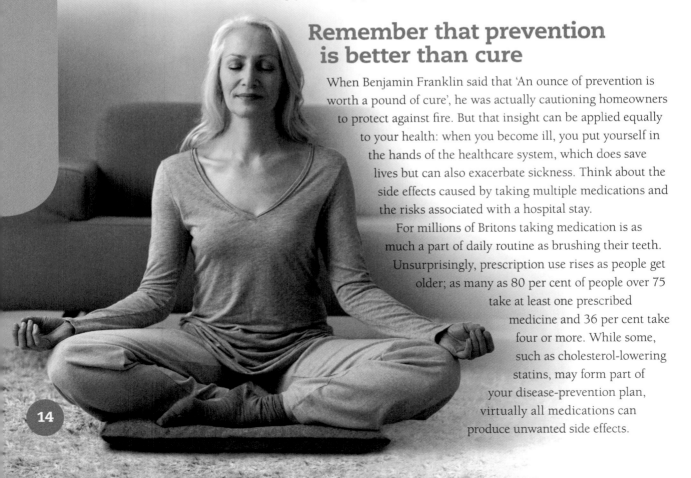

Remember that prevention is better than cure

When Benjamin Franklin said that 'An ounce of prevention is worth a pound of cure', he was actually cautioning homeowners to protect against fire. But that insight can be applied equally to your health: when you become ill, you put yourself in the hands of the healthcare system, which does save lives but can also exacerbate sickness. Think about the side effects caused by taking multiple medications and the risks associated with a hospital stay.

For millions of Britons taking medication is as much a part of daily routine as brushing their teeth. Unsurprisingly, prescription use rises as people get older; as many as 80 per cent of people over 75 take at least one prescribed medicine and 36 per cent take four or more. While some, such as cholesterol-lowering statins, may form part of your disease-prevention plan, virtually all medications can produce unwanted side effects.

14

One example is medication for high blood pressure, a condition that affects about a billion people worldwide. Only about a third of people who are prescribed medication for this condition are able to bring their blood pressure into the safe zone. One well-documented reason is that many people stop taking medication, often as a result of side effects. One study found that nearly 70 per cent of people taking calcium-channel blockers developed unpleasant side effects.

A 2008 analysis concluded that there was little proof that widely used antidepressants such as fluoxetine (Prozac) and paroxetine (Seroxat) offer any benefit to people with moderate depression. And another recent study showed that the cholesterol-lowering drug ezetimibe (Ezetrol) may not keep arteries clear of life-threatening plaque. Meanwhile, regular exercise, a happy personal life and a healthy, balanced diet appear to help prevent both depression and high cholesterol in many people.

It's been said that a hospital is no place for sick people, and it's true. In the UK, one study showed that an average of 9 per cent of hospital patients acquire an infection during their stay. Simple urinary tract infections are among the most common, but hospitals the world over are increasingly plagued by 'super-bugs' such as MRSA (methicillin-resistant *Staphylococcus aureus*), an infection immune to most antibiotics, which can cause pneumonia and other life-threatening infections.In 2007, an estimated 0.2 per cent of all deaths in Australia were caused by complications arising from medical or surgical care.

All this news could make even the most die-hard couch potato skip the takeaway, walk for an extra 10 minutes, and take other steps to avoid the risk of a heart attack, which would necessitate a stay in hospital.

Decide to be healthy

That's the sum of it: good health is a goal you can either reach for or ignore. Only you can decide for yourself whether or not your health is a priority. If you don't make any effort to eat well, exercise or control stress, you've decided that it's not, even if you don't think about it that way. But it's never too late to change your mind.

When asked about other significant causes of chronic disease, one doctor wrote, 'Risky behaviour, even when the person understands the risks', which accounts for many cases of poor health. Most of us know what it takes to stay healthy; we just don't always do it.

Then and now

Available statistics from 1900 show that British people were most likely to die from a respiratory or infectious diseases. But improved hygiene and sanitation later prevented many premature deaths from diseases such as dysentery. Today, the diseases that kill us are often linked to the way we live.

Top 4 causes of death in 1900	Top 4 causes of death in 2011
1. Respiratory diseases	1. Cancer
2. Infectious disease	2. Ischaemic heart disease
3. Cancer	3. Respiratory diseases
4. Diarrhoea/dysentery	4. Stroke

Source:ONS/BMJ

The solution for changing old, bad habits isn't always obvious. One doctor polled for the survey suggested: 'Rely on your inner strength to change your ways'. And the source of that strength will be different for everyone. Perhaps your grandchildren make you want to live a longer, healthier life. Maybe you can use the 'you can do it' attitude that made you a success in your career to help transform your lifestyle. Or think of a friend or relative who has struggled with the difficulties of ill health. You may know first-hand the toll that being sick takes on your mental wellbeing, and that may be motivation enough to make changes in your life. Consider the health problems your parents had and promise yourself that you will try to avoid them. Your health, to a large extent, is up to you, although it's also true that certain diseases are unavoidable for some people.

*Only **you** can decide for yourself whether or not **your health** is a priority*

The bulk of this book is geared towards helping you reduce your risk for conditions you're worried about or may be susceptible to. Following the advice in *Key steps to disease prevention* starting on page 60 will go a long way towards helping you stay healthy, but for detailed risk-reduction strategies for specific conditions, turn to the entry for that disease or major symptom in Part Two.

Working with your doctor

Understandably, prevention may be neglected in favour of urgent treatment in busy doctors' surgeries, so it's up to you to take charge. Historically, healthcare systems have been focused on the care and cure of diseases after they have manifested themselves – care that is sometimes delivered too

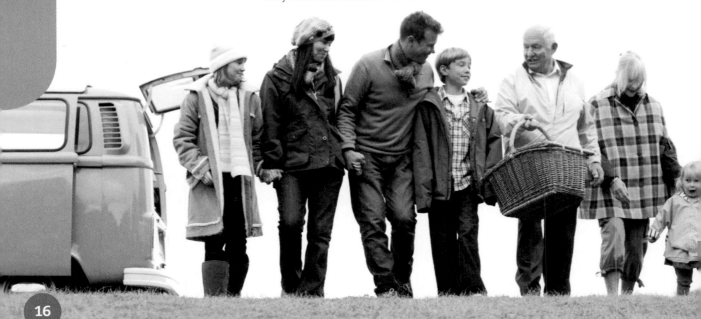

16

late. In the past, there has been far too little emphasis on preventing diseases in the first place.Studies show that many doctors have failed to give even the most obvious prevention advice, such as telling overweight patients to lose weight or encouraging patients who smoke to quit.

In fact, preventive medicine has become an increasingly important part of general practice in the UK. A recent study found that most British GPs rated it as very important and spend 10 per cent to 30 per cent of each consultation on it. But GPs are also busy dealing with acute illness and packed waiting rooms. As GP Dr Brian Gaffney, medical director of NHS Direct recently told *Pulse* magazine, 'We know as GPs we can't cope with demand for our practice appointments.'

Fortunately, the NHS also provides many services to promote preventive medicine and self-care, including diet and exercise schemes, smoking cessation clinics, screening services and immunisation clinics, often carried out by teams within the practices. So, increasingly, it's up to you as a patient to ask and find out what preventive services are available and to play a part in understanding the importance of prevention, and make sure it's on the agenda.

Whenever you walk into your doctor's surgery, have a list of questions or problems to discuss, with the pressing preventive issues at the top. Try to raise your concerns early on, rather than waiting until the end of an appointment to ask questions. Busy doctors can quickly become frustrated with people who say, 'By the way, Doctor', with one foot out the door.

If you're already coping with a chronic condition, your doctor may need to spend most or all of your visit discussing medications and other treatments. If you run out of time and don't get to talk about exercise, diet or other protective steps you could be taking, make another appointment to discuss this solely – or ask for a referral to a practice nurse or some other NHS service that might be able to help. Making time to discuss these issues is an essential element of your medical consultations and could be crucial to your recovery and future good health.

It's up to you

Rates of chronic disease are rising fast, so it's important to remember that prevention is mainly about the things you yourself do outside your doctor's surgery – what you make for dinner, how much time you spend being active in a positive way, whether you're an angry or a happy person. As one doctor from the Disease Prevention Survey put it, 'Don't simply wait for health professionals to correct your health problems after they become obvious', because there is no one who can prevent disease and debilitating major symptoms better than individuals can themselves.

It is quite clear that an ounce of prevention is, indeed, worth a pound of cure. If you want to stay healthy throughout life – for many more years ahead – then the time to start taking control of your health is now.

Vaccines for adults

No matter how much you exercise and watch what you eat, any plan for disease-proofing your body needs a shot or two in the arm – literally, in some cases.

Flu jabs
The most obvious form of defence against disease you can seek in a doctor's surgery is a flu jab. In addition to the chills, aches and other miserable symptoms brought on by influenza, the condition can lead to life-threatening complications such as pneumonia. A flu jab cuts your risk by up to 90 per cent. If you haven't discussed vaccinations with your doctor before now, don't assume that you're up to date.

Other vaccines
You may also be eligible for one of several newer vaccines that guard against conditions such as pneumococcal disease, cervical cancer and shingles.

Quiz: is your health on track?

It's tempting to blame many health issues on genetic predisposition, but in most cases it's the way we live our day-to-day lives that ultimately determines what happens to our bodies and whether or not we develop health problems that can deplete our energy and general zest for living.

The Reader's Digest Disease Prevention Survey polled more than 100 specialist doctors and, among other questions, asked them how beneficial or harmful they believed certain habits to be. Take this quiz to find out how they would rate your current health profile. If your lifestyle needs modifying to improve your odds of living disease-free, make sure you read *Key steps to disease prevention*, starting on page 60, for practical advice on what you can do.

Good health habits

For each healthy habit you claim, note down the number of allotted 'smiley faces' in the far right column.

○ Regularly eat five servings of fruit and vegetables daily	☺☺☺☺☺	
○ Have two or more glasses of skimmed milk or small pots of low-fat yoghurt daily	☺☺☺	
○ Have no more than 4 units (men) or 3 units (women) of alcohol on any day	☺☺☺	
○ Get 20 to 30 minutes of moderate aerobic exercise on most days	☺☺☺☺☺	
○ Do strength training two or three times a week	☺☺☺☺	
○ Meditate or practise another stress-relief technique regularly	☺☺☺☺	
○ Always wash your hands after using the toilet and before cooking	☺☺☺☺☺	
○ Brush your teeth twice daily and floss (or use an interdental brush) daily	☺☺☺☺	
○ Get an annual flu jab if your GP advises it	☺☺☺☺	
○ Have your blood pressure checked annually or as advised by your GP	☺☺☺☺	
○ Have your cholesterol levels checked annually or as advised by your GP	☺☺☺	

YOUR FINAL SCORE

Add up your bad and good health habits, then subtract the total number of bad habits from the total good habits to get your final score, then see below to interpret the results.

Over 20: Excellent
Congratulations. You're living a life that will help to keep you disease-free.

14 to 20: Good Your lifestyle is reasonably healthy. Look for at least one more good habit to adopt and at least one bad habit to lose.

8 to 13: Average You're not doing badly, but there's still room for improvement. Look for a few more good habits to adopt and a few bad ones to lose.

0 to 7: Worrying You're getting by with a lifestyle that is healthy in part, but there's still room for improvement. Look carefully to see where you missed out on smiley faces and collected too many frowns.

-1 to -7: Dangerous It's time to take your health more seriously, before you're dealing with treating disease rather than preventing it. Some unhealthy habits are probably dragging down your score; look back to see where you can improve it.

-8 or lower: Very dangerous You're not looking to improve your health, and are clinging to some harmful habits. Start by making just one positive change at a time. Every step counts.

Bad health habits

For each bad habit you have, note down the allotted number of 'sad faces' in the far right column.

Regularly eat foods containing trans fat (hydrogenated oil)	☹☹☹	
Regularly eat packaged goods, canned soups, chips and other processed foods high in sodium	☹☹☹☹	
Add salt to food at most meals	☹☹☹	
Eat out (or have takeaways) more than three times a week	☹☹☹☹	
Regularly drink more than 4 units (men) or 3 units (women) of alcohol on most days of the week	☹☹☹	
Eat white bread, white rice or white pasta at most meals	☹☹☹	
Have a dessert after your evening meal on most nights	☹☹☹	
Smoke regularly	☹☹☹☹☹	
Smoke an occasional cigarette	☹☹☹☹	
Don't have regular contact with others	☹☹☹☹☹	
Live with frequent and uncontrolled stress	☹☹☹☹	
Are more than 15kg (33lb) overweight	☹☹☹☹	
Get less than 7 hours of sleep a night	☹☹☹	

☺   —   ☹   =

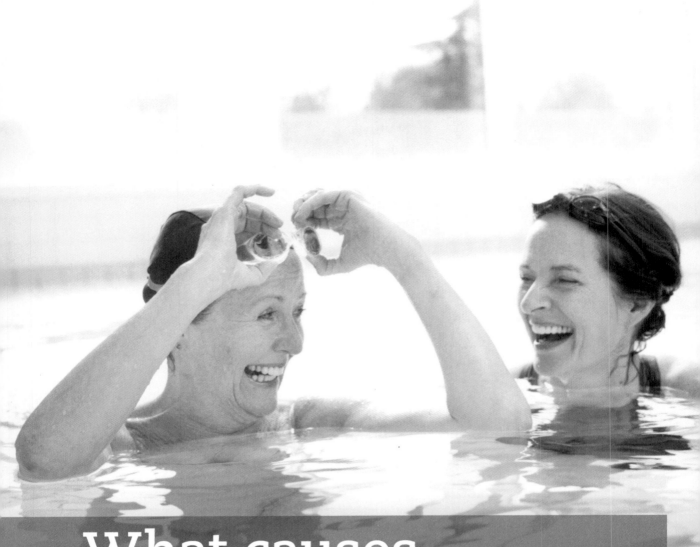

What causes disease?

The Disease Prevention Survey results revealed what more than 100 specialist doctors believed to be the basic causes of disease. Here the top six culprits are revealed and the ways in which they cause serious disease is explained, together with key prevention strategies to help you to combat or even reverse their ill effects.

The inside story

As far as the human body goes, for every effect there is a cause. And for every symptom you experience there is a pathological process going on within your body, or in the brain, that can be studied. Not all of these processes are fully understood, especially ones involving the brain, but for the most common major diseases we have a clear idea of the overall picture, and of what happens to the organs and cells involved.

In this chapter, the top six pathological processes leading to chronic disease are looked at in detail so that you can get a better idea of what's going on inside your body. These processes are caused, to a large extent, by our lifestyle choices and they, in turn, lead to disease. One of the most significant of these processes is high blood pressure, which increases the risk of heart attack and stroke, among many other problems.

Changing bad habits will improve physical health and also **preserve** your memory and mental clarity.

Intra-abdominal fat is linked to diabetes and colon cancer; depression increases the risk of heart disease and cancer; insulin resistance contributes to a variety of cardiovascular and other disorders; and a bad cholesterol ratio can spell disaster for blood circulation. Inflammation is a process that can increase your risk of developing a host of chronic conditions, including Alzheimer's disease.

On the following pages, you'll discover what causes these pathological processes, find out what happens inside your body and learn why they can be so damaging to your health. Practical prevention strategies from top medical experts will give you the information you need to start making positive changes to reduce your risk of developing these disease-causing problems in the first place, and improving, or even reversing, their negative effects if one or more of them is already active in your body.

If you need another reason to get active and eat healthily, remember that it's not only your major organs that can be affected, it's also your brain and its ability to function normally. Changing bad habits will improve physical health and also preserve your memory and mental clarity.

Jogging, swimming and other forms of aerobic exercise – essential to any disease-prevention plan – appear to protect the brain, too. One study of nearly 19,000 women found that the most active participants were the least likely to show signs of memory loss or clouded thinking. Studying, reading and other mental challenges are also linked to a lower risk of dementia. And the same is true of coping with emotional stress.

EMERGENCY PHONE NUMBERS

✚ Ambulance	999 or 112
✚ Poisons advice (NHS Direct)	0845 4647

CAUSE 1
Hypertension

Blood pressure is the force of blood against the walls of your arteries. If your arteries are healthy, they expand and contract easily with every heartbeat, keeping pressure low. But if blood vessels grow stiff, they don't expand as easily and blood pressure rises, just as a wide, lazy river becomes a raging torrent when channelled into a narrow valley. Stiff blood vessels are both a cause and an effect of high blood pressure (hypertension). Pre-hypertension begins at a reading of 120/80 mmHg; hypertension begins at 140/90 mmHg.

1 High blood pressure makes the layer of muscle inside blood vessel walls grow thicker. This narrows the arteries, raising the risk that a blood clot will completely block an artery and cause a heart attack or stroke.

LDL cholesterol

White blood cell

Plaque build-up

2 Fast-moving blood damages the delicate layer of cells that line artery walls. Damaged artery walls are magnets for white blood cells and LDL cholesterol, which accumulate and form heart-threatening plaque.

What causes it?

Family history, advancing age, diabetes and being male all increase risk. So do smoking, being overweight, stress, lack of exercise, eating foods high in salt and saturated fat, and skimping on fruit, vegetables and dairy products. What is more, certain ethnic groups are at increased risk. Many risk factors contribute to high blood pressure in part by reducing production of nitric oxide, a chemical that makes blood vessels flexible.

3 High blood pressure can make blood vessels in your brain grow narrow and weak, raising your risk of two kinds of stroke. A blood clot can block blood flow (below left), causing an ischaemic stroke, or an artery may rupture (below right), causing a haemorrhagic stroke.

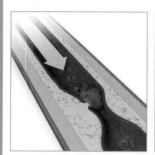 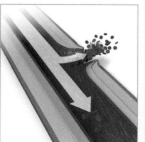

4 As arteries narrow, the heart works harder and the left ventricle grows bigger. But a bigger heart can't expand fully or fill completely with blood, so it becomes less efficient at pumping, raising your risk of a heart attack, congestive heart failure and other life-threatening heart conditions.

Why is it dangerous?

High blood pressure makes artery walls thicker, narrower, stiffer and weaker, which means less blood, oxygen and fewer nutrients get to your organs. And blood clots are more likely to get stuck in narrowed arteries, which can trigger a heart attack, a stroke or blockage of a blood vessel (thrombosis) in the leg. Blood vessel damage can also raise your risk of dementia, kidney failure, vision problems and even blindness.

Top prevention strategies

- Stop smoking if you haven't done so already.
- Exercise to lower blood pressure and lose weight.
- Avoid high-sodium processed foods and don't add extra salt to food.
- Eat more low-fat dairy products and foods high in potassium – fruit, vegetables, nuts and seeds.

23

CAUSE 2
Intra-abdominal fat

Fat packed deep within the abdomen, in and around your internal organs. Women with a waistline measurement of more than 88cm (34½in) and men with a measurement of more than 102cm (40in) are likely to have it. (For people of Asian descent, risk rises with measurements over 80cm/31½in for women and 95cm/34½in for men.) A large waist measurement is dangerous even if your body weight is within the healthy range for your height. To measure your waist, wrap a tape measure snugly around your mid-section at about belly-button height.

What causes it?

Eating too many fatty foods, being sedentary and spending too much time doing activities that keep you sitting down, such as working at a desk and driving. In other words, a diet high in calories and a life devoid of exercise. Chronic stress plays a role, too, especially for women, since the stress hormone cortisol directs your body to store more fat in your abdomen.

Why is it dangerous?

Unlike the relatively harmless fat on your buttocks, hips, thighs and even just under the skin at your waist, intra-abdominal fat churns out substances that raise your risk of diabetes, high blood pressure, heart attack, stroke, colon cancer and even memory problems. These include inflammatory compounds that make blood stickier as well as free fatty acids that prompt your liver to produce more blood glucose and LDL ('bad') cholesterol.

Top prevention strategies

- Eat more fruit, vegetables and whole grains, and less saturated fat.
- Exercise to lower blood pressure and lose weight.
- Find time to relax every day.
- Get enough good quality sleep, for example, by treating snoring problems.

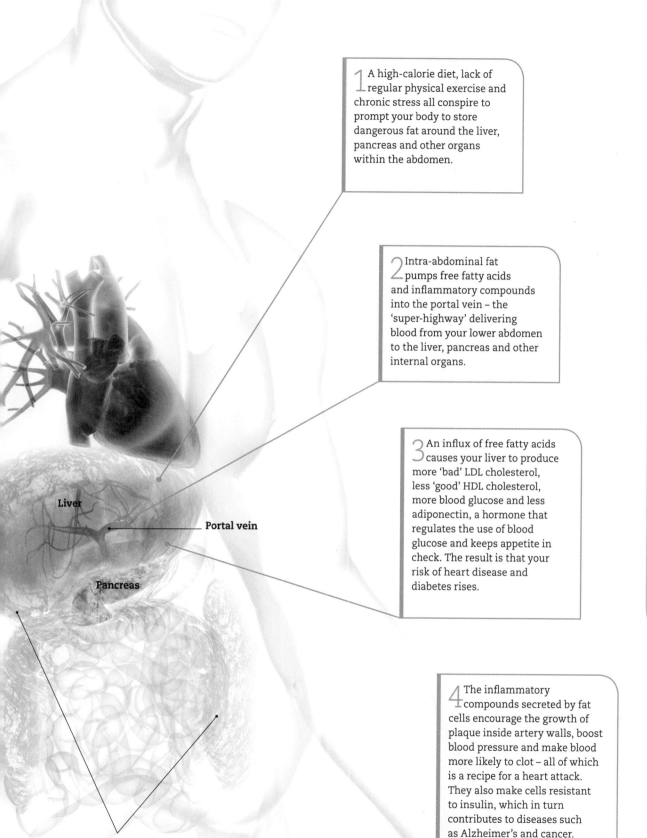

1 A high-calorie diet, lack of regular physical exercise and chronic stress all conspire to prompt your body to store dangerous fat around the liver, pancreas and other organs within the abdomen.

2 Intra-abdominal fat pumps free fatty acids and inflammatory compounds into the portal vein – the 'super-highway' delivering blood from your lower abdomen to the liver, pancreas and other internal organs.

3 An influx of free fatty acids causes your liver to produce more 'bad' LDL cholesterol, less 'good' HDL cholesterol, more blood glucose and less adiponectin, a hormone that regulates the use of blood glucose and keeps appetite in check. The result is that your risk of heart disease and diabetes rises.

4 The inflammatory compounds secreted by fat cells encourage the growth of plaque inside artery walls, boost blood pressure and make blood more likely to clot – all of which is a recipe for a heart attack. They also make cells resistant to insulin, which in turn contributes to diseases such as Alzheimer's and cancer.

Liver

Portal vein

Pancreas

Intra-abdominal fat

25

CAUSE 3
Depression

More than a passing low mood, depression interferes with your life, relationships, sense of yourself and health. It ranges from dysthymia – low-level depression that can last for years – to major depression, which can make working, performing daily activities and relating to your spouse, family and friends nearly impossible. Another type is seasonal affective disorder, which occurs only during certain times of the year (usually winter).

1 Depression releases a hormone called ACTH that increases levels of the stress hormone cortisol in the body. Extra cortisol may be the reason people with depression have higher rates of diabetes, because it reduces production of insulin in the pancreas, allowing blood glucose to rise. Cortisol also prompts the body to store more abdominal fat, which is a risk factor for many chronic diseases.

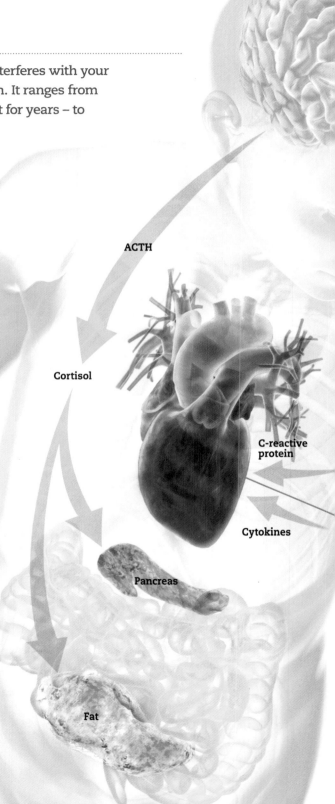

ACTH

Cortisol

C-reactive protein

Cytokines

Pancreas

Fat

26

What causes it?

Often a combination of genetics, chronic stress and difficult life experiences. Levels of the brain chemicals serotonin, dopamine and noradrenaline, which brain cells use to communicate with each other, may be out of balance. And areas of the brain that regulate mood, thought, sleep, appetite and behaviour may function abnormally.

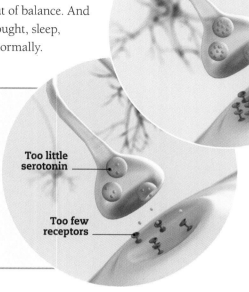

Serotonin returns to source cell

Too little serotonin

Too few receptors

2 If you are depressed, you may have abnormally low levels of the brain chemical serotonin. The brain may not produce enough serotonin, brain cells may not have enough receptors to receive it, or it may bounce back instead of being delivered from cell to cell.

3 People with depression may have higher levels of C-reactive protein, an inflammatory compound associated with increased heart attack risk. Depression also increases the release of other inflammatory compounds, called cytokines, that fuel the deposition of heart-threatening plaque in artery walls.

4 Depression raises the risk of osteoporosis and bone fractures. Research is continuing into the precise mechanism that underlies this link.

Why is it dangerous?

Serious depression may lead to suicide. In addition to this risk, depression often coexists with diabetes, heart disease, stroke, cancer and other major health conditions, making symptoms of these illnesses more severe and more difficult to manage. The combination can be fatal: people with diabetes and depression face a higher risk of dying from heart disease. According to new evidence, depression may even help trigger diabetes heart disease and osteoporosis by raising levels of inflammatory compounds and stress hormones.

Top prevention strategies

- Seek professional help as early as possible.
- Exercise regularly; studies show it can help prevent or lift depression.
- Relieve stress every day in whatever way you find works best for you.
- Cultivate a positive attitude.
- Connect with family and friends for social support whenever you can.

CAUSE 4
Insulin resistance

When you eat, some of the food is turned into glucose (a form of sugar), the body's main source of fuel, and is absorbed into the bloodstream. The pancreas responds by secreting the hormone insulin, which triggers cells throughout the body to allow glucose to enter. But when cells are insulin-resistant, they turn partially 'deaf' to insulin's signals. The pancreas turns up the volume by churning out more and more insulin.

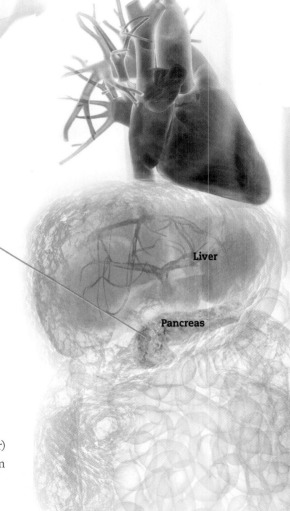

1 After a meal or snack, the pancreas secretes insulin to help glucose to enter cells. The insulin finds its way to various cells in the body, especially muscle cells, which burn glucose for energy.

Liver

Pancreas

What causes it?

Scientists aren't exactly sure, but genetics, advancing age, lack of exercise and excess weight (especially intra-abdominal fat) play key roles. Diets high in saturated fat and simple carbohydrates (such as sugar) also contribute, as do chronic infections (such as gum disease), which release inflammatory chemicals that interfere with chemical signals from insulin.

Why is it dangerous?

High insulin levels can damage blood vessels and trigger the liver to produce more heart-threatening triglycerides and LDL ('bad') cholesterol and less HDL ('good') cholesterol. They also increase the risk of blood clots and prompt the body to retain more sodium, raising blood pressure. Excess insulin may even spur the growth of some cancers and contribute to Alzheimer's disease. If your pancreas can't keep pace with your body's need for extra insulin, blood glucose levels may begin to rise after years or even decades of insulin resistance, resulting in diabetes.

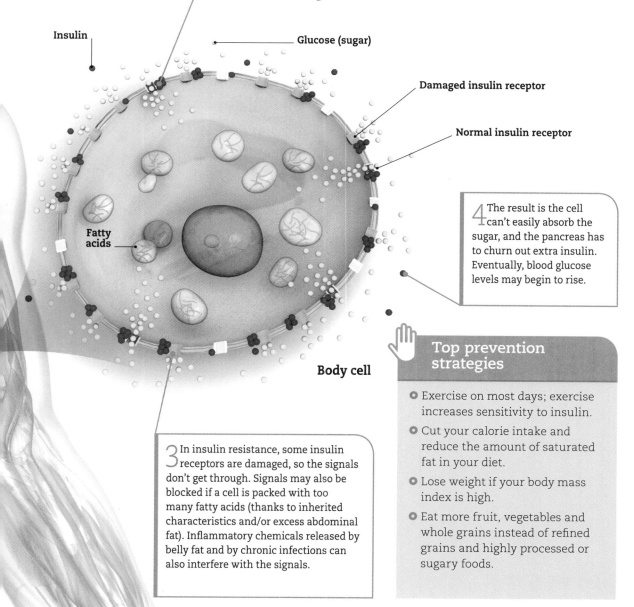

2 Insulin binds to receptors on the cell, which triggers a series of chemical signals that allow molecules of glucose to be transported into the cell.

Insulin

Glucose (sugar)

Damaged insulin receptor

Normal insulin receptor

Fatty acids

4 The result is the cell can't easily absorb the sugar, and the pancreas has to churn out extra insulin. Eventually, blood glucose levels may begin to rise.

Body cell

3 In insulin resistance, some insulin receptors are damaged, so the signals don't get through. Signals may also be blocked if a cell is packed with too many fatty acids (thanks to inherited characteristics and/or excess abdominal fat). Inflammatory chemicals released by belly fat and by chronic infections can also interfere with the signals.

Top prevention strategies

- Exercise on most days; exercise increases sensitivity to insulin.
- Cut your calorie intake and reduce the amount of saturated fat in your diet.
- Lose weight if your body mass index is high.
- Eat more fruit, vegetables and whole grains instead of refined grains and highly processed or sugary foods.

CAUSE 5
Bad cholesterol balance

There are two main types of cholesterol in your body: 'bad' LDL cholesterol, which clogs arteries and 'good' HDL, which acts as a vacuum cleaner, taking the damaging LDL cholesterol to the liver for disposal. Optimal LDL levels are under 4.0mmol/l; optimal HDL levels are over 1.0mmol/l. The lower your LDL and the higher your HDL, the better.

1 Smoking, a diet rich in saturated and hydrogenated fats, being overweight and not exercising lead to high levels of LDL in the bloodstream. The same factors, along with a lack of 'good' fats in the diet, contribute to low levels of HDL.

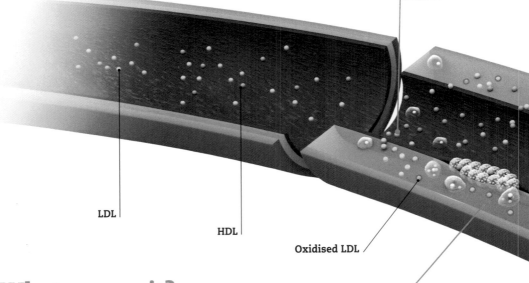

LDL

HDL

Oxidised LDL

What causes it?

A diet high in saturated fat gives your liver too much of the raw material it needs for producing LDL and reduces its ability to remove excess LDL from the bloodstream. Eating hydrogenated fats, smoking, being overweight and lack of exercise can also raise LDL and depress HDL. Skimping on monounsaturated fats (in olive oil, nuts and avocados) and soluble fibre (in oats, barley, legumes, pulses and pears) also has an impact on your ratio.

2 Trouble starts when extra LDL particles move out of the bloodstream and into artery walls. There LDL can be damaged by a process called oxidation, attracting white blood cells to accumulate.

Why is it dangerous?

LDL normally moves through artery walls and into cells, where it's put to good use. But excess LDL gets 'stuck' in artery walls, beginning the formation of artery-narrowing plaque. HDL can clean up this LDL, but if HDL levels are low, it can't get the job done, putting you at risk of a heart attack or stroke.

3 HDL is your bloodstream's clean-up crew, removing LDL from circulation and returning it to the liver for elimination or re-use. HDL can even extract cholesterol from plaque in artery walls. But if levels are low, the LDL remains.

4 The combination of LDL and white blood cells in artery walls eventually leads to the dangerous build-up of plaque. Areas of plaque may then burst, leading to the formation of a blood clot (thrombus) that can stop the flow of blood to your heart or brain.

Liver

Plaque

Blood clot

White blood cell

Top prevention strategies

- Stop smoking if you haven't done so already.
- Eat less saturated fat and fewer hydrogenated oils (which give rise to trans fats).
- Eat more soluble fibre (from oats, barley and legumes) and good fats (from fish, nuts and olive or rapeseed oil).
- Do more brisk walking.
- Have a maximum of two units of alcohol daily.

31

CAUSE 6
Inflammation

Inflammation is a side effect of the immune system at work. When you have an injury or infection, immune-system cells and chemicals rush to the site to kill germs and repair damaged tissue. You can see inflammation in action when the skin around a cut becomes red and swollen. In the short term, the process can promote healing and is therefore beneficial, but when the body is constantly barraged by inflammation – due to ongoing low-grade infections or 'injuries' from smoking and other irritants – it ceases to help and starts to harm.

What causes it?

Chronic inflammation can be triggered by allergens, toxins and radiation, but also by medical conditions such as rheumatoid arthritis; infections such as untreated gum disease or stomach ulcers, which are caused by bacterial infection; or microscopic injuries such as damage to artery walls caused by smoking, high blood pressure or high cholesterol. Another culprit is intra-abdominal fat, which secretes inflammatory chemicals. Stress, anger, lack of exercise and a diet high in fast foods and hydrogenated fats also increase inflammation.

32

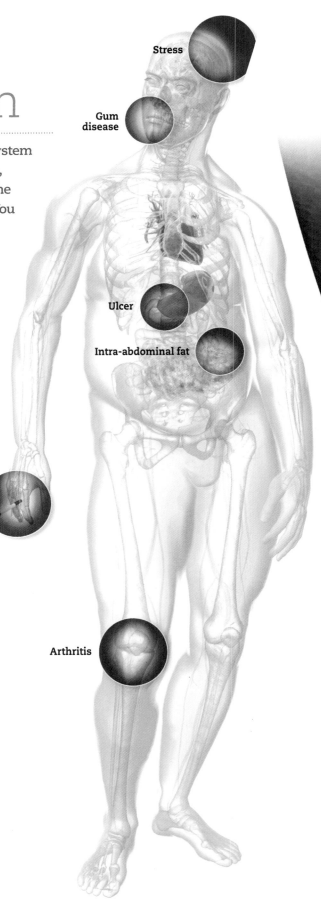

Stress

Gum disease

Ulcer

Intra-abdominal fat

Smoking

Arthritis

1 Blood levels of inflammatory chemicals called cytokines rise in response to smoking, bacteria, intra-abdominal fat and other stressors to the body. Cytokines alert the body that something is wrong and set off a chain of events in the body that causes inflammation.

Why is it dangerous?

It accelerates the formation of plaque in artery walls and then makes that plaque less stable and more likely to burst open and block an artery. Chronic inflammation also contributes to insulin resistance and raises your risk of a whole host of chronic diseases, including diabetes, Alzheimer's disease, lung disease, osteoporosis and even cancer.

Oxidised LDL

White blood cell

Plaque

Inflammation

Cytokines

Blood clot

Tissue factor

LDL

3 White blood cells release more cytokines that eat away at the protective cap covering the plaque. Eventually, the plaque may burst open and spill its contents into the bloodstream. A distress signal sent by white blood cells, called tissue factor, triggers a clotting response. If a blood clot blocks the artery, a heart attack or stroke can be the consequence.

Fatty streak

2 White blood cells rush to the site of the infection or injury – such as artery walls damaged by oxidised cholesterol (LDL) particles. When LDL burrows into artery walls, the immune cells engulf them in order to dispose of them. But if there's too much LDL, the white blood cells become overstuffed, collect in the artery wall and form plaque that narrows the artery.

Top prevention strategies

- Stop smoking as it inflames artery walls.
- Eat more oily fish, fruit and vegetables, and less fried food and hydrogenated oils.
- Sleep at least 7 hours a night.
- Exercise regularly.
- Treat any chronic infections – for example, gum disease or gastric ulcers.

33

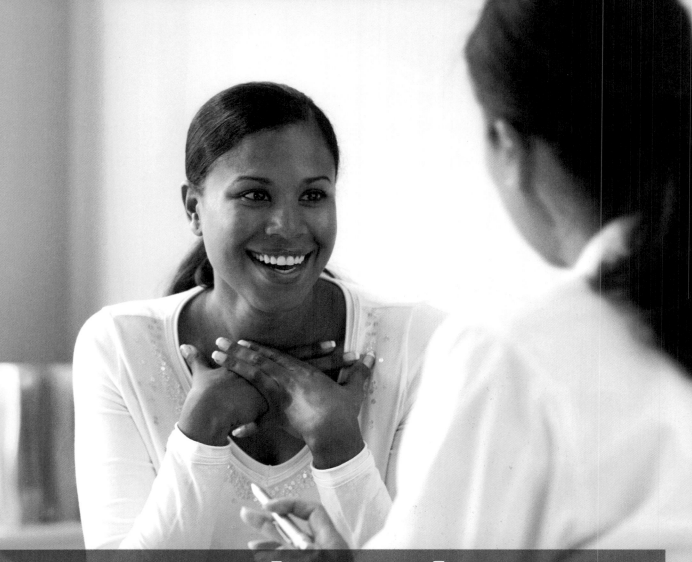

Know the early warning signs

While the majority of aches, pains and other symptoms signal minor ailments, some may indicate the onset of a serious health problem, and early diagnosis and treatment can be vital. In the tables in this chapter you'll find common symptoms that may be the first sign of impending trouble and learn what action to take.

Symptoms you should never ignore

The tables on the following pages are designed to provide a guide to the possible cause of your symptoms and advise what steps you should take, whether self-help, a phone call or visit to your GP, or a call for an ambulance (for emergency numbers, see page 21). Reading all the descriptions of symptom combinations will help you to find the explanation that most closely fits your case. However, you should always consult your doctor whenever a symptom is worrying you, regardless of whether or not it is listed in this section. If you need to go to hospital, take all your regular medications with you – including over-the-counter medicines and alternative remedies – or take a list of them.

Abdominal pain (sudden onset)

Description	Possible causes	Response
Sudden onset of severe, constant pain, at first around the navel, then settling in the right lower abdomen, possibly accompanied by fever or diarrhoea.	An acute abdominal condition such as appendicitis.	Go to the hospital for rapid assessment and treatment. Appendicitis must be treated quickly or the appendix will rupture and leak infected fluid into other parts of the abdomen. Surgery may be required.
Sudden pain accompanied by bloody diarrhoea, blood in the stools or vomiting blood.	A serious condition causing bleeding in the digestive tract.	Go straight to the nearest hospital A&E department.
Sudden, severe, colicky, gripping pain in the right upper abdomen, possibly radiating to the back.	Gallstones or inflammation of the gall bladder, especially if pain starts after a meal.	Make an appointment to see your doctor without delay. If the pain is not relieved by over-the-counter painkillers, seek urgent medical advice.
Sudden pain below your navel that radiates to either side.	A bowel disorder, a urinary tract infection or (in women) pelvic inflammatory disease.	Call your doctor, who may order diagnostic tests or advise you to go to the A&E department.
Sharp, colicky pain (initially in the mid to lower back), that then radiates round on one side and down to the groin.	Kidney stones or, if accompanied by fever, a kidney or bladder infection.	Increase your water intake and call your doctor. Most kidney stones eventually pass on their own, although in rare cases surgery is necessary. If you also have a fever, call your doctor without delay.
Sudden tearing abdominal and back pain that may be accompanied by lightheadedness.	A ruptured or leaking aortic aneurysm, especially in an older person who smokes or has high blood pressure.	Call an ambulance immediately.

Abdominal pain (recurrent)

Description	Possible causes	Response
A burning sensation just below the breastbone, particularly after a large meal.	Heartburn (acid reflux).	Take over-the-counter antacids and avoid large greasy meals. If pain persists, in spite of these measures, see your GP. Do this as a matter of urgency if you are over 55 or are losing weight.
Mild pain or discomfort that comes on slowly and continues or recurs for weeks or months, possibly accompanied by diarrhoea, constipation, bloating or flatulence.	A chronic ailment such as lactose intolerance, irritable bowel syndrome, peptic ulcers, food intolerance, Crohn's disease, coeliac disease or ulcerative colitis.	See your doctor, who may refer you to a gastroenterologist for diagnostic tests.

Back pain

Description	Possible causes	Response
Back pain accompanied by fever or chills in someone whose immune system is suppressed (e.g. by drug treatment) or has had a recent bacterial infection, back surgery, epidural/spinal anaesthesia, or who injects drugs for any reason.	Serious infection.	Call your doctor immediately or go to the nearest A&E department.
Sudden onset of severe back pain in someone who has osteoporosis.	Fracture, especially if there has been a recent injury or fall.	Call your doctor immediately.
Recurrent back pain accompanied by weight loss, sensory changes, leg weakness, bladder or bowel dysfunction, or a history of cancer.	Compression of the nerves in the spine by a serious condition such as a tumour.	Call your doctor; if there are sensory changes, leg weakness or bladder or bowel dysfunction, go to the nearest A&E department immediately, as urgent treatment may be necessary to restore function.

Black or bloody stools

Description	Possible causes	Response
Black or tarry stools accompanied by a burning pain in the upper abdomen.	An ulcer in the upper gastrointestinal tract.	Consult your doctor without delay. You may need to have an urgent endoscopy for visual inspection and to take tissue samples for biopsy.
Maroon or black stools with no other symptoms.	Consuming black liquorice, blueberries, lead, iron pills, tomatoes or spinach, or possibly bleeding in the digestive tract.	If you've consumed any of these substances, wait 24 hours to see if stool colour returns to normal. If not, call NHS Direct or your doctor. If you've ingested lead or iron, or if you have not eaten any of these items, call your doctor promptly.
Blood lightly coating stools and/or just on toilet paper or in the toilet pan accompanied by pain while moving your bowels.	Anal fissures (tears around the anus) or haemorrhoids (dilated blood vessels in swollen tissue within the rectum and anal canal).	Over-the-counter haemorrhoid creams or ointments can bring relief; surgical treatment may be necessary for persistent haemorrhoids. If bleeding continues, see your doctor.
Bloody diarrhoea, or blood in the stool with sudden abdominal pain, perhaps accompanied by vomiting.	A serious abdominal condition causing bleeding in the digestive tract.	Call an ambulance or go straight to the nearest A&E department.
Blood mixed up with stools accompanied by discomfort in the lower abdomen and other digestive-tract symptoms, such as flatulence, constipation or diarrhoea.	A serious condition such as ulcerative colitis, Crohn's disease, diverticular disease, a tumour or polyps.	See your doctor, who will refer you to a gastroenterologist for tests and treatment.

Blood in the urine

Description	Possible causes	Response
Pink, red or brownish urine, accompanied by pain in the central part of the lower back or in the pelvic area, burning during urination, or a frequent strong urge to urinate.	A bladder infection.	See your doctor, who may arrange for analysis of a urine sample. Treatment of such infections is usually an oral antibiotic.
Blood in the urine accompanied by fever and back pain possibly on one side.	Kidney stones or, if you also have a fever, a kidney infection.	See your doctor promptly. Many kidney stones pass out of the body naturally. If this doesn't happen, they may need to be surgically removed or shattered with shock waves. If you have an infection, antibiotics will probably be prescribed.
In men, blood in the urine accompanied by difficulty urinating or a strong need to urinate often.	Prostate enlargement.	See your doctor, who will order diagnostic ultrasound or other imaging tests. Treatment may include medication, laser therapy or surgery.
Blood in the urine with no other symptoms.	A kidney disorder or urinary tract cancer.	See your doctor, who will refer you for diagnostic imaging tests, such as ultrasound or CT scans.

Changes in appetite

Description	Possible causes	Response
Reduced appetite accompanied by fatigue, hair thinning, dry skin, decreased tolerance of cold, weight gain or puffiness of the face.	Hypothyroidism (underactive thyroid gland).	See your doctor, who will order a diagnostic blood test. If your thyroid is underactive, you will usually be prescribed thyroid hormone replacement medication.
Reduced appetite accompanied by a change in bowel habit, fatigue, nausea, blood in stools, or vomiting.	A chronic inflammatory condition or infection of the digestive tract or cancer.	See your doctor, who may order tests to determine the cause and appropriate treatment.
Appetite changes after starting a new medication.	Many medications can cause changes in appetite.	Ask you doctor if this could be the reason for your symptoms, and whether a different medication should be substituted.
Increased appetite accompanied by insomnia, excessive thirst, increased sweating, more frequent bowel movements or hair loss.	Hyperthyroidism (overactive thyroid gland).	See your doctor, who will order diagnostic blood tests. If your thyroid is overactive, treatment may include drugs or radioiodine therapy to slow it down or surgical removal of excess thyroid tissue.
Increased appetite accompanied by excessive thirst, fatigue, increased urination, frequent infections or poor wound healing.	Type 1 or Type 2 diabetes.	See your doctor, who will order a test to measure your blood glucose. Treatment depends on several factors, including the type of diabetes, age at onset and severity.

Chest pain

Description	Possible causes	Response
Crushing, squeezing, tightening pressure on your chest that comes on suddenly; may be accompanied by pain that radiates from your chest to your jaw, back, neck, shoulders or arm (particularly the left arm); may also be accompanied by nausea, racing pulse or shortness of breath.	Heart attack.	Call an ambulance immediately. If your doctor has prescribed medication to take during an angina attack, take the suggested dose. After you have called an ambulance, chew a standard aspirin (300mg) or four low-dose (75mg) aspirin tablets straightaway.
Recurrent squeezing, tightening pain in the centre of the chest, that may radiate to the arms, jaw, back or teeth and worsens with exertion and eases on rest.	Angina, which occurs when the heart muscle is not getting enough blood or oxygen.	If this is the first such attack, call an ambulance or get someone to drive you to the nearest A&E department immediately for diagnosis and treatment. If you have been diagnosed with angina, take your emergency medication but seek immediate help if this does not relieve symptoms within a few minutes.
Pain accompanied by shortness of breath, coughing or wheezing.	Asthma or, if you also have a fever or feel generally unwell, a chest infection.	If you have an asthma inhaler, use it, then make an urgent appointment with your doctor. If you have difficulty breathing, go straight to the nearest A&E department. If you can't complete a sentence when talking, call an ambulance.
Sharp pain that worsens when you cough or take a deep breath and that may be accompanied by flu-like symptoms.	A lung condition such as pneumonia, pleurisy, a blood clot in the lung, a collapsed lung or inflammation of rib-cage cartilage.	Make an urgent appointment with your doctor, or, if you have difficulty breathing, go straight to the nearest A&E department. If you can't complete a sentence when talking, call an ambulance
Burning pain accompanied by gastrointestinal symptoms such as indigestion or heartburn.	An ulcer, pancreatic disease or an inflamed gall bladder.	See your doctor, who may recommend diagnostic tests or refer you to a gastroenterologist.
Pain accompanied by feelings of anxiety, racing pulse or shortness of breath.	Panic attack.	Breathe deeply and try to relax. If symptoms persist, call your doctor. Panic attack symptoms can mimic those of a more serious condition such as a heart attack. If it's your first panic attack, call your doctor or go to the nearest A&E department for assessment.

Confusion or memory loss

Description	Possible causes	Response
Sudden confusion that is accompanied by blurred vision, slurred speech, sudden numbness on one side of the body or sudden severe headache.	Stroke or transient ischaemic attack (TIA).	Call an ambulance immediately. Prompt treatment can save your life, reduce damage to your brain and lower your risk of permanent disability.
Sudden confusion or memory loss after an accident or blow to the head.	Head injury or concussion.	Go to the nearest A&E department immediately.
Confusion that comes on quite suddenly and may be accompanied by hunger or lightheadedness.	Low blood glucose.	Have a sweet snack or drink. If you have diabetes, talk to your doctor about treatment adjustment.
In the elderly, gradual memory loss or confusion that doesn't worsen quickly or interfere with everyday life.	Normal age-related memory loss.	Keep your mind active with crossword puzzles and other mental challenges. Use a detailed appointment diary, always put keys and other items in the same place and repeat a person's name to yourself several times when you meet.
In the elderly, gradual memory loss or confusion that starts to worsen quickly and interferes with everyday activities.	Alzheimer's disease, a brain tumour, underactive thyroid gland, any chronic disease and vitamin B_{12} deficiency.	Consult your doctor, who will determine what tests and treatment are needed.
Confusion that comes on gradually after a period of vomiting, diarrhoea or significant exposure to heat or sunlight.	Dehydration.	Rehydrate by sipping water frequently. If dehydration is caused by vomiting or diarrhoea, choose clear fluids or an over-the-counter electrolyte solution. Call your doctor if you can't keep liquids down or confusion persists.
Memory loss or confusion after starting a new medication.	A drug side effect.	Talk with your doctor about whether a different medication should be substituted. Side effects sometimes disappear after a few days or weeks of taking a medication.

Constipation

Description	Possible causes	Response
Occasional constipation that may be accompanied by bloating, a feeling of fullness and the need to strain to have a bowel movement.	Poor diet (low in fibre and high in fat), dehydration (low fluid intake), not enough exercise or too much alcohol or caffeine.	Symptoms usually clear up once you resume a healthy diet with plenty of fibre and fluids. Natural fibre supplements can also ease symptoms; always drink plenty of water if you take them.
Constipation after starting a new medication.	A side effect of medications such as painkillers, antacids that contain aluminium and calcium, calcium-channel blockers, drugs for Parkinson's disease, antispasmodics, antidepressants, iron supplements, diuretics and anticonvulsants.	Talk with your doctor about whether a different medication should be substituted. Side effects sometimes disappear after a few days or weeks of taking a medication.
Constipation that occurs regularly, is accompanied by abdominal pain and bloating and that tends to occur at times of stress, and may alternate with episodes of diarrhoea.	Irritable bowel syndrome.	See your doctor, who may order tests to rule out a more serious condition and may prescribe medication, fibre supplements, physical activity or stress reduction techniques, to help reduce symptoms.
Constipation during or after travel or other lifestyle changes.	A temporary reaction to change.	Symptoms should clear up on their own.
Recurrent constipation accompanied by bloating, flatulence or pain.	A disease or condition of the colon or rectum, such as diverticular disease, tumours or scar tissue in the intestines.	See your doctor, who may arrange for you to undergo diagnostic tests.
Constipation accompanied by excessive thirst, increased urination, fatigue, depression, weight gain or headache.	A metabolic or endocrine disorder such as diabetes, hypothyroidism (underactive thyroid gland) or hypercalcaemia (too much calcium in the blood).	See your doctor, who may arrange for you to undergo diagnostic tests.

Cough

Description	Possible causes	Response
A cough accompanied by repeated throat clearing, nasal discharge or excessive phlegm.	Allergy or mucus congestion following a cold.	See your doctor, who may prescribe allergy medication or refer you to a specialist for diagnosis and treatment.
A dry cough that may be worse at night, after exercise or during strong emotion, and that may be accompanied by wheezy breathing.	Asthma.	See your doctor, who may prescribe a bronchodilator, corticosteroid inhaler or other medication to control asthma.
A cough after starting to take an ACE inhibitor (a type of drug for high blood pressure).	A drug side effect; these medications cause dry cough in 5 to 10 per cent of those who take them.	Talk to your doctor about whether another medication should be substituted.
A long-standing cough that produces catarrh every day, is accompanied by shortness of breath and is worse on exertion.	Chronic obstructive pulmonary disease, a condition that includes chronic bronchitis and emphysema and is almost always caused by smoking.	See your doctor, who may do a test to measure lung capacity and order a chest X-ray. There is no cure, but symptoms can be treated and further lung damage prevented.
A long-standing cough accompanied by bouts of heartburn and/or regurgitation of stomach acid, especially at night.	Gastro-oesophageal reflux disease (GORD).	See your doctor, who will prescribe antacids and medications that inhibit stomach acid production, and may recommend gastroscopy to assess damage to the oesophagus.
A recurrent cough that has worsened over time perhaps accompanied by fatigue, chest pain, coughing up blood, hoarseness or shortness of breath.	A chronic respiratory condition or lung cancer.	See your doctor urgently, who will order blood tests, a chest X-ray and, if necessary, specialist referral.

Diarrhoea

Description	Possible causes	Response
Diarrhoea that comes on suddenly for no apparent reason and that may be accompanied by fever, vomiting, cramping pains or headache.	Viral gastroenteritis.	Symptoms usually clear up on their own within a few days. During that time, stay well hydrated. Drink clear, decaffeinated fluids or an over-the-counter electrolyte solution throughout the day.
Diarrhoea that always occurs after eating specific foods.	Food allergy or intolerance.	Eliminate the trigger food from your diet and talk to your doctor about whether allergy tests may be warranted.
Diarrhoea that starts 2 to 6 hours after a meal consumed while travelling overseas, or that also affects those who have eaten the same meal.	A bacterial infection caused by spoiled, undercooked or contaminated food; most cases of food poisoning are due to common bacteria such as staphylococcus or E. coli.	Symptoms usually clear up on their own within 48 hours. Drink plenty, but avoid solid food until your stools return to normal. Call your doctor if symptoms last longer than two or three days or if you're unable to stay hydrated; you may need intravenous fluids. If you may have eaten contaminated mushrooms or shellfish, go straight to the nearest A&E department.
Diarrhoea while taking medications.	A side effect of medications such as antibiotics, diuretics, laxatives containing magnesium or anti-cancer drugs.	Talk with your doctor. If you've been taking an antibiotic, eat yoghurt with active cultures to replenish the 'good' bacteria in your gut.
Diarrhoea that lasts longer than four weeks.	A chronic condition such as lactose intolerance, Crohn's disease, ulcerative colitis, irritable bowel syndrome or coeliac disease (intolerance to gluten – a protein found in wheat, rye and barley).	See your doctor, who may refer you to a gastroenterologist and/or dietitian.

Dizziness

Description	Possible causes	Response
Dizziness accompanied by blurred vision, slurred speech, sudden numbness on one side of the body or sudden severe headache.	Stroke or transient ischaemic attack (TIA).	Go to the nearest A&E department immediately. Prompt treatment can save your life and reduce your risk of permanent disability.
Sudden severe dizziness accompanied by chest pain, racing pulse, shortness of breath, sweating or pain.	Heart attack or irregular heartbeat.	Call an ambulance immediately. If your doctor has prescribed medication to take during an angina attack, take the suggested dose. After you have called an ambulance, chew a standard aspirin (300mg) or four low-dose (75mg) aspirin tablets straightaway.
Dizziness accompanied by dry mouth, thirst, dark urine and reduced urination.	Dehydration.	Rehydrate with caffeine-free drinks or an over-the-counter electrolyte solution. Call your doctor if you can't keep liquids down and dizziness persists.
Dizziness accompanied by earache, reduced ability to hear and fever.	An ear infection.	See your doctor to confirm the diagnosis. While many ear infections clear up on their own, you may be prescribed antibiotics for a bacterial infection. Use an over-the-counter painkiller or a heated pad to reduce pain.
Dizziness triggered by standing up or moving suddenly.	Postural hypotension caused by transient low blood pressure.	Sit or lie still until the dizziness passes. Avoid moving quickly.
Dizziness and feelings of faintness after starting a new medication.	A side effect of various drugs, especially those for diabetes, high blood pressure, depression and anxiety.	Talk with your doctor about whether a different medication should be substituted. Side effects sometimes disappear after a few days or weeks of taking a medication.
Dizziness accompanied by extreme anxiety, racing pulse or shortness of breath.	Panic attack.	Breathe deeply and try to relax. If symptoms persist, call your doctor. Frequent panic attacks can be treated with therapy, medication and relaxation techniques such as meditation. If it is your first panic attack, go at once to the nearest A&E department to exclude a more serious condition.

Excessive thirst

Description	Possible causes	Response
Thirst accompanied by decreased urination, appetite loss or fatigue.	Kidney failure is a possibility.	Consult your doctor as soon as possible. A thorough physical examination and tests may be needed to confirm the diagnosis and determine treatment.
Thirst that is accompanied by insomnia, unexplained weight loss, increased sweating, more frequent bowel movements or hair loss.	Hyperthyroidism (overactive thyroid gland) or other hormone imbalance.	See your doctor, who will order diagnostic blood tests. If your thyroid is overactive, treatment may include drugs or radioiodine therapy to slow it down or surgical removal of excess thyroid tissue.
Thirst after starting a new medication.	A side effect of medications such as antihistamines, diuretics, some antidepressants, anticancer drugs and steroids.	Talk to your doctor, but don't stop your medication without medical advice. Check the package inserts or ask your pharmacist for advice on whether to, or how much to, increase your fluid intake.
Thirst accompanied by increased urination, unexplained weight loss, increased hunger or blurred vision.	Uncontrolled diabetes of either Type 1 or Type 2.	See your doctor, who may order a test to measure your blood glucose levels.

Fatigue

Description	Possible causes	Response
Sudden fatigue accompanied by fever, headache, sore throat or muscle aches.	A viral illness such as flu.	Rest and take over-the-counter painkillers while your body fights off the virus.
Long-standing fatigue accompanied by loss of interest in favourite activities, unintentional weight changes, irritability, feelings of hopelessness, forgetfulness, low mood and tearfulness, or trouble concentrating.	Depression, which may co-exist with anxiety.	Seek support from friends and family and see your doctor, who may refer you to a mental health professional. Depression can be treated with therapy, medication or both.
Fatigue while taking medication.	A side effect of medications such as beta-blockers, antihistamines, anti-anxiety drugs, cough and cold remedies, and some antidepressants.	Ask your doctor or pharmacist if fatigue is a common side effect of any of the medications you take. If the answer is yes, talk to your doctor about whether a different medication should be substituted.
Fatigue accompanied by unexplained weight gain, dry skin, hair loss, change in sleep patterns, constipation or depression.	Hypothyroidism (underactive thyroid gland).	See your doctor, who may order a diagnostic blood test. If your thyroid is underactive, you can be treated with thyroid hormone replacement medication.
Severe, persistent, unexplained fatigue accompanied by muscle aches, sore throat, poor sleep or difficulty concentrating.	Chronic fatigue syndrome (CFS) also known as ME (myalgic encephalomyelitis).	See your doctor, who will rule out other possible causes. A variety of treatments including medication and exercise and psychological therapies can help to ease symptoms. Ask your GP for referral to a specialist CFS service for expert help.
Fatigue lasting more than two weeks with no other symptoms.	A problem such a long-standing infection, allergies, a sleep disorder such as sleep apnoea, anaemia, diabetes or kidney disease.	See your doctor, who may order diagnostic tests or refer you to a specialist.

Fever

Description	Possible causes	Response
A high fever (39.5°C/103°F or higher); may be accompanied by confusion, a stiff neck, difficulty breathing, hallucinations or convulsions.	A viral or bacterial infection such as pneumonia, meningitis, a kidney infection or other serious condition.	Go to the nearest A&E department. If the person seems lethargic or unresponsive, call an ambulance. Paracetamol or ibuprofen can reduce the fever, as can bathing in lukewarm water. Keep hydrated by drinking water or an over-the-counter electrolyte solution.
A moderate fever (38.5°C to 39.5°C/101.5°F to 103°F), accompanied by nasal discharge, sore throat, cough, earache, vomiting or diarrhoea.	A viral or bacterial infection such as a cold, flu, strep throat, an ear infection or bronchitis.	Paracetamol or ibuprofen can reduce the fever. If your fever is above 39°C (102°F) or lasts for longer than three days, call your doctor. If you have a bacterial infection, your doctor may prescribe an antibiotic. Stay hydrated by drinking plenty of fluids.
A moderate fever (38.5°C to 39.5°C/101.5°F to 103°F), accompanied by painful or frequent urination.	A urinary tract infection.	Consult your doctor, who may prescribe an antibiotic. Drink plenty of clear fluids.
A mild fever that occurs after a vaccination.	A side effect of the immune response to any vaccine.	Fever usually subsides in a day or two; take ibuprofen or paracetamol to lower temperature and reduce discomfort.
An increase in body temperature after exposure to heat, sun or intense exercise, perhaps accompanied by rapid pulse, nausea and disorientation.	Heatstroke or heat exhaustion.	Move to a cool place then spray yourself with and drink plenty of cool water. If symptoms are extreme (temperature of 39°C/102°F or higher), call an ambulance.
A recurrent fever that occurs with other unexplained symptoms, such as weight loss, muscle or joint aches, or abdominal pain.	A wide variety of conditions and diseases, such as ulcerative colitis, Crohn's disease, lupus, HIV/AIDS or rheumatoid arthritis.	See your doctor, who may arrange for you to have diagnostic tests.
A small increase in body temperature (0.5°C to 1°C/1°F to 2°F) with no other symptoms.	Exercise, heat, heavy clothing, intense emotion.	Normal body temperature is about 37°C (98.6°F). In adults and children over the age of six, a variation below and above that figure of up to 1.5°C (0.8°F) is normal. To reduce temperature, remove excess clothing, loosen tight clothing, drink fluids or bathe in lukewarm water.

Headache

Description	Possible causes	Response
Severe headache that becomes progressively worse; may be accompanied by fever, blurred vision, confusion, numbness on one side of the body or loss of consciousness.	A serious condition affecting the brain or the tissues surrounding it, such as meningitis, stroke, blood clots, temporal arteritis or an aneurysm.	Call an ambulance immediately. Urgent assessment in hospital is necessary. Prompt treatment can save your life, reduce damage to your brain and your risk of permanent disability.
Dull pain in the head, neck or shoulders that comes on gradually and may feel like a vice around your forehead, temples or back of your head and neck.	Tension headache; can be triggered by stress, fatigue, anger or depression, or can have no identifiable trigger.	Take aspirin, ibuprofen or paracetamol. Consult your doctor if pain persists.
Throbbing pain that comes on several days after consuming a large amount of caffeine or sudden cessation of your regular coffee intake.	Caffeine withdrawal.	Reduce or eliminate caffeine intake – the headaches will cease after a few days. Take an over-the-counter painkiller.
Throbbing pain that may be accompanied by nausea and sensitivity to light and sound; possibly preceded by flashing lights, blind spots or tingling in the arm or face prior to headache but without fever.	Migraine; occurs more commonly in women and can be triggered by menstruation, ovulation or the menopause.	Migraines can last from a few hours to several days. Take an over-the-counter painkiller immediately or a prescription migraine medication, if you have one, and lie down in a darkened room. If you have more than two migraines a month, see your doctor, who may recommend preventive medication. If this is your first headache of this type, do not take any medication and call your doctor immediately.
Sudden sharp, severe pain on one side of the head, possibly around the eye.	Cluster headache, which may be accompanied by excessive sweating and nasal congestion. Ninety per cent of sufferers are men.	These headaches may last anywhere from a few minutes to several hours but are likely to recur later that day. See your doctor, who may prescribe medication to treat them. There are also preventive medicines that help ward off attacks. Avoid alcohol.

Nausea and vomiting (sudden onset)

Description	Possible causes	Response
Nausea or vomiting that has come on suddenly; perhaps accompanied by pain around your navel, fever, loss of appetite or pressure to have a bowel movement.	An acute abdominal condition such as appendicitis.	Go to the nearest A&E department or call an ambulance. Suspected appendicitis must be assessed and treated quickly to avoid the risk that the appendix will rupture and leak infected fluid into other parts of the abdomen.
Nausea or vomiting accompanied by crushing, squeezing, tightening pain in your chest that comes on suddenly; pain that radiates from your chest to your jaw, back, neck, shoulders or arm, particularly your left arm; racing pulse; or shortness of breath.	Heart attack.	Call an ambulance immediately. If your doctor has prescribed medication to take during an angina attack, take the suggested dose. After you have called an ambulance, chew a standard aspirin (300mg) or four low-dose (75mg) aspirin tablets straightaway.
Nausea or vomiting that starts 2 to 6 hours after a meal.	A bacterial infection caused by spoiled, undercooked or contaminated food; most cases of food poisoning are due to common bacteria such as staphylococcus or E. coli.	Symptoms usually clear up on their own within 12 to 48 hours. Call your doctor if symptoms last longer than three days or if you're unable keep down fluids. If you may have eaten contaminated mushrooms or shellfish, go to the nearest A&E department.
Nausea or vomiting after an accident, sports injury or blow to the head.	Concussion or brain injury.	See your doctor without delay. If symptoms continue to worsen, call an ambulance.
Nausea or vomiting accompanied by black or tarry stools, a burning sensation in the upper abdomen or indigestion.	An ulcer in the upper gastrointestinal tract or gastro-oesophageal reflux disease (GORD).	See your doctor urgently. Diagnostic tests in hospital are likely to be needed and, if blood loss has made you anaemic, you may need to be admitted to hospital for a blood transfusion.
Nausea and vomiting after starting a new medication.	A drug side effect.	Talk to your doctor about whether a different drug should be substituted. Side effects sometimes disappear after a few days or weeks of taking a medication.

Nausea and vomiting (recurrent)

Description	Possible causes	Response
Nausea or vomiting accompanied by throbbing headache on one or both sides of the head and sensitivity to light and sound; possibly accompanied by flashing lights, blind spots or tingling in the arm or face prior to head pain.	Migraine.	If this is the first time you've experienced these symptoms, call your doctor immediately. If you've had migraines in the past, take an over-the-counter painkiller or a prescription migraine medication if you have one, and lie down in a darkened room. If symptoms do not subside within a few hours, call your doctor. If you have more than two migraines a month, see your doctor, who may recommend preventive medication.
Recurrent nausea or vomiting accompanied by sudden pain in your upper right abdomen, especially during or just after a meal.	Gallstones or gall bladder inflammation.	See your doctor, who may arrange for you to have diagnostic tests.
Recurrent nausea or vomiting accompanied by other unexplained symptoms, such as fatigue, pain or weight changes.	A chronic gastrointestinal condition; cancer is a possibility.	See your doctor, who may arrange for you to have diagnosic tests.
Nausea or vomiting after eating specific foods.	Food allergy or intolerance.	Eliminate the trigger food from your diet and talk to your doctor about whether allergy tests are appropriate.
Nausea or vomiting accompanied by excessive thirst, fatigue, increased urination or poor wound healing.	Poorly controlled diabetes.	See your doctor for advice on how to get your diabetes under control.
Nausea and vomiting in women in early pregnancy.	Morning sickness.	See your doctor. In severe cases treatment may be needed to ensure you and your baby receive adequate nutrients and fluid.
Nausea or vomiting that has recurred for weeks or months; possibly accompanied by pain or discomfort in the abdomen, diarrhoea, constipation, bloating, flatulence and other gastrointestinal symptoms.	A chronic condition such as lactose intolerance, irritable bowel syndrome, peptic ulcer, food allergy, Crohn's disease, ulcerative colitis or coeliac disease.	See your doctor, who may refer you to a gastroenterologist for investigations and treatment.
Nausea and vomiting accompanied by chest pain, excessive thirst, increased or decreased urination, appetite loss, swelling or numbness in the hands or feet, muscle cramps, trouble concentrating, shortness of breath or dizziness.	Heart, liver or kidney failure.	Consult your doctor urgently. A thorough physical examination and diagnostic tests can determine the existence and extent of these serious conditions.

Numbness and tingling

Description	Possible causes	Response
Numbness or tingling that has come on suddenly and affects one side of the body; possibly accompanied by dizziness, blurred vision, headache or confusion.	Stroke or transient ischaemic attack (TIA).	Go to the nearest A&E department immediately. Prompt treatment can save your life and reduce your risk of permanent disability.
Numbness and tingling along the arm or down the back of the leg.	An injury to a nerve in the neck or back.	If the symptoms occurred following an injury or fall, go to your nearest A&E department immediately. In other cases, see your doctor.
Pain in the lower back radiating to the buttock or down the back of the leg that may include numbness in the leg or foot.	Sciatica caused by pressure on a spinal nerve root from a herniated disc in the back.	See your doctor. Avoid activity that hurts, but don't avoid all exercise or the muscles around the disc will weaken. Over-the-counter painkillers and physiotherapy can also help.
Numbness or tingling in the hand, wrist and fingers that develops over time and may be worse at night; possibly accompanied by loss of feeling in the fingers.	Carpal tunnel syndrome, which is often caused by overuse of the hands for repetitive motion.	See your doctor. Treatment options include wrist splinting, stretching exercises, non-steroidal anti-inflammatory drugs, corticosteroids and, in some cases, surgery.
In people with diabetes, numbness and tingling in the feet; possibly accompanied by a reduced ability to feel pain, heat or cold; loss of balance; or sharp pains that worsen at night.	Diabetic neuropathy.	See your doctor. There is no cure, but symptoms can be managed with medication. To prevent progression, keep your blood glucose and blood pressure under control and take your diabetes medication as prescribed.
Numbness or tingling that comes on gradually in your fingers, hands and lower extremities; possibly accompanied by fatigue or muscle weakness anywhere in the body.	Abnormal levels of calcium, potassium, sodium or vitamin B_{12}.	Consult your doctor who may order diagnostic tests.

Painful urination

Description	Possible causes	Response
A burning sensation during urination accompanied by fever over 38.5°C (101°F) and back pain.	A kidney infection.	See your doctor without delay. An antibiotic is likely to be prescribed.
A burning sensation during urination; perhaps accompanied by a frequent need to urinate.	An infection of the lower urinary tract (cystitis).	See your doctor, who may arrange for a urine test. Treatment is usually with antibiotics.
In women, itching and burning during urination accompanied by a thick, white vaginal discharge.	A yeast (candida) infection (also known as thrush) that commonly occurs after antibiotic treatment.	See your doctor, who may collect a specimen from your vagina to check for the presence of yeast. Antifungal treatment can be prescribed and is also available over the counter.
Painful urination after starting a new medication.	A side effect of medications such as ibuprofen and some antidepressants, osteoporosis drugs and anticancer drugs.	Talk to your doctor about whether a different medication should be substituted. Side effects sometimes disappear after a few days or weeks of taking a medication.
In women, pain or pressure in the lower abdomen with difficulty emptying the bladder completely.	An enlarged womb or ovary pressing against the bladder.	See your doctor, who may order tests such as an ultrasound to clarify the cause and refer you for appropriate treatment.
Pain on urination, perhaps preceded by severe pain in the back and side and accompanied by a frequent need to urinate or inability to urinate.	Kidney stones.	See your doctor, who will arrange appropriate imaging investigations. Many kidney stones pass on their own. If they don't pass, they may need to be surgically removed or shattered with shock waves.
Painful urination possibly accompanied by sores, blisters, scabs or pustules in the genital area; painful intercourse; or unusual discharge from the vagina or penis.	A sexually transmitted infection such as genital herpes, syphilis or gonorrhoea.	Attend a local GUM (genito-urinary medicine) clinic, which will maintain confidentiality; prompt treatment can often prevent more serious symptoms. Avoid intercourse until you've been given the 'all clear'.

Shortness of breath

Description	Possible causes	Response
Sudden shortness of breath accompanied by chest pain or pressure; pain that radiates outward from the chest.	A heart attack, arrhythmia or a blood clot that travels from the legs towards the heart.	Call an ambulance immediately. If your doctor has prescribed medication to take during an angina attack, take the suggested dose. After you have called an ambulance, chew a standard aspirin (300mg) or four low-dose (75mg) aspirin tablets straightaway.
Sudden shortness of breath immediately after choking on a piece of food or other foreign object.	Airway obstruction.	If the person is choking, slap them between the shoulder blades or, if you know how, perform the Heimlich manoeuvre. Otherwise, call an ambulance or take the person to the nearest A&E department.
Sudden shortness of breath hours or a few days after inhaling a piece of food, liquid or other foreign object.	Lung infection caused by aspiration of a foreign object.	See your doctor as a matter of urgency or go to the nearest A&E department. If infection is present, antibiotics may be prescribed.
Sudden shortness of breath after exposure to an allergen such as nuts, shellfish or eggs; may be accompanied by swelling of the tongue or itching, a rash, or reddened skin.	Anaphylactic shock.	Call an ambulance immediately. Use an EpiPen if your doctor has prescribed one.
Shortness of breath after exposure to a known trigger such as dust, pollen or pet dander.	Asthma or an environmental allergy.	Use an inhaler if you have one; or take an antihistamine. Seek medical help urgently if this does not provide relief.
Shortness of breath before, during or after a stressful or anxiety-provoking experience; may be accompanied by sweating, nausea, chest pain or tightness in your throat.	Panic attack.	If this is your first panic attack, go to the nearest A&E department. If you are breathing rapidly, breathe through pursed lips (as if you were going to blow out a candle) or cover your mouth and one nostril and breathe through the other nostril. If attacks continue, see your doctor.
Shortness of breath that has come on gradually and is accompanied by fever or cold or flu symptoms.	Bronchitis or pneumonia.	See your doctor, who may order a chest X-ray and treat with antibiotics. Hospital admission may be advised in severe cases.
Shortness of breath that has come on gradually over a period of weeks or months.	A chronic respiratory illness such as asthma, chronic obstructive pulmonary disease, emphysema or a tumour.	See your doctor, who may arrange for you to have diagnostic tests.

Skin lesions and rashes

Description	Possible causes	Response
A rash that doesn't fade when pressed under a glass; accompanied by a fever or headache.	Meningitis or septicaemia.	Go to the nearest A&E department immediately.
A rash that doesn't fade when pressed under a glass; without other symptoms.	Low platelet count.	See your doctor promptly. A blood test may be necessary to confirm the diagnosis.
Mouth ulcers.	Medication reaction, low white cell count or viral infection, vitamin C, B_{12} or folic acid deficiency.	See your doctor, who may order blood tests.
A mole that changes shape, size or colour, or is bleeding.	Mole changes can be a symptom of skin cancer.	See your doctor promptly. Early diagnosis is important for effective treatment.
Rash with fluid-filled spots.	Chickenpox, shingles, impetigo, allergic reaction or, occasionally, an autoimmune skin disease.	See your doctor for diagnosis and treatment.
Unexplained bruises.	Bleeding disorder, liver problems, medication side effects.	See your doctor promptly.
Skin ulcer that doesn't heal.	Infection, circulation problem, or possibly skin cancer.	See your doctor for investigation and treatment.

Unintentional weight gain

Description	Possible causes	Response
Weight gain accompanied by fatigue, hair loss, dry skin, decreased cold tolerance or constipation.	Hypothyroidism (underactive thyroid gland).	See your doctor, who may order a diagnostic blood test. If your thyroid is underactive, treatment is thyroid hormone replacement medication.
Weight gain after starting a new medication.	A side effect of some medications, including corticosteroids, lithium, antipsychotics, and some antidepressants.	Talk to your doctor about whether a different medication should be substituted.
In women, gradual weight gain possibly accompanied by irregular or nonexistent periods, excess hair growth, acne or infertility.	Polycystic ovary syndrome.	See your doctor, who may arrange investigations to clarify the diagnosis and refer you to a specialist for treatment.
Weight gain accompanied by sadness, fatigue, loss of interest in enjoyable activities, or thoughts of suicide.	Depression.	See your doctor, who may refer you to a mental health professional for medication, therapy or both.
Weight gain after quitting smoking.	Snacking as a displacement activity, improved general appetite, better absorption of nutrients in the gut and the slowing of metabolism that comes with smoking cessation.	Suck on sugarless sweets or chew sugarless gum, snack on raw vegetables, drink plenty of water and start an exercise programme.
Weight gain accompanied by excessive thirst, fatigue, increased urination or poor wound healing.	Type 2 diabetes.	See your doctor, who will order a test to measure your blood glucose levels.
Gradual weight gain with no other symptoms.	An increase in calorie intake or a decrease in exercise or energy output.	Eat less and get more exercise. As you get older, you tend to use less energy; therefore your calorie needs usually decrease.

Unintentional weight loss

Description	Possible causes	Response
Weight loss accompanied by insomnia, unusual thirst, increased sweating, increased bowel movements and hair loss.	Hyperthyroidism (overactive thyroid gland) or other hormone imbalance.	See your doctor, who may order a diagnostic blood test. If your thyroid is overactive, prescription medication can slow it down.
Weight loss after starting a new medication.	A side effect of some drugs, including sedatives, SSRI antidepressants and narcotic painkillers.	Talk to your doctor about whether a different medication should be substituted.
Weight loss during a period of high stress or anxiety.	Anxiety or intense stress.	Look for ways to change whatever is causing the stress or anxiety. Relaxation techniques such as meditation, yoga and visualisation may help you cope. Longer-lasting anxiety can be treated with therapy, medication or both.
Weight loss accompanied by feelings of sadness, fatigue, loss of interest in enjoyable activities or thoughts of suicide.	Depression.	See your doctor, who may recommend medication, therapy or both.
Weight loss accompanied by gastrointestinal complaints such as bloating, flatulence, constipation or diarrhoea.	Coeliac disease, an autoimmune disorder in which the gluten in wheat, rye and barley damages the intestines and reduces the body's ability to absorb nutrients.	See your doctor, who may order a diagnostic blood test or gastroscopy. Switching to a gluten-free diet for life is the only treatment for coeliac disease.
Weight loss accompanied by recurrent abdominal pain and loose stools.	Ulcerative colitis or Crohn's disease, which prevent digestion and absorption of some nutrients in the food you eat.	See your doctor, who may recommend dietary changes, surgery or medication that reduces inflammation.
Weight loss accompanied by excessive thirst, fatigue, increased urination or poor wound healing.	Type 1 diabetes.	See your doctor, who may order a test to measure your blood glucose levels.
Weight loss with no other symptoms.	A chronic bowel condition or cancer.	See your doctor, who will arrange for you to have diagnostic tests.

Vaginal bleeding or discharge

Description	Possible causes	Response
Greyish white, fishy-smelling vaginal discharge.	Bacterial vaginosis, an inflammation of the vagina caused by bacteria.	See your doctor, who will prescribe antibiotics; these can clear up the symptoms within a few days.
Yellow or greenish bubbly discharge with a foul odour; perhaps accompanied by genital soreness or irritation.	Gonorrhoea, trichomoniasis or another sexually transmitted infection.	Attend a GUM (genito-urinary medicine, clinic), which will maintain confidentiality; antibiotics will be prescribed. Avoid intercourse until the infection clears up. Encourage your partner to attend, too.
Thick white discharge; may be accompanied by soreness and itching.	A yeast (candida) infection (also known as thrush), which may occur during or after antibiotic treatment.	See your doctor, who may collect a specimen from your vagina to check for the presence of yeast. Antifungal treatment can be prescribed and is also available over the counter.
Abnormal discharge accompanied by fever or pain in the pelvic or lower abdominal area.	Pelvic inflammatory disease, an inflammation or infection of the ovaries, fallopian tubes or uterus.	See your doctor without delay. Prompt treatment with antibiotics can prevent lasting damage to your reproductive system that could contribute to infertility, ectopic pregnancy and other reproductive disorders.
Bleeding during pregnancy.	A miscarriage, ectopic pregnancy or other serious complication.	Call your doctor immediately or go to the nearest A&E department. If you are in severe pain, call an ambulance.
Bleeding after intercourse.	A sexually transmitted infection, cervical erosion, cancer of the cervix or dry vaginal walls caused by lack of oestrogen.	See your doctor, who will refer you for diagnostic investigations.
Bleeding between menstrual periods after having an IUCD fitted or when taking the contraceptive pill.	Both these methods of contraception may cause irregular vaginal bleeding.	See your doctor, who may recommend a change in contraceptive method or a different contraceptive pill.
Bleeding between menstrual periods for no obvious reason.	Hormonal imbalance that may be caused by a condition such as polycystic ovary syndrome; cancer of the uterus or cervix.	See your doctor, who will arrange investigations and specialist referral if necessary.

Vision loss

Description	Possible causes	Response
Sudden loss of vision that has occurred after an accident, sports injury, chemical burn or contact with irritant substance.	An injury to the retina, cornea or nerves, including corneal abrasion and torn retina.	Sudden vision loss is always an emergency. Go to the nearest A&E department immediately.
A sudden change in vision accompanied by confusion, slurred speech, sudden numbness on one side of the body or sudden severe headache.	Stroke or transient ischaemic attack (TIA).	Call an ambulance immediately. Prompt treatment can save your life and reduce your risk of permanent disability.
In those of the age of 40, a gradual reduction in the ability to focus on nearby objects.	Presbyopia, an age-related change in vision.	Take this opportunity to have your eyes checked by an optician, but you can buy reading glasses from a pharmacy.
Blurred vision with dryness, irritation or a gritty feeling in the eyes.	Dry eyes, which often occurs in women during the menopause.	See your doctor, who may prescribe eyedrops or recommend an over-the-counter preparation.
Blurred vision and dry eyes after starting a new medication.	A side effect of medications such as diuretics, beta-blockers, antihistamines, sleeping pills and some painkillers.	Talk to your doctor about whether a different medication should be substituted. Side effects sometimes disappear after a few days or weeks of taking a new medication.
In people with diabetes, blurred or spotty vision.	Diabetic retinopathy, in which blood vessels in the retina are damaged.	See your doctor. Surgery (laser or conventional) can reduce loss of vision.
In older people, blurred, cloudy vision; may be accompanied by faded appearance of colours, glare or halos around lights, poor night vision, or double vision.	Cataracts, a condition in which the eye's lens is clouded by clumps of protein.	See your doctor. Clouded lenses can be surgically removed and replaced with artificial ones, improving vision in 90 per cent of cases.
Blank spots in your field of vision possibly accompanied by blurred vision, loss of peripheral vision, eye pain, headache and rainbow-coloured halos around lights.	Glaucoma, a disease caused by pressure within the eye that damages the optic nerve.	See your doctor. Surgery and medication (eyedrops or tablets) can slow glaucoma's progression but can't bring back lost vision. Go straight to the nearest A&E department if your eye is also red and/or painful.
Blurriness or loss of central vision; may be accompanied by straight lines appearing wavy, difficulty recognising faces and the need for extra light while reading.	Age-related macular degeneration, a disease that occurs when the macula – the central part of the eye – breaks down or is damaged.	See your doctor. Treatments include laser surgery, photodynamic therapy (medication combined with light therapy) and medications that are injected into the eye. Treatment can't restore lost vision but may delay further loss.

Wounds that won't heal

Description	Possible causes	Response
Cuts or bruises that heal unusually slowly but do not appear infected.	Weakened immunity, which can be caused by poor nutrition, vitamin deficiency, steroid drugs or cancer treatment.	See your doctor, who may recommend vitamin supplementation or changes in steroid use; advice from a dietitian may be useful.
A wound that is swollen, red or hot, or has pus or red lines radiating from it; may be accompanied by fever.	Cellulitis (a bacterial infection of the skin) or a foreign object in the wound.	See your doctor without delay, who may prescribe an antibiotic. If symptoms are worsening quickly, go to the nearest A&E department.
Poor wound healing accompanied by excessive thirst, increased urination, unexplained weight loss, increased hunger or blurred vision.	Undiagnosed or poorly controlled diabetes.	See your doctor, who will order a test to measure your blood glucose levels. If you have diabetes that is poorly controlled, you may need to change your regular treatment regime.
In people with diabetes, poor wound healing in the feet; may be accompanied by a reduced ability to feel pain, heat or cold; loss of balance; or sharp pains that worsen at night.	Diabetic neuropathy.	See your doctor. There is no cure, but symptoms can be managed with medication. To prevent progression, keep your blood glucose and blood pressure under control and take your diabetes medication as prescribed.
Sores on the legs or feet that won't heal accompanied by cold feet, leg or foot pain or numbness, or changes in the toenails or amount of hair on the legs or feet.	Peripheral arterial disease, a restriction of blood flow in the arteries of the leg caused by accumulation of arterial plaque.	See your doctor. Circulation can be improved with exercise, quitting smoking and a heart-healthy diet; in some cases, medication or surgery is needed.
A sore in the mouth or on the lip or skin that doesn't heal.	Vitamin deficiency may be the cause, but oral cancer or skin cancer are also possibilities.	See your doctor, who may order diagnostic tests.

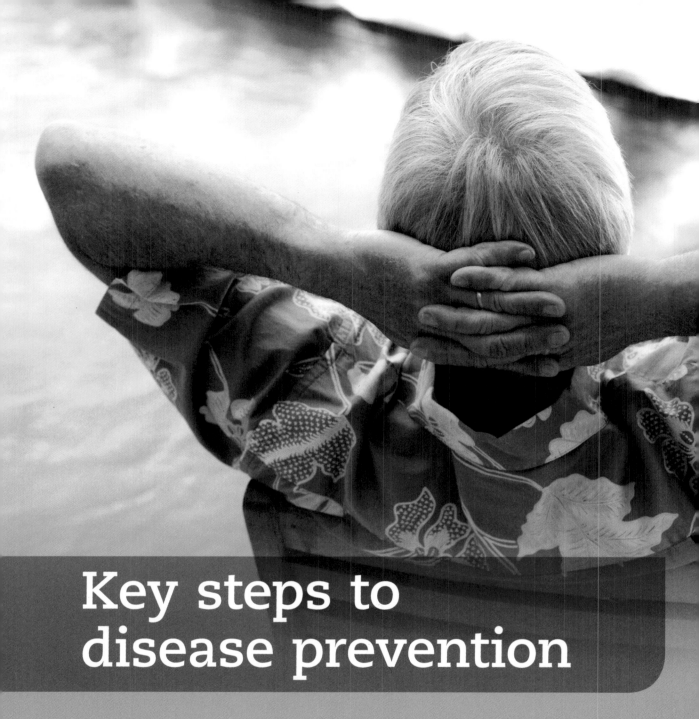

Key steps to disease prevention

When preventive medicine specialists were asked what really helps to prevent disease, their answers were surprising, and offered new perspectives on health. While exercising, better diet and quitting smoking are still seen as vital, the survey also showed that a stress-free, purposeful life can make a big contribution.

Getting organised

Now that you've read about the main causes of disease and completed the quiz on pages 18–19, it's worth looking more closely at the key steps that are going to put your health back on track – and keep it on track. By following the steps outlined in this chapter, you'll lower your risk of many major diseases, from cardiovascular disease and stroke to Type 2 diabetes and lung cancer, and ensure that health issues are not going to become an obstacle to your enjoyment of life. Even if your quiz score was good, there's still room for improvement. But if your score was lower than it should be, then you'll want to make sure you start incorporating all of the steps outlined on the following pages, to reap the maximum health benefits.

All 12 key steps are important lifestyle measures that most of us can manage, but the top three – quitting smoking, getting at least 30 minutes of light exercise on most days, eating at least five servings of fruit and vegetables daily – can drastically reduce your risk of disease. Giving up smoking was rated highest in the Reader's Digest Disease Prevention Survey. As most smokers and ex-smokers know, quitting is one of the most challenging things they'll ever do. The book outlines five easy ways to make breaking the habit a successful enterprise.

For other people, making time for regular physical activity is what's hardest to achieve. Our bodies need movement – exercise builds strong muscles, bones and joints. We also need to burn calories in order to maintain a healthy weight and to prevent obesity and the complications arising from it. Exercise also plays an important role in our mental and emotional health. Each of the key steps works in combination with the others.

Getting started usually happens once you get organised, but how do you do that? Make a list of the key steps that aren't already part of your everyday life, then read through each of those steps, noting down what the advice on offer is. For example, if you still smoke and have tried quitting a number of times, talk to your GP about the possibility of taking medication to help you succeed. By approaching lifestyle changes in an organised way, you'll boost your chances of sticking to them in the long run.

What is risk?

Risk is the chance that something might happen in a set time frame. In health terms, that chance can be high (catching at least one cold each winter) or low (getting pancreatic cancer).

For some conditions, you may be able to affect personal risk. For example, the average chance of getting a disease might be 5 per cent (1 in 20), but you can halve that risk to 2.5 per cent (1 in 40) by making certain changes in your lifestyle. This can be described as an 'absolute risk reduction' of 2.5 percentage points. Alternatively, the same scenario could be described in terms of a 'relative risk reduction' of 50 per cent, because you are now 50 per cent less likely to contract that disease than you would otherwise have been.

Throughout this book relative risk reduction is used, partly because this is easier for researchers to calculate, but also in the hope that the larger, more dramatic numbers will motivate you to act on the advice of medical experts in order to see a significant improvement in your overall health outcomes.

STEP 1
Get 30 minutes of light exercise on most days

In the short amount of time it takes to watch many TV programmes, you could cut your risk of diabetes by 34 per cent, of stroke by 20 per cent, of a hip fracture by 41 per cent and of dying over the next few years by half – and at the same time sharpen your thinking skills, reduce your waistline and improve your general sense of wellbeing.

How? By exercising regularly. The Disease Prevention Survey panel of experts ranked exercise high on their list of health-enhancing changes. If you are a smoker, quitting is likely to be your priority (see page 66), but for most of us just half an hour of light activity (a walk, a swim, working in the garden) on most days of the week will bring dramatic, body-wide benefits. Even if you have limited mobility, perhaps as a result of illness or carrying too much weight, you can still be active.

Three 10 minute walks are as ***beneficial*** as one 30 minute walk ...

However, the real question about exercise and health isn't whether it works, because most of us have heard that lecture at least 1,000 times before. Rather, it is: why don't most of us do it?

The honest answer is many people have trouble motivating themselves to get up and out of the door, possibly because they're scared of 'exercise' with its pumping iron connotations, and also because it requires some effort. And sometimes sitting around all day (whether in a desk-bound job or reading, internet-surfing or watching TV can also make you feel tired, so the impetus to exercise isn't there.

If you've been putting it off until you're in the mood, forget it. Waiting for the perfect wave of enthusiasm to get you on your feet doesn't work. Instead, make a firm decision to do 10 minutes of exercise on a certain schedule. Regular exercisers say that simply getting out there – whether you feel motivated or not – creates the energy that gets you moving and buoys your mood. Just tell yourself you'll walk for just 10 minutes, then once you get started, 10 minutes will soon become 20 minutes and eventually 30 minutes.

Walking or cycling is an excellent way to start It's also important to engage in physical activities that strengthen your muscles and build bones, such as working with hand weights or elastic exercise bands, doing moves like sit-ups and push-ups, using the strength machines at the gym, or even working hard in the garden. You begin losing muscle mass in your thirties, and as a result your body burns fewer calories every day – making it tougher to maintain a healthy weight. Some strength training can reverse this trend and boost your energy levels. It's worth investing a little time and energy learning how to do the right strength-training exercises for your age and fitness level by having sessions with a personal trainer or taking a class at a local gym. Try getting in the right frame of mind with these ideas.

Anything is better than nothing If you don't have time for a 30 minute walk or a 45 minute gym workout, then use the 5, 10 or 15 minutes you do have. Numerous health studies show that three 10 minute walks burn off energy just as effectively as one 30 minute walk and may be even better at things such as keeping blood pressure lower and healthier all day. Dancing, walking rather than driving and using the stairs instead of the lift can all boost cardiovascular health just as effectively as a formal work-out.

Willpower is not the answer If you're like most people, willpower alone won't get you up every day for that 7am walk, or pull you away from the day's work for those sit-ups. Instead, set an exercise 'date' – a regular walking or jogging time with a friend, a class at the gym or even an appointment with your personal trainer, then write it in pen in your diary.

It should be enjoyable It's no wonder many people think they dislike exercise – how much fun is it to sit in the living room pedalling an exercise bike that's going nowhere? If you're a competitive person, consider taking up squash or tennis. Or if you're social, try to schedule walks with different friends or join a spin or water aerobics class. Exercise isn't just a means to an end; it's part of your life, so it shouldn't feel like a drag.

Opportunities are everywhere The stairs next to the escalator, the dog with a lead in his mouth – these are golden opportunities to fit more exercise into your day. Fifty years ago, our parents and grandparents burned far more calories per day than we do today, not by running marathons but through a host of daily activities that we've since engineered out of our lives, from walking to the bus stop to washing the dishes. It's up to you to create a new trend.

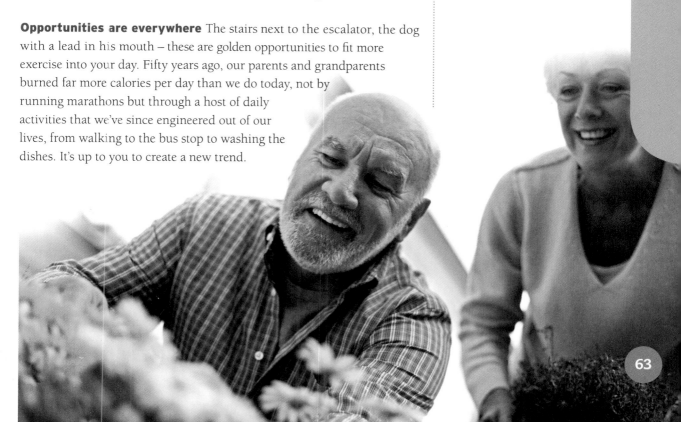

Step 2
Eat at least five servings of fruit and vegetables daily

If everyone followed the simple advice of health experts by eating at least five servings of fruit and vegetables a day, there would undoubtedly be emptier hospitals and doctors' surgeries, shorter queues at the pharmacy and far fewer of the major diseases that disable and kill millions each year around the world.

The fact is, we are designed to eat these foods in volume every day. Our bodies are meant to be flooded on a daily basis by the health-giving chemicals called antioxidants, which protect cells from damage. And we need them now more than ever. Modern life triggers the production of more free radicals in our bodies than previously – thanks in large part to fried foods (and simply overeating), more air pollution and the fact that we're living longer, along with environmental damage such as the thinning atmosphere, which could also be a contributing factor.

Free radicals are atoms or groups of atoms with an odd number of electrons. They form naturally when we digest food, convert blood glucose into energy or are exposed to sunlight or pollution. Free radicals destroy cell walls or, even worse, DNA itself. The result is an increased cancer risk, high levels of cholesterol that's more likely to burrow into artery walls, and damaged cartilage that isn't able to cushion joints properly. Your body uses the antioxidants in fruit and vegetables to neutralise these free radicals before they harm cells. If you shortchange yourself by not getting enough of them in your diet, then you're essentially allowing rogue elements to wreak havoc in your body.

What's a serving?

It's easier than you think to get five servings of fruit and vegetables a day. You can get one by starting your morning with fruit juice, and three or four more by having a big salad at lunch. Below are examples of a single serving:

Fruit
- 1 medium-sized fruit (apple, pear, orange, banana) two smaller pieces (plums, satsumas, apricots)
- 3 tbsp (fresh fruit salad, cooked or canned fruit)
- 30g dried fruit
- 1 small glass (150ml) fruit juice

Vegetables
- 3 heaped tbsp cooked fresh or frozen vegetables (carrots, peas, beans, pulses etc.)
- 4 heaped tbsp green vegetables (kale, spinach, greens etc.)
- medium portion (1 dessert bowlful) of mixed salad (lettuce, cucumber, tomatoes)

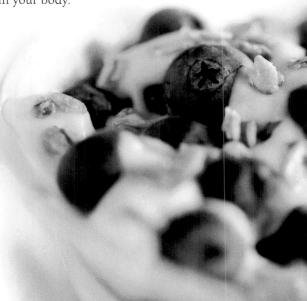

Fruit is simple to eat and it can transform a meal. Think about adding grapes to a chicken salad or giving a burst of sharp sweetness by including a few berries in your morning cereal. With a little creativity, vegetables can be just as delicious – ripe tomatoes dressed with basil, roasted courgettes or sweet potatoes with a pinch of cinnamon or nutmeg.

Putting fresh, healthy food on your plate doesn't have to take longer than picking up fast-food or tossing a frozen meal into the microwave, and it's more than worth it for the health gain. And thanks to the convenience of prewashed and pre-cut fresh vegetables that are available in most supermarkets, you'll be surprised at how easy it can be to put a meal together quickly. Try these strategies to reach your daily target.

Assign specific servings to each meal For example, you might always have a small glass of freshly squeezed orange juice plus a handful of berries at breakfast, start lunch with a salad (three servings of vegetables), have fruit as a snack and have another two servings of vegetables with dinner. That's more than five servings right there.

Aim to always have two colours of fruit or vegetables on your plate At breakfast have a strawberry and melon compote or a fresh fruit smoothie, add carrots and black beans (pulses count as vegetables) to your salad at lunch, top pasta with tomatoes and steamed broccoli at dinner, and snack on berries and bananas. This scheme provides two servings per meal.

Double each vegetable portion you'd normally eat This is a good approach if you're already eating several servings a day.

Stock up on ready-to-use produce Try cans of fruit in natural juice (not syrup), frozen plain (no sauce) vegetables and frozen berries – flash-frozen produce retains most of its nutrients – and pre-sliced, pre-trimmed vegetables. And look for pre-washed salad leaf mixes.

Keep salads interesting Plain green salads can be boring so add a variety of toppings. Try toasted sesame seeds, a few olives, roasted beetroot, peppers, chillies or even a few raspberries or orange segments.

New reasons to eat less

Big portions and high-fat, high-calorie, processed foods are the number-one enemies of good health. Excess weight puts you at higher risk of heart disease and diabetes. But research also links obesity to an increased risk of cancer, too. Not surprisingly, cutting back on overeating is a top priority.

Eating too much not only puts on visible weight, it also crowds internal organs with hidden fat that fuels the development of major disease processes. What's more digestion creates destructive particles called free radicals that play a role in a host of health problems, from joint pain to cancer. More food, more digestion, more free radicals. Eating just enough is a challenge in today's world, but it can be done. Here's how:

Dole out single servings Don't serve platters of food or sit near an open bag of snacks.

Eat at home Women who eat out five times a week or more consume up to a thousand more calories each day than those who don't.

Bulk up your meals with extra vegetables These add fibre, water and volume to your meal – three factors that make you feel fuller while you're eating fewer calories. Researchers say this strategy also stretches the stomach wall, activating 'fullness receptors'.

Eat only until you're 80 per cent full Leave the table when you still have room for a little more instead of finishing everything. Within 20 minutes – the time it take your brain to register your food intake – you'll feel satisfied.

STEP 3
Quit smoking

Most health-conscious people no longer smoke or never did. If you still smoke, nothing else offers anything close to the health benefits you'll get from quitting. When the book's panel of preventive medicine experts ranked the habits they considered most detrimental to wellbeing, 99 per cent put smoking first on the list, ahead of other well-known threats such as being significantly overweight or not getting enough sleep.

It's not news that cigarettes (as well as cigars and pipes) are lethal. Around the world, tobacco kills 5.4 million people annually thanks to lung cancer, breast cancer, heart attack, stroke, diabetes, progressive lung diseases and hundreds of other health problems it triggers or makes worse. And we now know why it's so difficult to quit: in terms of addictive power, experts put nicotine in the same class as heroin and cocaine. So if you've tried to quit smoking before and it hasn't worked, don't blame yourself – and don't give up. It can take as many as five or more attempts. And you don't have to go it alone; in fact, the latest research shows that using several strategies to help you quit, such as nicotine replacement and support from your doctor, can double or even triple your chances of succeeding.

*Nicotine-replacement nasal sprays can **increase quit rates** by 12 to 16 per cent*

Quitting gives your health an immediate boost. Within 8 hours, levels of toxic carbon monoxide gas in your bloodstream drop to normal. Within a day, your heart attack risk begins to fall. Over your first smoke-free year, your circulation will improve, your senses of taste and smell will sharpen, and you'll have fewer lung infections, cough less and have less sinus congestion. After just a year, your odds of developing heart disease drop by half. And the payoffs mount with each smoke-free year: after four years, your chance of having a heart attack falls to that of someone who has never smoked. After 10 years, your lung cancer risk drops to nearly that of a nonsmoker, and your odds of developing cancers of the mouth, throat, oesophagus, bladder and kidney decrease significantly, too. To help yourself quit successfully, try these strategies.

Line up help before your quit date After you smoke that last cigarette, a relapse can occur very quickly. Within two days, half of all people light up again; by the end of the first week, two-thirds are back to smoking. Help at the right moment can be crucial. Before your quit date, set up an appointment with your doctor, a cognitive behavioural therapist or a smoking-cessation support group for your first smoke-free week. Or plan to call a telephone quitline. All of these resources can offer tailored advice to help you cope with specific challenges, such as what to do if you've

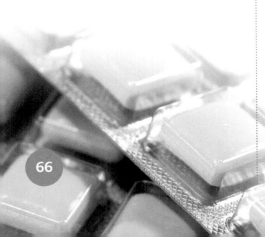

always had a cigarette after dinner (schedule an activity for that time – mow the lawn or take an evening walk with a friend), or smoked when life threw a few challenges your way. In one US study, 43 per cent of people who used a telephone quitline were still smoke free after nine months compared to just 5 per cent who didn't. In the UK, you can call the NHS Stop Smoking Helpline on 0800 022 4 332 or visit www.smokefree.nhs.uk.

Consider a behavioural therapy programme or support group
When researchers at Oxford University in the UK reviewed 55 smoking-cessation studies, they found that people who joined therapy groups doubled their odds of succeeding, compared to those who tried to kick the habit by themselves.

Use the correct nicotine-replacement dose Chewing gum, patches, lozenges, sprays and inhalers containing nicotine can all be helpful. They all release nicotine very slowly into the bloodstream, easing symptoms of withdrawal without all the other toxins in cigarette smoke.

Studies find that the patch increases quit rates by about 7 per cent compared to a placebo, the gum and inhaler by about 8 per cent, and the nasal spray by 12 to 16 per cent. But make sure you're getting enough. If you smoke more than 10 cigarettes a day, for example, choose a higher-dose (usually 21mg) patch. And if you have your first cigarette within half an hour of waking up in the morning, start the day with a 4mg lozenge rather than a 2mg dose.

If you still have cravings, using a patch plus a faster-acting product such as gum, lozenges or a spray or inhaler can further boost your chances of succeeding, according to experts.

Use medications to help you There's a choice of two prescription medications to help you quit smoking: bupropion (Zyban) and varenicline (Champix). They are not addictive and work by reducing cravings, although doctors are not sure how they do this, but both medications significantly increase your chances of quitting and staying smoke free. Varenicline is taken for at least 12 weeks and the commonest side effect is nausea (it can't be used by pregnant women, but they can use nicotine-replacement therapy). Bupropion is taken for at least seven weeks and the commonest side effect is headache. It is not suitable for anyone who has had a seizure (fit) or is at risk of seizures. Before prescribing either medication, your doctor will need to know your full health history and your regular medications.

Schedule exercise Exercising three times a week may work even better than a behavioural therapy programme. In one study, nearly 20 per cent of those who exercised were still smoke free after a year compared to 11 per cent of the therapy group. Counselling plus exercise is an even better idea.

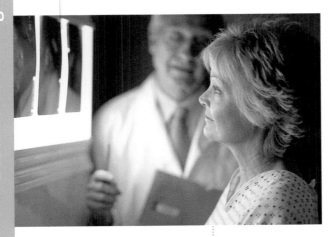

STEP 4
Get recommended screening tests

Left to their own devices, some invisible health problems turn into big ones. A slightly raised blood glucose level becomes full-blown diabetes; pre-hypertension becomes high blood pressure; suspicious-looking cells become cancer. Your best defence is to catch these problems early on, when they can be most easily reversed and even cured.

There's no doubt that a healthy lifestyle is the best way to prevent most major medical problems from developing in the first place, but trouble can still arise in the healthiest of bodies. That's why the specialists consulted by Reader's Digest ranked the recommended screening tests highly on their list of 'prescriptions' for staying disease free.

Unfortunately, some people ignore these important tests, which are readily available. Laziness, lack of time, fear of finding out that something's wrong or the mistaken conviction that you really don't need the screenings because you're feeling fit and healthy can cause you to not get tested – but you could seriously regret this later on.

See the table on the page opposite for a list of common screening tests and when to get them.

Get a check-up during a routine GP visit Next time you see your doctor, take the opportunity to ask if you should have simple screening tests such as cholesterol, blood pressure and blood glucose checks. If you are aged between 40 and 75, the NHS offers a series of routine tests every five years to check your risk of developing heart disease, stroke, kidney disease or Type 2 diabetes.

Hate going to the doctor? Ask your spouse or a good friend to go along with you when you're having, for example, blood tests for cholesterol levels. You can also offer to be each other's support team when it's time for specialised screening, such as for breast or prostate cancer.

Speak up about your family history Make sure your GP knows about any relevant family history. If a close relative has had a stroke or heart attack or has been diagnosed with cancer or diabetes, it's important to let your doctor know, in case you are vulnerable, too.

Mention depression Doctors should be on the look-out for signs of depression. If you're constantly overwhelmed by feelings of sadness or hopelessness, tell your doctor. There are treatment options that may help.

The screening tests you may need

	Test	When to get it
Women	Mammogram	If you have a family history of breast cancer, ask your doctor when you need to have this X-ray. Otherwise, you will be invited for screening every two years from 50 to 70 and you are encouraged to have a mammogram every three years after the age of 70.
	Cervical smear	Between the ages of 25 and 49 every three years; from 50 to 64 every five years. If your last test showed any abnormalities, you may need more frequent screening.
Men	Prostate specific antigen (PSA test)	This test may be advised if you have symptoms or risk factors for prostate cancer. However, there are risks, so talk to your doctor about the pros and cons of the test.
	Digital rectal examination	Every year from the age of 50 (45 if you have a family history of prostate cancer).
Everyone	Dental examination	Every six months.
	Blood pressure reading	Every five years between the ages of 40 and 75; more frequently if you have diabetes or risk factors for cardiovascular disease.
	Cholesterol test	Every five years between the ages of 40 and 75; more frequently if you have raised blood cholesterol levels.
	Blood glucose test	Every five years between the ages of 40 and 75; more frequently if you have risk factors for diabetes or if symptoms suggest you may have high blood glucose.
	Eye examination	Every year for those with a family history of glaucoma or if symptoms suggest a problem with your eyesight.
	Faecal occult blood test (for bowel cancer)	Offered to those between the ages of 60 and 75 every two years. People at high risk may need more frequent testing from a younger age.
	Weight	Every two years; more often if you have diabetes, cardiovascular disease, gout, liver or gall bladder disease, or are an indigenous person.

Ask about vaccinations Aside from a yearly flu vaccine, if you're aged 65 or older or have reduced immunity, you should ask about the advisability of a pneumonia vaccine.

Take charge Don't rely on a reminder from your doctor; keep a record of the tests and vaccinations you've had and when the next is due.

STEP 5
Get at least 7 to 8 hours sleep a night

Blame it on insomnia, our infatuation with caffeine, shift work, TV, DVDs or the internet; whatever the cause, we've become sleep-deprived. And we're paying the price with higher rates of obesity, diabetes, depression, anxiety and some forms of cancer – all partly due to a lack of sleep.

Researchers are beginning to suspect that sleep deprivation exerts its far-reaching effects on the body by disrupting levels of key hormones and proteins. These include the appetite-regulating hormones ghrelin and leptin, which is why lack of sleep contributes to weight gain; stress hormones, such as cortisol, that raise blood glucose and blood pressure (a reason lack of sleep makes diabetes worse); and proteins involved in chronic inflammation, a condition in which the immune system remains on high alert, raising the risk of heart disease, stroke, cancer and diabetes. Lack of sleep also seems to reduce levels of melatonin, which is a hormone that may help to protect our bodies against cancer.

If you have insomnia or you're a heavy snorer and often wake up exhausted, turn to *Insomnia* and *Snoring*, on pages 232 and 296, respectively. Many of us are our own worst enemies when it comes to getting enough sleep. If that's you, put these three simple strategies to work in order to get 7 to 8 hours of deep, refreshing sleep every night.

1 Pick your perfect bedtime, then stick to it for two weeks Count back 8 hours from the time you have to get up in the morning. This is your new, non-negotiable lights-out time. Subtract another half an hour: this is your new 'get into bed' time. Subtract another half an hour to find the time when you should start relaxing, getting your mind and body ready for sleep before turning in. Here's an example: if you have to be up at 6.30am, you'll need to start relaxing by 9.30pm, get into bed by 10pm and turn out the lights by 10.30pm.

2 Turn off all electronics Half an hour before you get into bed, turn off the TV, computer and mobile phone. Politely tell anyone who phones that you'll talk to them tomorrow (or better yet, screen your calls and return non-urgent messages in the morning). Have a shower or bath and climb into clean, comfortable nightwear. Brush your teeth, comb your hair, do a few minutes of gentle stretching or deep breathing, then read a few pages of your book. And don't snack during this wind-down time.

3 When it's time, turn out the lights If you've trained yourself to fight back fatigue and keep on going, you may be tempted to stay up just a little later. But make a habit of simply turning out the lights when it's time to sleep. It will soon become a habit in itself and you'll feel much better for it.

STEP 6
Know your blood pressure reading

Simply knowing what your blood pressure is could cut your risk of heart attack, stroke, kidney failure or blindness. If you don't know what your reading is, you may not know whether you're developing high blood pressure, the disease that nearly every doctor in the survey said has the greatest potential for causing chronic disease. And if you don't know your blood pressure is creeping up over the years, you can't take steps to bring it back down, leaving the door open for years of damage to occur.

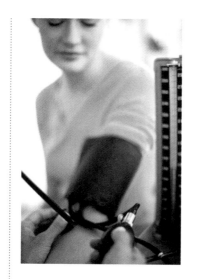

You can't feel high blood pressure, but it wreaks havoc on your cardiovascular system – thickening heart muscle, promoting the growth of plaque in artery walls, rupturing blood vessels in your brain, tearing vessels in your eyes, weakening your kidneys and even raising your risk of dementia. You should have your blood pressure checked regularly. Ask for a reading when you visit your GP and be sure to record the results.

Until just a few years ago, doctors thought you were in the clear if your blood pressure was below 140/90 mmHg. Now we know the risk of heart disease and stroke begins to rise when blood pressure is as low as 115/75 mmHg. Having a reading between 120/80 and 140/90 mmHg – raises your risk of dying from heart disease by 58 per cent, making this 'little' problem more deadly than smoking.

More than one in four adults have what's called pre-hypertension and 90 per cent of us will develop high blood pressure after the age of 55. According to studies, some doctors opt to 'wait and see' what develops when their patients' pressures start creeping up. So it's up to you to keep tabs on your own blood pressure and to take action if it starts rising, even if your reading is still within the normal range.

Live a healthy blood-pressure lifestyle At breakfast, lunch and dinner, you can choose the power foods that fight hypertension. One top eating strategy recommended by the British Heart Foundation is to ensure that fruit and vegetables make up around one third of your diet, starchy foods (preferably whole grain) another third, while the last third should come from protein foods. Keep your intake of sodium (salt) low, too. Quitting smoking, treating obstructive sleep apnoea and getting regular exercise can all help.

Ask about medication Medication for raised blood pressure can play a big part. Some doctors are beginning to prescribe blood pressure-lowering drugs even to people in the pre-hypertensive category if they have other risk factors for heart disease or kidney problems.

What the numbers mean

120/80 mmHg or lower	Optimal
Below 130/85 mmHg	Normal
130–139/85–95 mmHg	High normal
Over 140/90 mmHg	High blood pressure

STEP 7
Cut back on saturated fat

Steering clear of fast-food and fatty meats, butter and full-fat milk and cheeses could lower your LDL ('bad') cholesterol by an impressive 10 per cent. This medication-free measure could, in turn, cut your risk of having a heart attack by as much as 20 per cent. That's not a bad return on a sensible food investment, which is why it is highly recommended for anyone wanting to make healthy dietary modifications.

These days, experts say that getting LDL cholesterol levels down as low as possible is essential (below 3.5 mmol/l for most people and as low as 2.5 mmol/l if you have diabetes or have had a heart attack or stroke). The best way to do this is to cut back on the amount of saturated fat you eat as this is the body's raw material for manufacturing LDL.

*Lower 'bad' **cholesterol** by 10 per cent; lower **heart attack** risk by 20 per cent*

Your goal is to keep your saturated fat intake at less than 10 per cent of the total calories you eat. That's no more than 20g for women eating the recommended 2,000kcal a day, or 30g for men eating the recommended 2,500kcal. You can see that there's no room for butter, at 7g of saturated fat per tablespoon; double cream, at about 3.5g per tablespoon; or full-fat cheddar cheese, at 6.5g per 30g (about one slice). Here are more suggestions for reducing your intake.

Buy low-fat or skimmed milk and dairy products Choosing skimmed rather than full-fat milk saves you more than 4g of saturated fat per glass (200ml), and having low-fat cheese will save 3.5g per slice. If you don't like low-fat cheese, try soft cheeses, such as goat's cheese, which are naturally a little lower in saturated fat than hard cheeses. Or choose a strong-flavoured cheese such as Parmesan and use less of it in dishes.

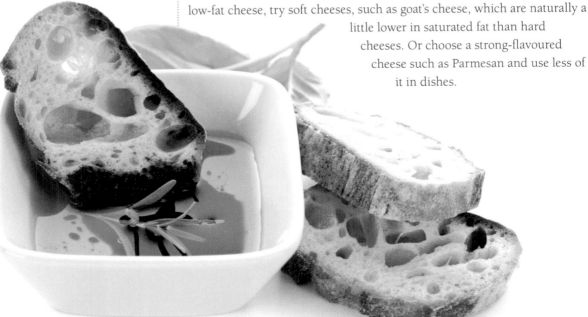

Replace butter with something healthier If you like to spread margarine on your bread, choose a brand enriched with plant sterols, such as Benecol or Flora pro.activ, which can help to reduce 'bad' cholesterol. Or dip your bread in olive oil, or use a little mashed avocado as a spread instead of butter or margarine.

Opt for fish and chicken Most cancer experts agree that a high intake of red (beef, lamb or pork) or processed (ham, bacon, sausage, salami) meat per day can raise your risk of bowel cancer. Fish, skinless chicken and turkey are healthier protein choices.

Keep it lean If possible, avoid beef mince, which may have a high fat content, and choose cuts of meat that have been trimmed and have very little visible fat (marbling). A 90g piece of grilled sirloin has about 1.5g of saturated fat. If you do cook with beef mince, opt for the leanest grade. The World Cancer Research Funds suggests you should limit the amount of cooked red meat you eat per week to 500g (700-750g raw meat).

Steer clear of tropical oils Coconut, palm and palm kernel oil are rich in saturated fat, and appear in some commercial baked goods such as biscuits and crackers. Some food manufacturers are using these oils at the same time they remove transfats (partially hydrogenated vegetable oils linked to higher risk of heart disease). So if the label says 'no trans fats', check the ingredients list for tropical oils and look at the nutrition panel to see what the overall saturated fat content is.

Swap bad fat for good Choose fish – in particular, oily fish such as mackerel, salmon, sardines or tuna, which are high in health-boosting omega-3 fatty acids – over red meat. Try a fish burger instead of a beef burger. Instead of butter, use olive oil. Olive, flaxseed (linseed) and rapeseed oils (high in omega-3 fatty acids) are a better choice for cooking oil than sunflower or corn oils. And instead of snacking on crisps, cake or biscuits, have a small handful of walnuts or almonds, which

Can carbohydrates keep you disease free?

Many people are cutting down on their carbohydrate intake to keep their weight in check. But is that a good idea? It depends.

Most experts agree that carbohydrates in the form of sugary drinks, shop-bought baked goods such as muffins, packaged snacks and confectionery make blood glucose and blood fats (such as triglycerides) soar, raising your risk of Type 2 diabetes, heart disease and even some cancers.

Instead, stock up on 'smart carbs' – whole grains such as oats, barley, whole-grain bread and brown rice, as well as fruit and vegetables, and pulses – and you'll fortify your body with very powerful disease-fighting compounds. The following strategies can help you to replace refined carbohydrates with more healthy alternatives.

- **Look for breads and cereals with the word 'whole' in the first ingredient**

- **Minimise your intake of 'white' foods**
  White potatoes, white pasta and white rice make blood glucose soar; in comparison, whole-grain carbohydrate side dishes such as barley, quinoa and brown rice keep it lower and steadier.

- **Have pulses for dinner a few nights a week**
  Rinse canned beans, peas or lentils to reduce excess sodium (salt). Then add them to soups, salads, casseroles or pasta dishes, or enjoy them with your favourite seasonings as a side dish.

- **Drink unsweetened herb tea or water**
  Besides containing hundreds of empty calories, sugary drinks (even one can a day) have been linked to a higher risk of diabetes, heart disease and obesity, so it's best to avoid them.

STEP 8
Reduce chronic stress

Our bodies are reasonably adept at dealing with short-term stress. If you swerve to avoid a car accident, a burst of adrenaline occurs before your mind has time to fully process what happened. But living with chronic stress is another story altogether, one with surprising health implications. It increases levels of cortisol and other stress hormones and leaves them set on 'high' for days, weeks, months and sometimes even years on end.

The result is often tension headaches, insomnia, disrupted digestion, the list goes on. Researchers are finding links between this kind of stress and higher blood glucose levels, dangerous intra-abdominal fat and possibly even a higher risk of certain cancers. So it's no wonder that living with uncontrolled stress is potentially more destructive than major disease triggers such as being a couple of stones overweight or eating too many processed foods on a regular basis.

All of us have stress in our lives, whether it's the result of a dramatic event such as divorce or a major illness, or the low-level frustrations that come with a busy job, a tense home life, financial worries or regrets about the roads not taken in life. 'Quick fixes' such as a bubble bath, a hot cup of tea or a good cry are all very nice, but it's more important to get to the bottom of what's causing your stress. The best place to start is by being completely open and honest with yourself about what's bothering you, before looking for solutions.

Admit to yourself what's really stressing you Whatever it is, it deserves your attention and respect. Once you bring it out into the open, you can start dealing with it rather than letting it eat away at you on the inside. Don't downplay the issues that are gnawing away at you, even if they seem commonplace. When US researchers at Pace University quizzed people over the age of 50 about the biggest sources of stress in their lives, a decreasing circle of friends, slowing down physically, diminishing time left to spend with children and grandchildren, regret over earlier life choices, physical pain, memory problems, and the headache of growing red tape (filling out tax or other official forms, for example) were issues that appeared on the list.

*Find a **relaxation technique** you like and use it **every day***

Once you've identified the things that are really worry you, write them down, leaving room beside each one to note whether it's something you can't really change and need to accept (such as a milestone birthday coming up) or something you do have some control over. If it's the latter, allow yourself some time to think, then list a few concrete steps you can take to start addressing it. Introducing even one small improvement into your life can make you feel remarkably better by finally giving you a sense of control.

Ask for help where you need it It's human nature: people are often unwilling to ask for help. Or they assume there's nowhere to turn, when often there are resources available. Financial planners, relationship counsellors, life coaches, your doctor or a trusted adviser from your faith community, if you have one, are good resources that can help you

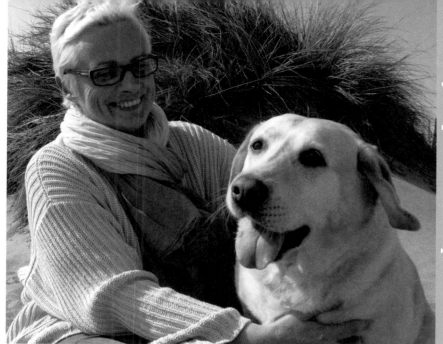

address specific problems in your life. And friends, relatives, neighbours or even acquaintances are usually willing to help out with small tasks if you have the courage to reach out. It's just as likely that they could use your help in return, too.

Build, or rebuild, a social network Loss is a theme that occurred again and again when the Pace University researchers asked people about larger stressors. Their advice was to rebuild a web of caring connections through community groups, volunteering and church groups or other religious organisations. Don't depend on a small, close-knit circle of friends – now is the time to branch out. Scientific journals are now supplying evidence that having friends around can actually change the biochemistry of your brain – by pumping up feelings of joy and wellbeing that bolster immunity, for example – while being lonely puts you at increased risk of an earlier death, high blood pressure, depression and even accidents at home and on the road.

Learn and practise relaxing Most of us aren't very aware of our bodies. If our muscles are tensed or our breathing is faster and shallower than it should be, we don't manage to notice, let alone make the connection to stress. A good solution is to find a relaxation technique you like and use it every day, regardless of how you feel that day. You can try formal meditation and mindfulness-based stress reduction (see http://www. livingmindfully.co.uk/ or http://mbct.co.uk/), yoga and breathing exercises (inhale slowly for four counts, pause for one to two counts, exhale for seven to eight counts, pause for one to two counts, and inhale again).

The health benefits of relaxation include better weight control, lower blood glucose, stronger immunity, less depression, an easing of chronic pain and even faster recovery from the serious skin condition psoriasis.

Step 9
Seek treatment for depression

Depression isn't simply low spirits. It's a common, serious illness that puts your health in danger – the Disease Prevention Survey's medical experts ranked it as more dangerous than having high cholesterol. It's linked to an increased risk of diabetes, heart disease and a host of other serious health conditions. Having depression plus diabetes and heart disease (a common combination) increases your risk of early death by as much as 30 per cent.

It's not clear why depression accompanies so many serious health problems. Some experts are beginning to suspect that stress hormones and changes in the nervous system play important roles. What is clear, though, is that defeating depression is vital for good health.

Believing **you will** *recover fully must* **be your goal**

The trouble is often a case of people not getting the help they need. Thanks to archaic beliefs that this illness is a sign of weakness (or something you can 'tough out' on your own), and to doctors who fail to recognise or treat depression, millions of people plod along on their own. If that sounds like your situation, call your doctor today and make an appointment specifically to talk about this issue and to get help.

It's well recognised that depressed people find it extremely hard to believe that they will ever be able to feel completely better. But that belief has to be your own and your doctor's goal. Mental health experts now say that feeling a bit better isn't enough. You can, and should, feel as good as you felt before the depression began. However you choose to get there, call on the following three courageous qualities (and expect them of your doctor, too) on your journey towards feeling happier again.

Be patient Nearly 70 per cent of the 3,700 people in a recent landmark study of depression therapies eventually felt that their treatment had worked. Just 37 per cent got there with the first treatment they tried – an antidepressant. The rest needed as many as four different therapies before finding the right one for them. You won't know what works for you until you try – and keep trying until you hit on the right approach.

Have high expectations of treatment Expect to feel significantly better. If feelings of depression linger after giving a therapy a good try (usually 8 to 12 weeks), talk to your doctor about alternatives.

Be persistent Plenty of people stop taking antidepressants or going to therapy as soon as they begin to feel better, but many relapse. The reason is that a single episode of depression can last for 9 to 12 months. Stopping treatment too early leaves you at risk of a recurrence.

Step 10
Build emotional security

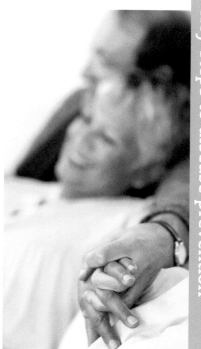

Scientific research is proving that positive, happy relationships literally change the biochemistry of your brain for the better, while loneliness raises your risk of problems such as high blood pressure, depression and even an early death. In fact, an overwhelming 79 per cent of the doctors polled in the Disease Prevention Survey said that social isolation is extremely detrimental to health. When you're alone for too long, levels of the stress hormone cortisol rise, increasing your odds of developing heart disease, high blood pressure, depression and sleep problems.

Studies also show that a strong core belief system and the support of a friendly community (whether it be religious or some other group that offers communal support) can cut stress, boost immunity, improve your chances of recovering from illness and even reduce chronic pain. The Disease Prevention Survey ranked meditating or embracing a higher sense of purpose as more important to disease prevention than diet tweaks such as consuming more omega-3 fatty acids or eating less sugar. Here are some easy ways that you can improve your health by staying connected socially.

Reach out Plenty of people are shy but would actually be delighted if you called with an invitation to a film or to have dinner together. Thinking that you need an elaborate plan or a perfectly clean house before you can issue an invitation only postpones your own and their happiness.

Have physical contact more often Sit closer to your spouse or partner, hold hands more often – and while you're at it, make love more often. Studies show that these physical connections buffer stress and even cut heart attack risk. If you don't have a life partner, hug the younger people in your life or a pet. Having a pet can have profound health benefits.

Expand your network Relying only on a small group of old friends could be a recipe for loneliness. Invest in your future health by reaching out to a new person this week.

Reconnect with your religion If you've let this dimension of life languish, it may be time to re-connect with your faith.

Revive your inner self through music, art or nature Immersion in the arts and nature are stimulating ways to stay focused in the moment.

Give back Volunteering can be highly rewarding. If you don't want to do it formally, look for small ways to help others. Perhaps older neighbours could use a hand with shopping or gardening, for example.

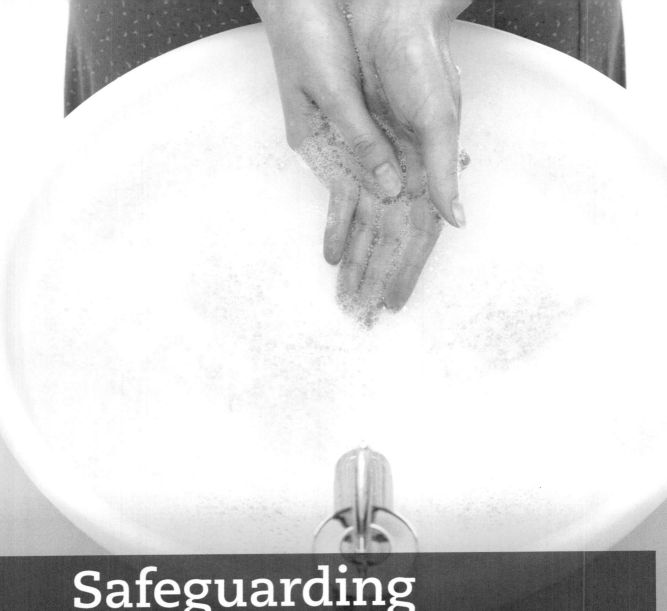

Safeguarding your health

Follow even just a few of the steps outlined in the previous chapter, and you'll be reducing your risk of major diseases such as heart disease, diabetes and cancer. But you also need to consider protection against threats lurking outside your body, from germs and toxins to spoiled food, all of which can make you ill.

Create a healthy home environment

Your house could well be a haven for more than just yourself and your family. Allergens such as dust and mould, as well as toxic gases, are all found in most homes in varying degrees. Experts estimate that people spend around 80 to 90 per cent of their time indoors, and most of that at home, so why not make your home environment as healthy as possible? No home can ever be truly 'clean', which is not usually a problem, but make sure you address any major issues within the home that may threaten your health, to avoid making you or your family unwell. Here are the three top priorities you need to focus on:

1. Clear the air

Modern homes are well sealed, so you'd think they'd be practically pollution-free. In fact, just the opposite is true: indoor air is often more polluted than the air outside. Take these steps to ensure that the air you breathe isn't undermining your efforts to live a healthy, disease-free life.

What to do

Wage war on dust House-dust mites trigger allergy and asthma attacks, but dust itself is a 'repository of pollutants', according to experts who have studied it extensively. It's a carrier of countless toxins, including pesticides, flame retardants, volatile organic compounds – VOCs, (emitted as gases by everything from paints and varnishes to cleaning products) – and more. If you live in a dusty house these contaminants enter your body every time you breathe or eat food to which the particles have adhered. You also absorb the dust through your skin.

Battling dust doesn't necessarily mean vacuuming more often – in fact, vacuuming raises clouds of dust and other allergens, even if you use a vacuum cleaner fitted with an HEPA (high efficiency particulate air) filter. Instead, replace carpets with hard flooring wherever possible and dust floors and surfaces with a damp mop or cloth. (For more tips on counteracting dust problems see *Allergies*, starting on page 96.)

Minimise mould If you have a stuffy nose, irritated throat, coughing and wheezing, it could be attributable to a mould allergy. You may not even realise that your home has become a mould repository, but old carpets, damp garages and even stacks of old newspapers are very likely to harbour mould spores. Here's how to prevent mould and mould-related health problems:

HELPS PREVENT
- Allergy and asthma attacks
- Chronic bronchitis
- Lung cancer
- Nervous system disorders
- Developmental and reproductive disorders

Before ripping up your carpets read this

Wooden flooring is popular and recommended for reducing allergy and asthma symptoms. However, some floor finishes used in the 1950s and 60s may contain polychlorinated biphenyls (PCBs), which have been shown to retard development in foetuses and young children, and could contribute to your cancer risk.

As people rip up carpet in older homes and refinish floorboards, those chemicals are released into the air. In one US study, researchers detected PCBs in the indoor air of a third of homes tested. The highest concentrations in homes and in the blood of their residents were found in places in which the floorboards had just been sanded and refinished.

If you're planning to refinish your floorboards, use a process that captures the dust so it doesn't go into the air, and make sure you and your family vacate the house during that time.

○ Go to a hardware shop and buy a hydrometer to measure the humidity in your home. Aim to keep indoor humidity levels between 40 and 60 per cent. Use a dehumidifier in any excessively damp or humid areas.
○ Make sure that extractor fans in your kitchen, bathroom and utility room are functioning properly and are vented to the outside.
○ Fix any leaking roofs, windows or pipes.
○ Repair air ducts if you find a build-up of mould, dirt or moisture inside, or if insects or rodents have taken up residence in them. Keeping air filters clean and fixing leaks are the first steps – not duct cleaning, which may not even help.
○ Remove mould with a bleach solution made using a cup of bleach added to 4 litres of water.
○ Use mould-inhibiting paint in your home.
○ Avoid carpeting your bathrooms or kitchen.

Go green when building or remodelling Furniture, paints, adhesives, ceiling tiles and carpeting are major sources of VOCs such as formaldehyde. These compounds have been linked with fatigue, concentration problems, sore throats, runny noses and even cancer. Most of these products are available in VOC-free forms; ask your decorator the next time you're having work done in your house.

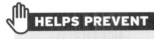

HELPS PREVENT
○ Viral and bacterial infections

2. Fight germs in key places

Charles Gerba, a microbiologist and professor at the University of Arizona in the USA, notes that 'if you have the right germs in the right place and the right amount, you can get sick from anything you touch'. You'll never get rid of all the germs in your house for the simple fact that bacteria are by far the most numerous organisms on Earth – so it's pointless to think that you can. Instead, choose your battles strategically.

What to do

Microwave your cellulose kitchen sponges A kitchen sponge, or squeegee, can contain more germs than any other object in your house. When US researchers tested common methods of disinfecting sponges – soaking them in bleach or lemon juice, microwaving or washing them in the dishwasher – they found that microwaving for a minute destroyed the most germs, followed by washing in the dishwasher; bleaching came third. Ensure a sponge is damp before microwaving; otherwise it could catch fire.

Scrub the sink After the sponge, the kitchen sink is the second dirtiest place in your house (even worse than the toilet). Keep a spray bottle of cleaner handy and clean the sink after each use, then wipe and rinse clean with hot water.

Beware of mixing chemical 'cocktails' In your enthusiasm for hygiene, make sure you never mix bleach with an ammonia-based product, as this creates toxic vapours that can seriously damage your lungs and eyes.

Buy a new chopping board Older chopping boards, regardless of whether they are made of wood or plastic, are likely to harbour bacteria, including salmonella, wherever the knife has cut deeply into the surface. If yours has seen better days, buy a new one (and choose wood). When researchers smeared bacteria onto plastic and wooden cutting boards, they found that the bacteria grew deep within the pores of the wooden boards. And while that may sound revolting, those bacteria stayed there and didn't re-emerge, so they were harmless unless the board was scarred by a knife. The plastic boards, however, retained germs on their surface for hours. Clean wooden chopping boards in a sink of hot soapy water and microwave them for 1 minute (if they fit in) every few days to completely destroy any remaining germs.

*A kitchen sponge may contain **more germs** than any object in the house*

Protect your toothbrush Store your toothbrush in an upright position after each use so the water drains away from the bristles; don't store a wet toothbrush in a closed case. If you're still worried about germs, dunk brushes in an antimicrobial mouthwash. Studies show that a 20 minute soak can eliminate germs. Don't re-use the disinfection liquid or soak more than one brush in it at a time. If you've had a cold or flu, replace your toothbrush after you recover to prevent reinfection.

Take care when changing nappies Every time a baby's nappy is changed bacteria are transmitted to surfaces in the room, no matter how careful you think you're being. Use an easy-clean changing table or mat and wash your hands thoroughly with soap and water after every nappy change.

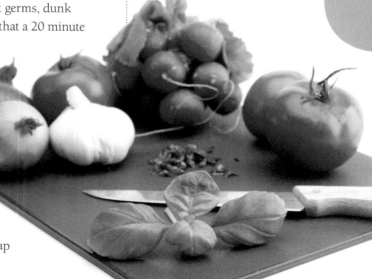

Wipe down 'sick' surfaces You can't disinfect every surface in your house, but even if you could, it wouldn't make much difference. If a member of your family has been ill, though, it might make sense to wipe down surfaces that everyone touches all the time – doorknobs, light switches, telephone handsets, TV remote controllers – with disinfectant. Disinfectants don't kill all viruses (they mainly work against bacteria), but they may kill some. Experts recommend a solution of 1 part bleach to 10 parts water, which effectively kills bacteria and some viruses. Leave it on the surface for 10 to 20 seconds before wiping dry.

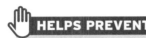

HELPS PREVENT
- Diarrhoea
- Food poisoning

3. Keep your food safe

Food should make you healthy, not unwell. If you're careful about how handle food, you'll be much less likely to come down with diarrhoea, vomiting or worse. Don't rely on your senses to judge safety – you can't see germs, and a food can smell perfectly OK even when it's contaminated.

What to do

Thaw properly The best option is to defrost items in the fridge overnight. But if you're in a hurry, put the frozen item in a plastic bag and immerse it in cold water, changing the water every 30 minutes. Otherwise, use the microwave oven on the defrost setting. Be ready to cook the food as soon as it's thawed.

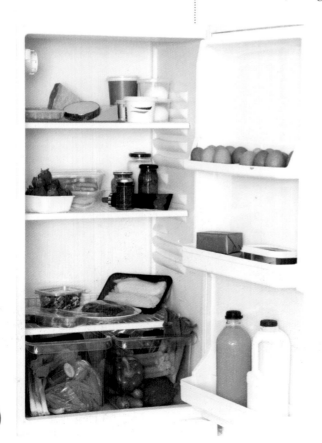

Use a meat thermometer Poultry should reach 71°C/160°F (white meat); 75°C/170°F (dark meat), beef (rare) 60°C/140°F-80°C/175°F (well done); pork at least 80°C /175°F; and mince 70°C /160°F.

Take your fridge's temperature Most fridges come with a built-in thermometer, but if yours doesn't, buy an appliance thermometer from a hardware shop and check that the fridge is at 5°C or below and the freezer at -18°C or below.

Purge your larder Any highly acidic canned foods such as tomatoes, grapefruit and pineapple should be stored for no longer than 18 months; other canned foods can be kept for two to five years if the can is still in good condition.

Wash, wash, wash Whether it's a bunch of grapes or an orange, always rinse fresh fruit and vegetables before cooking or eating. Remove and discard the outer leaves of lettuce or cabbage.

82

Travelling disease free

Norovirus has become known as the scourge of cruise-ship holidays, just as viruses caught during plane travel are also known to put a damper on holidays overseas. Don't allow your holiday – or a business trip – to be wrecked by illness or accidents. The goal is to remain disease free whether you're at home or in a four-star hotel in an exotic location. Here are the three key steps to preventing a holiday disaster:

1. Use 'plane' common sense

Not only is catching a virus on a plane upsetting, it's all too common, thanks to packed aeroplanes, germs that settle on every surface you touch and stale recirculated air (the result of airlines trying to save fuel by not allowing in as much fresh air from outside). Protect yourself with some travel-savvy advice.

HELPS PREVENT
- Blood clots
- Respiratory illnesses
- Stomach complaints
- Influenza
- Dehydration

What to do

Take a bottle of water The cabin air in planes is incredibly dry, which puts you at added risk for picking up an infection, since you need moisture in your mucous membranes (nose, throat and eyes) to help repel viruses and bacteria. Avoid salty snacks and alcohol, which are dehydrating, and drink lots of water. Just make sure the water is bottled, whether you take it with you or get it on the plane. The US Environment Protection Agency tested 158 passenger planes and found that the unbottled drinking water offered in nearly 13 per cent of them was infected with coliform bacteria, the presence of which is often used as an indicator of poor water quality.

Stand up and walk every 2 hours Walking around and stimulating your circulation helps to prevent the formation of blood clots in your legs that can occur after sitting for several hours. It's easiest to get up as often as you like if you've booked an aisle seat. If getting out of your seat often is too disruptive, exercise every half an hour by raising your shoulders and shrugging them forward and back, dropping your chin and nodding yes and no, drawing circles with your toes, and pressing up onto the balls of your feet 10 times in a row. And always try to avoid sitting with your legs crossed.

*Walking around **helps to prevent** the formation of **blood clots** in your legs*

Take your own pillow and blanket People who have compromised immunity, perhaps because they are undergoing chemotherapy treatment, may want to use their own, rather than those supplied by airlines, which some suggest cut corners when it comes to deep-cleaning these products. You can buy inflatable pillows and lightweight travel blankets from travel shops at most airports.

Buy a pack of antibacterial wipes at the airport Similarly, if you need to take extra hygiene precautions, use wipes to clean your seatbelt, tray table and armrests, as well as the button that turns on the light. Also, take the wipes with you to the bathroom to clean the handles when opening the door and flushing the toilet.

HELPS PREVENT

- Traveller's diarrhoea
- Blisters
- Motion sickness
- Sunburn
- Malaria

2. Pack your suitcase well

Sometimes it's the small things like blisters or sunburn that detract from a holiday's enjoyment. Other times it's the not-so-small things, such as a bad case of traveller's diarrhoea that leaves you stuck in a hotel for days. You can prevent a range of health problems by planning in advance.

What to do

Contact your GP's surgery at least two months before travelling to another continent Find out if you'll need vaccinations for the places you're travelling to and whether malaria tablets are advisable (if they are, start taking them as directed before leaving the country).

Take insect repellent and insect-blocking clothes Mosquitoes aren't just annoying; the mosquitoes in certain parts of the world can transmit diseases such as malaria and dengue fever. Ticks can cause tick-borne encephalitis. Use an insect repellent on any exposed skin to repel mosquitoes, ticks and fleas. Choose one that contains DEET or a newer pesticide called picaridin. Also take clothes to wear when the mosquitoes are out in force, including long-sleeved shirts, long trousers and closed shoes. If you're heading into heavy mosquito territory, apply insect repellent containing permethrin to clothing, shoes, tents, mosquito nets and other gear (but not to your skin). It works for five washes.

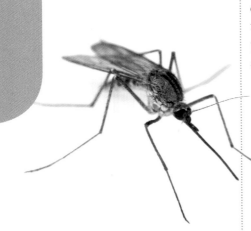

Screen out the sun Whether you're skiing in the Alps or embarking on a cruise of the Pacific, keep in mind that countries near the equator and at higher elevations receive more UV rays than other parts of the globe. What's more, snow and light-coloured sand reflect the sun, increasing your risk of sunburn. Even if you're not heading to the beach, use a high-SPF sun lotion (30 is plenty) that blocks both UVA and UVB rays, and reapply it every couple of hours.

Be ready for blisters Blisters are always unpleasant. If one becomes infected you have a bigger problem, especially if you have diabetes. Take shoes that are already broken in, along with a packet of moleskin (sold in pharmacies) and some travel scissors. As soon as you feel a 'hot spot' developing, cut a piece of moleskin large enough to cover the area and stick it on to prevent a full-blown blister developing. Or cover the area with an advanced blister-healing plaster, such as Compeed.

Pack flip flops for the shower If you plan to use the hotel pool or public showers, slip some rubber flip flops into your suitcase to protect your feet from athlete's foot. If you're planning to visit any rocky beaches, take some 'jelly' shoes along.

Prevent Delhi belly You can reduce the risk of traveller's diarrhoea by taking the usual precautions – avoiding tap water or ice, eating unpeeled raw fruit and vegetables, and so on. And you could pack some Pepto-Bismol, which can even be used to prevent diarrhoea. Studies show it can cut your risk by 65 per cent. Take two 262mg tablets at each meal and at bedtime. Do this daily for up to three weeks.

Don't forget travel sickness prevention Be sure to seek advice from a pharmacist on a suitable motion sickness medication; a variety of antihistamine products are available over the counter. The trick is to take the tablets well before you board a ship or begin a winding car ride.

Take steps against altitude sickness This can occur if you move rapidly from sea level to more than 1,800m (5,900ft). To avoid it, make your ascent gradually (for instance, spend the night at 1,200m/4,000ft) before continuing to your destination), slowly integrate physical activity (that 5 mile hike should wait a couple of days, until you've had a chance to acclimatise), and avoid alcohol and heavy meals. If you're prone to severe altitude sickness, talk to your doctor; there are medications (acetazolamide or dexamethasone) you can take to help prevent this problem.

3. Keep your hands clean

Next time you embark on a cruise, consider that in 2007 there were 23 outbreaks of norovirus infection, which causes severe stomach upsets (vomiting and diarrhoea), on 19 cruise ships, affecting about 3,000 passengers and crew members. Most involved person-to-person transmission, making hand washing, which studies find removes 99 per cent of the virus particles, crucial. No matter what your destination, how you are travelling or what you're doing, hand washing should be your number-one strategy for avoiding infections.

Before you go

Make sure you have had a complete course of tetanus immunisations (five in total). Also check which vaccinations are recommended for the areas in which you'll be travelling. You can search www.cdc.gov/travel/contentvaccinations.aspx by your destination country (this US website has useful information for all travellers, regardless of where you live). The only ones required are yellow fever vaccine for travel to certain countries in sub-Saharan Africa and tropical South America, and meningococcal vaccine for travel to Saudi Arabia during the religious festival, the Hajj.

HELPS PREVENT

- Diarrhoea
- Intestinal bugs
- Colds
- Other viral illnesses

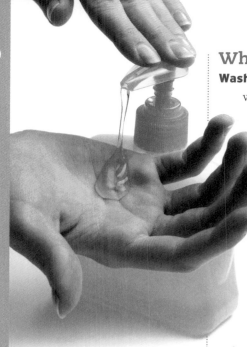

What to do

Wash with soap and hot water Wash long and often. Plain soap and hot water are fine; you don't need an antibacterial soap. Just make sure you wash for at least 20 seconds.

Use antibacterial hand wipes and gel sanitisers Whenever you have access to soap and water, wash your hands – it's more effective at removing germs than antibacterial products because it physically rinses them away. Hand sanitisers kill some, but not all germs. However, for times when you can't wash your hands, alcohol-based antibacterial gels and towelettes are a lot better than nothing. Choose a sanitiser containing 99.5 per cent ethanol.

Leave taps and door handles untouched It's not toilet seats in shared facilities, you have to worry about, it's the taps and door handles that are the dirtiest areas, so use a paper towel or hand wipe to turn the water on and off and to open the door when you leave.

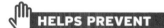
HELPS PREVENT
○ Accidents and injuries

4. Protect your physical safety

Traffic accidents are a leading non-natural cause of death for tourists. And throwing your back out trying to lift your suitcase, or tripping on a step or kerb and twisting your ankle will also spoil a holiday.

What to do

Forget about motorcycles and mopeds If you need convincing, just visit a local hospital and witness all the tourists who have sustained moped injuries. Use public transport, rent a car or hire a driver if you're not comfortable driving on strange roads. If you do rent a car, get a large one – it reduces your risk of sustaining injury if an accident does occur. And be sure to wear a seatbelt. If the car or taxi doesn't have them, look for another form of transport. It's not worth the risk.

Don't travel in overcrowded conditions Less developed countries are notorious for overfilled buses. If you don't have room to sit comfortably or if the bus or van seems top-heavy organise another ride, if possible.

Use rolling luggage It prevents back strain. And always lift with your legs, not your back (see *Back pain*, page 114).

Guard against heat exhaustion The temperatures in some countries can be overwhelming. Drink plenty of non-alcoholic fluids, wear light-coloured, lightweight clothing and a wide-brimmed hat and stay inside, preferably in an air-conditioned room, during the hottest part of the day.

Avoiding germs where you can

Call it the revenge of the germs. Less than a century after the introduction of antibiotics, the world is facing an onslaught of highly resilient bacteria – some of which are impervious to all but the most powerful of medications – not to mention viruses that are able to mutate, making current vaccinations ineffective. Short of wearing a spacesuit, here are the two key steps you can take to protect yourself:

1. Prevent staph infections

Staph is one of the most common types of bacteria on the planet. The infections aren't always serious; often they cause only minor skin problems. But methicillin-resistant *Staphylococcus aureus* (MRSA), a common strain of staph, can be fatal because it's resistant to even powerful antibiotics. In the elderly or those with weakened immune systems, MRSA infections can cause real trouble. People at increased risk include those who have recently had a stay in hospital, people who live in long-term care facilities and anyone who participates in contact sports such as football and martial arts.

HELPS PREVENT
- Potentially deadly infection from MRSA and other staph bacteria

What to do in everyday life

Wash your hands It's an often-repeated recommendation, but keeping your hands clean by washing with hot water and soap for at least 20 seconds is the best way to prevent MRSA. If there is a MRSA outbreak in your workplace or school, try using an antiseptic cleanser called Hibiscrub (available from most pharmacies). It contains chlorhexidine, which eradicates bacteria that proliferate on the skin.

Shower regularly This is particularly important after sports activities and other forms of physical exertion. Always use soap or a suitable skin cleanser.

Cover scrapes and cuts with a dressing Keep an area of broken skin covered until it's had a chance to heal, to keep out bacteria and avoid touching of other people's wounds or dressings.

Neither a borrower nor a lender be Don't share towels, razors, make-up, combs or brushes.

Protect yourself from avian flu

So far, there's no need to worry about contracting avian flu from people. It's spread from animals to people, not from person to person. Nevertheless, you should seek urgent medical advice if you have had close contact with anyone suspected of having avian flu as preventive antiviral treatment might be advisable. In addition, if you're travelling to a country that has had outbreaks of the disease, make sure you avoid direct contact with chickens, ducks or geese; poultry farms; live-animal markets; and surfaces that may be contaminated with poultry faeces.

The hygiene hypothesis

Much of the advice on these pages is aimed at preventing infection by minimising your contact with bacteria and viruses in the environment. In recent decades, there has been considerable publicity given to a theory generally known as the 'hygiene hypothesis', which proposes that over-cleanliness and a failure to allow the immune system of young children to be 'challenged' by exposure to germs has contributed to the increased prevalence of allergic conditions such as asthma, eczema and hayfever.

Many theories have been proposed to provide an explanation for this relationship, but so far the scientific community has not reached a consensus. So in practical terms, the best advice is to take sensible measures to avoid infectious organisms in the environment and in food as far as possible. But parents should not allow their concern about contact with 'germs' to prevent their young children exploring the world around them and having plenty of contact with other children. Getting the odd cold is part of growing up.

Create a barrier Use your own towel or clothing as a barrier between your skin and any gym equipment. And wipe the seats and handles of all equipment with an antibacterial solution or wipe before and after using it to avoid coming into contact with someone else's body fluids or passing on your own to the next person.

Use the hot setting Washing gym clothes and towels in a hot-wash in a machine will help to kill any bacteria that they may harbour.

What to do in a hospital

Make a few enquiries If you're due to have in-patient treatment in hospital, try to find out about its surgical infection rates and infection-control policy. Many hospitals include such information on their websites. NHS Choices also provides this information and allows you to compare your hospital infection rates with those of other hospitals. If you're not happy with the information you gain, discuss with your GP whether it is possible to find another hospital in which to have your treatment.

Shower pre-op It's very important to cleanse your skin thoroughly before any planned operation.

Stop smoking Give up smoking for at least four days before you're admitted to hospital, or as soon as you know you need to have surgery. People who smoke have three times the risk of infection compared to non-smokers, probably because smoking interferes with the delivery of oxygenated blood throughout the body, affecting the immune response.

Check your blood glucose If you have diabetes, your risk of infection is much higher than it is for someone without diabetes. Try to keep your blood glucose levels as stable as possible before being admitted to hospital and make sure they're checked regularly while you're there.

Remain vigilant Request that hospital staff who enter your room – even your doctor – wash their hands or use an antibacterial sanitiser before touching you. One study found that simply increasing hand washing among intensive care unit (ICU) staff by 25 per cent led to a 25 per cent drop in hospital-acquired infections in the ICU. Also ask your doctor or nurse to wipe off their stethoscope before using it on you. Stethoscopes can also be contaminated with MRSA and other bugs.

2. Protect yourself from flu

Flu kills thousands each year (most of them elderly). And that's just ordinary flu. Experts say it's only a matter of time before the big one hits – a flu pandemic reminiscent of the 1918–19 pandemic, which killed about 50 million people around the world. These strategies will help protect you whether there's a flu outbreak close to home or in a more distant location.

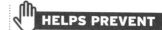

HELPS PREVENT
- Complications from flu
- Hospitalisation
- Death from the virus

What to do

Get vaccinated The effectiveness of flu vaccines varies from year to year, providing anywhere from 40 to 90 per cent protection against the strains of flu that are prevalent that year. If a flu virus suddenly mutates and a pandemic strikes, you'll get at least a little boost from having had a flu jab. The NHS has recommended that the following high-risk groups receive an annual flu vaccination: if you're 65 or over, you are pregnant, or if you have a serious heart or chest complaint (including asthma), serious kidney disease, diabetes, lowered immunity due to disease or treatment such as steroid medication or cancer treatment, or if you have ever had a stroke. Your GP may advise you to have a flu jab if you have serious liver disease, multiple sclerosis (MS) or some other diseases of the nervous system. People in these groups should also ask if they need a vaccine to protect against pneumonia.

Wash and wipe Flu viruses are usually spread from hand to mouth. Wash your hands as often as possible during flu outbreaks and wipe down surfaces with alcohol-based wipes or solution.

Dress like a surgeon You don't need the gown, but the mask could be helpful, especially when you're on a plane full of people coughing and sneezing. Buy an N95 face mask (available from pharmacies), which filters out about 95 per cent of virus-size particles.

Minimise the damage At the very first sign of flu, ask your doctor if you would benefit from one of the antiviral flu medicines, zanamivir (Relenza) and oseltamivir (Tamiflu). They can cut the flu short by a little over a day.

Influenza epidemics

During a serious outbreak of flu it's vital to know when to worry and what to do. Occasionally, a major mutation in the virus that causes flu produces a strain that isn't covered by vaccination. Sometimes this can cause serious illness, as with avian flu, and sometimes the illness is milder, as with swine flu. To protect yourself during a pandemic, take the following precautions:

- Cover your mouth and nose with a disposable tissue when you sneeze or cough, then bin it and wash your hands (and encourage others to do the same).
- Wash your hands regularly with soap and water or an alcohol-based product.
- Do not share personal items.

If you become ill, take the following precautions:

- Stay at home and avoid contact with others.
- Contact a doctor by phone rather going to the surgery in person.
- Rest, drink plenty of fluids, take over-the-counter painkillers such as paracetamol or ibuprofen, gargle with a glass of warm water to ease a sore throat, and use saline nose drops or spray or a decongestant to help clear a stuffy nose. Antibiotics are not effective against flu because it is caused by a virus and antibiotics fight bacteria.

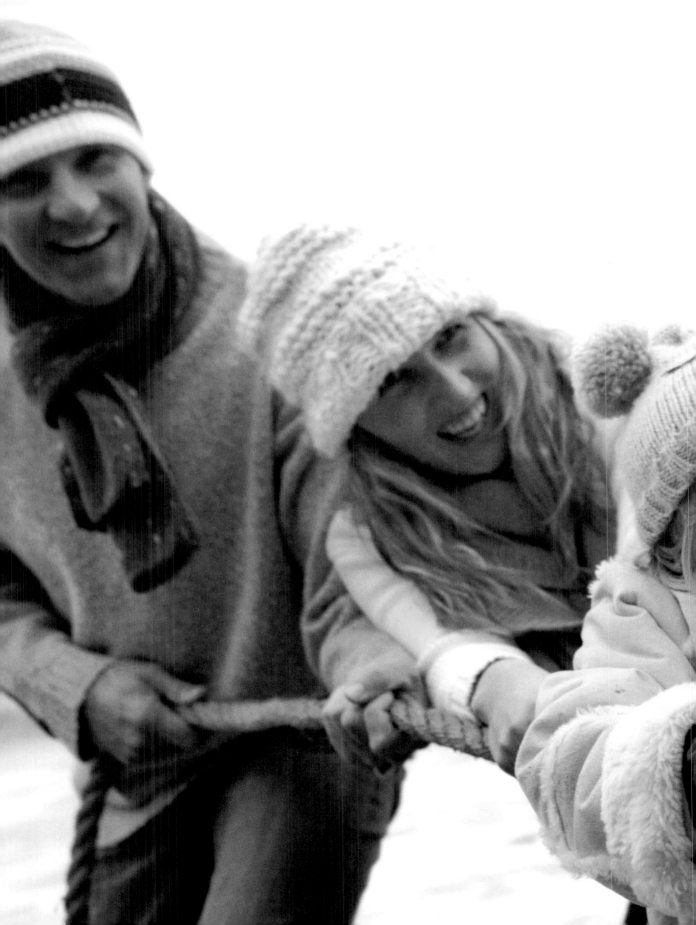

Disease Prevention A–Z

Find out how to protect yourself and your loved ones with expert advice and practical prevention plans for more than 90 common diseases and conditions.

Acne

Blackheads and bumps, pimples and cysts are a rite of passage for 90 per cent of teenagers. But studies show that up to 54 per cent of adults get acne, too. It's caused by everything from genetics to stress to hormones, and can initiate skin changes that clog pores, cause inflammation and provide acne bacteria with the perfect breeding ground. If you're prone to acne, these strategies can help prevent flare-ups, whether you're 14 or 44.

60%
The relative reduction in blemishes when people with acne used benzoyl peroxide preparations for four months.

What causes it

Heredity and hormones. The combination causes the production of excess oil by sebaceous glands in your skin, plus a build-up of dead skin cells. Together they clog pores, creating a breeding ground for acne-causing bacteria, which, in turn, can trigger an inflammatory response.

Symptoms to watch for

Tiny dark spots (blackheads) or small bumps (whiteheads). If clogged, pores become infected or inflamed, they turn red; white pus inside may be visible. Larger, tender bumps may signal a build-up of oil deep within pores. If these become infected, they're called cysts and can leave scars.

Key prevention strategies

Open your pores with products containing salicylic acid, resorcinol or lactic acid These ingredients are also called alpha-hydroxy acids and beta-hydroxy acids. Available in dozens of over-the-counter gels and creams, they prevent pores from clogging by breaking down the thick, gunky mix of skin cells and excess oil that starts the whole acne cycle. Some even act as gentle chemical peels to unblock pores that are already clogged. In one small US study of people with acne, salicylic acid was better than benzoyl peroxide for reducing the number of blackheads.

Stop bacteria with benzoyl peroxide This inexpensive, over-the-counter remedy is a proven bacteria-stopper that fights acne's top culprit, the bacterium *Propionibacterium acnes*. Its advantage over oral antibiotics and most antibiotic creams and gels is that it even works on strains of *P. acnes* that are resistant to the most widely used antibiotics for acne, such as tetracycline and erythromycin. Some experts estimate that bacteria are antibiotic resistant in at least half of all cases of acne.

In one UK study of 649 people with acne, 60 per cent of those who used benzoyl peroxide for 18 weeks saw a significant reduction in acne, while only 54 per cent of volunteers who took oral antibiotics saw an improvement. Benzoyl peroxide comes in several strengths; higher strengths are more likely to cause redness, irritation and even peeling. Start with a low dose and move up until you're happy with the results.

Ask about a retinoid cream Prescription-only creams and washes containing the vitamin A derivatives adapalene (Differin), isotretinoin (Isotrex gel) or tretinoin (Retin-A) speed the shedding of dead skin cells so they can't clog your pores. They may also cool inflammation, easing redness and swelling. When researchers reviewed studies involving 900 people with acne, they found that tretinoin reduced the number of pimples by about 54 per cent. Other research suggests that retinoids may clear up 70 per cent of blemishes.

Combine a pore-opening cream with an antibiotic cream

It's more effective than using an antibiotic cream alone. Your doctor can prescribe a combination cream that contains both an antibiotic and benzoyl peroxide. Another good duo is benzoyl peroxide plus an alpha- or beta-hydroxy acid or some types of retinoids. In a US study of 517 people with severe acne, 53 per cent of those who used both of these creams saw the number of blemishes halved after 12 weeks, compared to 35 per cent of those who used benzoyl peroxide or the retinoid adapalene alone. Benzoyl peroxide can deactivate tretinoin, so don't use them at the same time.

Prevention boosters

Light therapy It is said to work by killing bacteria and possibly reducing oil production. There are many types, including combined blue-red light therapy and pulsed-dye lasers. Studies suggest that light therapy can provide a temporary improvement in symptoms, but currently it is not readily available in the UK.

Low-dose oral contraceptive pills For women whose acne persists after trying many treatments, oral contraceptives can sometimes help. They can clear up skin by changing the hormone balance in a way that reduces the production of oil. This treatment is recommended only for women aged 35 years and younger, who have healthy blood pressure levels, don't smoke and don't suffer from migraines with auras.

Help for sensitive skin

Retinoid creams can be irritating, especially for people with sensitive skin. Here's a gentler alternative: a prescription cream containing azelaic acid (brand names include Finacea and Skinoren). In one German study, an alcohol-free azelaic acid gel reduced blemishes by 70 per cent after four months. Researchers also report that the cream can be just as effective as benzoyl peroxide and caused less irritation.

Latest thinking

Experts have said for years that highly sugary and fatty foods don't cause acne, but there is new research that suggests that diets generally high in sugar and refined carbohydrates may play a role. In a study of 43 young men with acne, those who followed a low-glycaemic diet – one that contains foods that have a gradual impact on blood sugar levels – had 23 per cent fewer blemishes after 12 weeks. Although this study is too small to be conclusive, it will certainly do your health no harm to eat plenty of fruit and vegetables, and choose whole-grain products when you eat foods such as rice and pasta; it may have an impact on your acne.

See also:

Step 2: *Fruit and vegetables,* page 64

Allergies

74%
The percentage of children who could avoid allergic rhinitis by eating fruit and vegetables at least twice a day.

Allergies appear to be seriously on the rise – hay fever, food allergies and allergies to dogs, cats or dust mites – and it's not your imagination. The incidence of allergies – including those that are adult-onset – has risen in developed countries. The reasons for this include too much time spent indoors, high levels of pollution and an overly clean environment during childhood – all of which can lead to a confused immune system. People with such allergies are three times more likely to develop asthma and to have sinusitis. Find out how to avoid an allergy attack.

What causes it

Your immune system overreacts to irritants such as dust, pollen, dander, mould, food proteins or insect venom, releasing inflammatory chemicals that trigger allergy symptoms.

Key prevention strategies

Wage war on dust and dust mites Think of dust as a repository for almost every allergen you can think of: dust mites, pet dander, insect droppings, pesticides and pollution from outside, for example. Modern homes are allergen traps. You'll need to make a big effort to reduce allergens enough to make a noticeable difference. Here's how to start:

- **Choose solid surfaces** Opt for hardwood, laminate, tile and vinyl for your floors, and as much non-upholstered furniture as possible. Carpets and fabrics harbour dust mites and attract pet dander, and grow mould when wet. One study found that the dust on walls, uncarpeted floors and bookshelves had little impact on the overall level of dust mites in the home compared to the dust found on carpets, upholstered furniture, duvets and mattresses and pillows.
- **Dry steam-clean your carpets** Vacuuming around the home does little to remove allergens. In fact, on old carpets, it may just bring more pet dander and dust mites to the surface. But dry steam cleaning, also known as vapour steam cleaning – not the same as regular steam cleaning – can reduce the number of dust mites for up to eight weeks. You can have it done professionally or buy a machine and do it yourself. Afterwards, finish by using a vacuum cleaner equipped with an HEPA (high efficiency particulate air) filter.
- **Encase your bedding** Always use hypoallergenic covers on your pillows, mattress and bed base.

A shot at permanent relief

The way to permanently prevent allergy attacks is to 'reboot' your immune system with immunotherapy – yes, allergy jabs. These injections, which you receive over a period of several months or years, contain increasingly larger doses of the substance to which you're allergic. Over time, your immune system learns to tolerate the allergen.

> **Carpets** *and fabrics harbour* **dust mites** *and attract pet dander.*

They prevent dust mites from accumulating in your bed. Wash all covers in hot water ($60°C$) once a week and dry them using a hot setting in a tumble-dryer to kill dust mites. If you don't use pillow covers, choose feather pillows, which studies have found to harbour far fewer dust mites than synthetic pillows do, probably because of the tighter weave on the covering, to stop feathers from escaping.

- **Vacuum your mattress – top and bottom** A Brazilian study compared dust mite bodies on the lower mattress surface (including the bed frame) and upper mattress surface and found more than three times as many dust mites on the lower surface. So flip the mattress monthly, vacuum each side and wipe down the bed frame with hot soapy water. To eradicate dust mites from a mattress, consider employing a specialised service that cleans and sterilises bedding: some companies will do the job onsite. Once a mattress has been sterilised, make sure you keep it wrapped in hypoallergenic coverings.
- **Clear out clutter** All those knick-knacks and piles of magazines lying around are magnets for dust and mould.

If you can't part with your pet, use an air purifier The truth is, there's scant proof that air purifiers can lessen allergy symptoms very much for most people. But if you buy one with an HEPA filter, use it in the bedroom and keep your pet out of the room, you will create a friendlier environment for your respiratory system. These filters are designed to remove airborne particles, including those coated with pet dander. One study on using air filters in the bedroom found that they significantly reduced cat allergens.

Another study evaluating the benefits of whole-house air cleaners fitted with HEPA filters found that they reduced levels of dog allergens by 75 per cent when the dog was allowed in the room and 90 per cent if the dog was kept out of the room.

Rinse your nasal passages daily Just as a rain shower rinses pollen from the air, a saline rinse washes allergens from your nasal passages. One study found that rinsing the nasal passages three times a day during

Symptoms to watch for

A runny nose and itchy eyes, particularly during high-pollen seasons; sneezing; hives (an itchy, red rash, also known as nettlerash or urticaria) and/or difficulty breathing after eating certain foods, such as peanuts or shellfish; and red, dry itchy skin.

Prevent allergies in children

Whether you're thinking about starting a family, are pregnant or already have children in the house, these measures could help to reduce their risk of developing allergies.

During pregnancy

1 **Follow a Mediterranean diet** That means one rich in whole grains, fruit and vegetables, and fish, with olive oil used as the primary fat. In one study, children whose mothers followed this type of diet were 82 per cent less likely to suffer from wheezing and 45 per cent less likely to have the skin rashes that predict childhood allergies.

2 **Take 1,000mg of fish oil a day** There is some evidence that taking supplements of this anti-inflammatory oil can reduce the risk of allergies in young children. Check with your doctor first.

3 **Take a probiotic supplement** Children whose mothers take supplements of these beneficial bacteria during pregnancy – and those who received probiotics as infants – appear to be less likely to develop eczema, an itchy skin condition that is a common precursor of allergies in children.

After birth

1 **Breastfeed for four to six months** This is the amount of time required to reduce the risk of all allergies in your child, probably by providing important immune system support.

2 **Discuss when to wean** It has been thought that babies who are weaned at six months or older may be less likely to develop food allergies – advice that is in line with UK health guidelines. However, British child experts have recently questioned the evidence citing studies that suggest that weaning breastfed babies earlier may actually protect against food allergies. Discuss this with your doctor or health visitor.

3 **Get a pet** Some studies suggest that exposing your infant to a cat or dog during the first year can help prevent allergies to common airborne allergens such as dust mites and pollen.

4 **Feed children plenty of fruit, vegetables and fish** Researchers who followed nearly 500 Greek children from the time their mothers became pregnant until the children reached the age of six found that diets high in these foods significantly reduced the risk of allergies and asthma. The children who ate fruit and vegetables at least twice a day were 74 per cent less likely to develop allergic rhinitis than those who ate them less often. Fruit and vegetables popular in Crete include grapes, oranges, tomatoes, aubergines, cucumbers and green beans. Eating an average of 60g (2oz) of oily fish daily also helped. Margarine, on the other hand, made allergies more likely, probably because the hydrogenated oils they contain can trigger inflammation.

the allergy season eased congestion, sneezing and itching and reduced the amount of antihistamines participants required. To make your own saline rinse, mix $\frac{1}{2}$ teaspoon salt, $\frac{1}{2}$ teaspoon bicarbonate of soda and 500ml (1 pint) warm tap water. To get it into your nose, use an infant ear bulb-syringe or a neti pot (a small container with a spout), available from most health food shops and pharmacies. Lean over a sink and turn your head so that your left nostril points downwards. Gently flush your right nostril with 250ml (5 teaspoons) of saline, which will drain out through your left nostril. When you're finished, gently blow your nose. Repeat with the other nostril.

Prevention boosters

Eat yoghurt every day US researchers at the University of California found that people who ate about 250g of yoghurt containing live, active cultures every day suffered allergy symptoms during the hay fever season on half as many days as people who didn't eat yoghurt. The researchers aren't sure why yoghurt helps, but it probably affects the immune system's response to allergens.

Eat more apples and drink more tea Apples with the peel on and green or black tea are excellent sources of quercetin. This powerful anti-oxidant inhibits the release of inflammatory chemicals from mast cells, the immune cells responsible for many common allergic reactions. Other good sources of quercetin include raw onions and red grapes.

Up your vitamin E intake You'll find this vitamin in spinach, wheatgerm, almonds, sunflower seeds and sweet potatoes. A German study on the dietary habits of 1,700 adults with and without hay fever found that those who ate foods rich in vitamin E had a 30 per cent lower incidence of hay fever than those whose diets were low in vitamin E.

Shut the windows A warm spring breeze seems just the thing to freshen up your house, but the problem is that it's filled with pollen. Keep the windows closed at times of year when the pollen count is high.

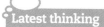

Latest thinking

UK researchers have discovered a protein called p110delta that plays a key role in triggering allergy attacks. Medications targeting it could prevent allergies, a massive improvement on existing allergy medications, which mostly reduce symptoms once the allergic reaction has occurred.

Alzheimer's disease

Alzheimer's disease was barely a dot on the horizon 50 years ago, because few people lived long enough to develop it. But with life expectancies creeping into the mid-seventies or older, Western populations are facing a potential epidemic of dementia. The good news is that scientists are learning more about it all the time. In the past decade, they've identified numerous biological and lifestyle risk factors for Alzheimer's, opening the door to potential preventive strategies.

60%
The difference in Alzheimer's risk between those who eat oily fish at least once a week and those who don't.

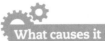
What causes it

Advancing age is the greatest risk factor, although an early form of the disease is linked to a genetic mutation. It's not clear what causes Alzheimer's, but it is associated with protein clumps, called amyloid plaques, in the brain, along with 'tangles' of brain cells. It's likely that these interfere with processing in the brain.

Key prevention strategies

Eat at least one meal of oily fish per week
You may know that salmon is heart healthy, but it could be just as good – or even better – for your brain. This added benefit is probably due to the omega-3 fatty acids, especially a type called DHA, which your brain is largely made up of. Low levels of omega-3s are linked to memory and learning problems, and even Alzheimer's disease.

DHA is thought to guard against the accumulation of beta amyloid proteins, which are the substances responsible for the sticky brain lesions, known as plaques, that are the hallmarks of Alzheimer's disease. Fish fats also counter inflammation, which may contribute to protein build-up in the brain. When scientists added DHA to the diets of mice bred to develop Alzheimer's disease, the mice had lower levels of brain plaques than those who weren't given the DHA.

One population study suggests that eating fish once a week or more even after the age of 65 can reduce your risk of developing Alzheimer's by 60 per cent compared to someone who eats less fish. If you don't like fish, talk to your doctor about taking 1,000 to 2,000mg of a fish oil supplement daily.

Exercise your brain Every time you challenge your brain to learn new information or attempt a new task (whether it's playing chess or just brushing your teeth with your non-dominant hand), you create new connections between brain cells, in effect strengthening your brain. Research suggests that daily mental stimulation could reduce Alzheimer's risk by as much as 47 or 75 per cent, depending on which study you look at. So get out those crossword puzzles and sudokus, and think about learning a new language or a musical instrument, too.

Walk 2 miles a day At a brisk pace, this should take you no more than 30 minutes, the amount of time required to cut your risk of Alzheimer's by 50 per cent, according to a Canadian study of about 10,000 people. Exercise probably has numerous benefits, including increased blood flow to the brain and increased production of a chemical called brain-derived neurotrophic factor (BDNF) – which encourages nerve cells in the brain to multiply and create more connections with each other.

Drugs that prevent disease

That same daily low-dose aspirin that some people take to protect themselves from heart attack may protect them from Alzheimer's disease, too.
In one study, people who took an NSAID (nonsteroidal anti-inflammatory drug), such as aspirin or ibuprofen, every day for two years or more were 80 per cent less likely to develop Alzheimer's than those who took an NSAID less often. Even people who took an NSAID for a month to two years reduced their risk by 17 per cent. Talk to your doctor about whether or not you should take a daily aspirin as there are potential side effects to consider.

Check the scales If you're obese, your risk of Alzheimer's is nearly twice that of someone whose weight is normal. For example, an analysis of several studies concluded that one in five cases of Alzheimer's disease in the USA was related to obesity. The link? For starters, carrying extra body fat – particularly around your waist – increases your risk of heart disease and diabetes, both of which make people more vulnerable to Alzheimer's. What's more, the fat itself releases inflammatory chemicals that may contribute to brain inflammation – and Alzheimer's.

Prevention boosters

Eat your spinach Despite what Popeye believed, it won't make your muscles strong, but what it could do is help you maintain healthy brain function. Spinach is an excellent source of folate, a B vitamin that helps keep levels of homocysteine – an amino acid – in check. This amino acid damages blood vessels and doubles the risk of Alzheimer's disease. Another B vitamin to look for is vitamin B_6 (niacin). Studies have found that a diet containing at least 17mg of vitamin B_6 a day reduces the risk of Alzheimer's disease by 70 per cent compared to a diet low in B_6. You can get 14mg from a 100g serving of cooked liver, 10mg from 110g peanuts and 13mg from 85g of chicken breast. Other great sources of B vitamins are pulses (beans, peas and lentils), fortified grains, nuts and wholemeal bread.

Have a glass of wine, with food, on most days One of the best studies of dementia in the world, the Canadian Study of Health and Aging, found that drinking a glass of wine a day reduced the risk of

Symptoms to watch for

Memory loss, difficulty planning or completing everyday tasks, forgetting simple words, or substituting unusual words in writing or speech; getting lost in familiar places; showing poor judgement, such as wearing shorts outdoors when it's freezing; having difficulty with abstract tasks such as adding up a column of numbers; putting things in unusual places; mood changes; and loss of initiative.

Got the gene?

Researchers have identified at least 20 genes and genetic abnormalities linked to Alzheimer's disease. The best known is the ApoE gene, which affects the concentration of apolipoprotein Apo(E) in the blood. Apo(E)'s job is to help remove excess cholesterol from the blood and carry it to the liver for processing. While you can be tested for the gene, there is no specific treatment and no certainty that carriers will develop the disease. So the best advice is to live your life to the full and also follow the tips here for reducing your overall risk.

Alzheimer's disease by 62 per cent in women and 51 per cent in all participants when men were included with the women. The benefit is probably due to something in the wine itself, since the protection afforded by wine was far greater than that from spirits or beer. However, it's important to remember that drinking more than this amount can be detrimental to your health.

Start drinking pomegranate juice People who drink the juice at least three times a week could reduce their risk of developing Alzheimer's disease by as much as 76 per cent compared to those who drink it less than once a week. Animal studies suggest that the high levels of antioxidants, called flavonoids, in pomegranates can neutralise free radicals – damaging molecules that attack cells and contribute to the formation of brain plaques. Pomegranate juice has already been shown to help prevent an Alzheimer's-like disease in mice.

Wear a helmet Protect your head while cycling, rollerskating, motorcycling, or when participating in any sport that may involve blows to the head. There's some evidence that sustaining a moderate or severe head injury increases your risk of Alzheimer's disease (up to 3.5 times as much if the injury is severe).

Prevent high cholesterol Although the theory is still controversial, population, animal and laboratory studies suggest a link between high cholesterol levels in midlife and Alzheimer's disease. High cholesterol levels interfere with the breakdown of the amyloid precursor protein (APP), which plays a major role in the development of Alzheimer's disease. (Follow the tips starting on page 216 for ways to keep your cholesterol under control.) There is also some evidence that using cholesterol-lowering statin medication may help prevent Alzheimer's, though it's too soon for doctors to start prescribing these medications as a preventive measure. The mechanism by which statins have an impact on Alzheimer's prevention may actually be unrelated to their ability to lower cholesterol and may instead result from their ability to reduce inflammation.

Drink some coffee If you enjoy a cup of coffee in the morning, don't give it up – it may be protecting your brain. According to recent research, caffeine appears to help protect the so-called blood–brain barrier from the harmful effects of high cholesterol, possibly reducing the risk of dementia. Other studies suggest that caffeine can help combat memory problems in older people.

Check your blood pressure

The link between Alzheimer's disease and heart disease grows clearer every year. New evidence suggests that high blood pressure may hasten the development of Alzheimer's in people with early memory loss. US researchers following 5,092 Utah women with mild dementia for three years found that those with systolic blood pressure readings (the top number) higher than 160mmHg declined 100 per cent faster than those with normal blood pressure. Those who also had angina, and/or had had a heart attack before their diagnosis, declined even faster. The good news is that a study in the same group of women found that taking medication to reduce high blood pressure reduced the risk of Alzheimer's. Check your blood pressure once a month; if it's higher than 120/80 mmHg, see your doctor. You may need to exercise more, change your diet or take medication to bring it down to the normal range.

Take steps to prevent diabetes Men who develop diabetes in midlife increase their risk of Alzheimer's disease by 150 per cent, according to one study. The risk remained irrespective of their blood pressure, cholesterol levels or weight and is probably linked to low levels of insulin. Interestingly, the risk was highest in people who did not have the so-called Alzheimer's gene. (See also *Diabetes*, page 156.)

Watch out for depression A study of 486 people found that those who had experienced depression severe enough to seek medical help were two and a half times more likely to develop Alzheimer's than those who had never suffered from the condition. The risk for those whose depression occurred before the age of 60 was four times higher. One theory is that depression results in the loss of cells in two areas of the brain that also are linked to Alzheimer's disease. (For more information, see *Depression* starting on page 152.)

Latest thinking

People with Down's syndrome usually develop Alzheimer's disease by the age of forty. Now researchers suspect that people without the syndrome who get Alzheimer's may develop a small number of the same chromosomal abnormalities throughout their lifetime. If true, it could one day mean new options for prevention, diagnosis and treatment.

See also:

Cause 4: Insulin resistance, page 28
Cause 5: Bad cholesterol balance, page 30

101

Anxiety

No matter what the cause, chronic anxiety is bad for your health. It makes your heart beat faster than it should and even makes your blood stickier, increasing your risk of a heart attack or stroke. If you're predisposed to anxiety, try these strategies to help you stay calm and quieten your mind.

50%
The amount by which you could reduce your stress levels by taking 3g of fish oil a day.

What causes it

Just about anything in life can cause anxiety. But if your anxiety is excessive or without reasonable cause and it disrupts your life, you may have a condition known as generalised anxiety disorder.

Symptoms to watch for

Restlessness, difficulty concentrating, irritability, trouble falling asleep, obsessive thoughts about something specific, racing heartbeat, shortness of breath and unusual sweating.

Key prevention strategies

Talk to someone Preferably a therapist trained in cognitive behavioural therapy (CBT). In this form of therapy, you learn to separate worry from reality and put your fears into better perspective. Studies find that, as a treatment for anxiety disorders, it works better than medication; other research finds that it can help prevent a full-blown anxiety disorder if it's employed early on.

Take a walk 'Feel-good' hormones are released during exercise, and one is the neurotransmitter known as gamma aminobutyric acid, or GABA. Studies find low levels of GABA in people with some anxiety disorders, particularly panic disorder. They also find that exercise, including yoga, can increase GABA levels. In one study 15 people were asked to walk for 30 minutes, then given a medication simulating a panic attack. Six had panic attacks after exercising, compared to 12 who had them when given the medication after resting.

Breathe calmly Many of the symptoms of anxiety attacks are caused by hyperventilation (over breathing). If the breathing rate is higher than the body physically needs, increased carbon dioxide is expelled in the breath, reducing the level of carbon dioxide (and its soluble counterpart, carbonic acid) in the blood. This makes the blood more alkaline, which affects the way that nerves and muscles work, causing light-headedness, loss of balance, tingling sensations often in the hands and round the mouth, then cramps in the hands and feet. Loss of consciousness can follow. Breathing then returns to the control of the body, rather than that of the mind, which allows the pH balance to return to normal.

If you are susceptible to panic attacks, take a class in relaxation: contact your local community centre, or talk to your doctor. Until then, try to focus deliberately on your breathing when you feel anxious. Take one deep breath as slowly as possible (count to five as you breathe in), watching your stomach (not your chest) inflate. Hold your breath for a few moments, then let it out, again counting to five. Repeat this five times.

Prevention boosters

Sip tea As if sipping tea weren't calming enough, UK researchers recently discovered that people who drink tea several times a day recovered faster from stressful situations that tend to increase heart rate and blood pressure. The tea drinkers' blood also showed lower levels of stress hormones. Antioxidants in tea may attach to the same receptors in the brain that anti-anxiety medications target.

Take brewer's yeast Brewer's yeast is an excellent source of biotin, also called inositol or vitamin B_7. In one study, taking 12-18g of an inositol supplement worked just as well as the antidepressant fluvoxamine (Faverin) for reducing the intensity and frequency of panic attacks. To reduce the frequency and severity of attacks, start taking a B-vitamin supplement that contains 12–18g of biotin. Try sprinkling a tablespoon of brewer's yeast over cereal or yoghurt. Peanut butter is also a good food source of biotin.

Take 3g fish oil daily There's intriguing evidence that fish oil can help relieve depression, and now it seems it may reduce stress as well. After three months, study participants who took 3g of fish oil a day reported feeling half as stressed as those who took a placebo. Check with your doctor before taking any supplement.

Drugs that prevent disease

If your heart races, your hands sweat and your mouth turns dry when you have to speak in front of people, talk to your doctor about taking a low dose of a beta-blocker. Beta-blockers, which include metoprolol (Betaloc or Lopressor) and propranolol (Inderal), block the effects of the stress hormone adrenaline, soothing the jitters of performance anxiety with few negative side effects.

Latest thinking

In people who have experienced a traumatic situation – for example, child abuse, war or rape – intervention through counselling and other non-medical approaches can prevent the development of an anxiety disorder.

See also:

Step 8: *Reduce chronic stress,* page 74

Arthritis

If you've ever seen people hobbling on arthritic hips or knees, or struggling to simply hold a butter knife with stiff, aching fingers, you know how arthritis can interfere with life. Osteoarthritis (OA) – in which the shock-absorbing cartilage between joint bones wears away – isn't inevitable. Although everything from genetics to joint injuries to age-related changes in cartilage-protecting enzymes plays a role. But there's also plenty of evidence that you can cut your risk significantly. Rheumatoid arthritis (RA), which occurs when the immune system attacks the tissues that protect bones, is less preventable, but there is plenty you can do to reduce its impact on your life.

30% The potential reduction in arthritis risk for women who exercise for an hour a week.

What causes it

For osteoarthritis, cartilage breakdown is the cause. Injuries, extra weight, genetics and muscle weakness can all contribute. Over time, cartilage may wear through in spots so that bones rub painfully against each other. Rheumatoid arthritis happens when your immune system attacks the lining of your joints (the synovium), leading to intense pain, swelling and joint deformities.

Key prevention strategies

Lose weight If you're carrying excess weight, here's yet one more reason to shed a few pounds: you'll put less pressure on your joints and thereby lower your risk of OA. Australian researchers maintain that osteoarthritis risk goes up 36 per cent for every 11lb (5kg) over your healthy weight range. Lose just 1lb (500g), on the other hand, and you'll put nearly 4½lb (2kg) less stress on your knees. Losing 11lb (5kg) if you're obese can cut your odds of developing the condition over the next 10 years by as much as 50 per cent. In another study, when US researchers at the Harvard Medical School checked the weight and health histories of 568 women with OA, they found that women with a higher body weight were twice as likely to need hip replacement surgery.

Exercise for at least an hour a week Until recently, doctors and scientists thought that a lifetime of exercising made people more vulnerable to osteoarthritis. But now researchers say that joint injuries, not exercise itself, account for the difference. In fact, there's growing evidence that exercise can prevent problems by building up muscles that protect joints.

In one Australian study of middle-aged and older women, those who got at least 2.5 hours of exercise per week cut their odds of developing arthritic joints by about 40 per cent. Exercising for just an hour a week lowered risk by about 30 per cent. And stretching exercises help, too.

Add strength training Strengthening your muscles by using any form of so-called resistance training (using light hand weights, elastic exercise bands, or machines at the gym or doing home exercises that use your

" *Tobacco* **smoke** *may provoke immune-system changes that lead to an* **attack on joints**. "

own body weight as resistance – think knee bends) may shield joints from damage. In one study, women with stronger thigh muscles had a 55 per cent lower risk of developing osteoarthritis of the knee and an amazing 64 per cent lower risk of osteoarthritis of the hips than women with weaker thigh muscles.

Getting stronger helps if you already have osteoarthritis, too. When Tufts University researchers tested a gentle, at-home strength-training programme for older men and women with moderate to severe knee osteoarthritis, the results surprised and pleased study volunteers. After 16 weeks, exercisers had 36 per cent less pain and 38 per cent less disability. (Try the *Joint strength* exercise routine, starting on page 330.)

Experts say gentle strength training can also reduce the pain and disability of rheumatoid arthritis. In a study from Finland, pain declined by 67 per cent and disability dropped by 50 per cent when people with mild RA followed a home strength-training programme for two years.

Prevention boosters

Don't smoke Women who smoked cigarettes raised their risk of developing RA by 30 per cent in one US study of 121,700 nurses. Smoking was shown to double the risk of the disease in another study of 30,000 women. According to Swedish researchers, tobacco smoke may provoke immune-system changes that lead to an attack on joints. The good news is that women who had quit smoking had no extra risk after about 10 years.

Get more vitamin D If you're running low on the 'sunshine vitamin', your joints may be at risk. Vitamin D, produced by your skin upon exposure to the sun, may help keep the immune system healthy and protect joints from wear-and-tear damage by strengthening nearby bone, too. When researchers studied men and women whose knees showed signs of osteoarthritis, those who took in above-average amounts of vitamin D from food and supplements were in better shape eight years later than those who didn't.

Symptoms to watch for

Pain, stiffness, tenderness and swelling in joints. Osteoarthritis most often affects the knees, hips, hands and spine. Rheumatoid arthritis usually begins in small joints in the hands and feet, then spreads to larger joints. In addition to pain and swelling, rheumatoid arthritis can cause fever, tiredness and weight loss.

Are glucosamine and chondroitin worth it?

This dynamic duo is taken by more people with osteoarthritis than any other 'joint' supplement. But a collection of recent research casts doubt on how well they work. Here's what you need to know to help make a choice:

What are they?

Both are components of human cartilage, the smooth covering on knee bones and other joints that acts as a shock absorber. In osteoarthritis, cartilage softens, cracks and wears out, allowing knee joints to rub together.

Glucosamine is thought to be involved in cartilage growth and repair; supplements are derived from the shells of crabs and lobsters. Chondroitin gives cartilage its elasticity; supplements are usually derived from animal cartilage.

The claim

Proponents of these supplements say that glucosamine and chondroitin relieve pain by maintaining cartilage so that joint bones don't grind against each other.

The research

There is conflicting data. Belgian researchers recently found that glucosamine had no effect on pain or joint deterioration in people with osteoarthritis in their hips. And a large US study of 1,583 people with osteoarthritis found that this combination didn't ease joint pain any better than placebos. But when researchers looked at the 20 per cent of study participants with moderate to severe arthritis pain, they found a benefit: 79 per cent of those taking the supplements (they took 500mg of glucosamine plus 400mg of chondroitin three times a day) had at least a 20 per cent reduction in pain, compared to 54 per cent taking placebos.

What about joint protection?

Other studies suggest that these supplements may help maintain 'joint space' – the distance between bones. (More joint space means less grinding, less damage and less pain.) In a Belgian study of more than 300 women with osteoarthritis, those who took glucosamine for three years showed no narrowing of the space between knee bones, while those taking a placebo saw the gap grow smaller. The glucosamine group also reported a 14 per cent improvement in pain and stiffness from the beginning to the end of the study, while the placebo group was a little worse by the end of the study period.

Are these supplements safe?

Yes. Long-term studies have found only mild side effects such as intestinal gas and softer bowel movements.

What should I take?

The US Arthritis Foundation suggests this pair may be worth a try. Take a supplement containing 500mg of glucosamine and 400mg of chondroitin sulphate three times a day. Try it for at least six weeks (some experts recommend three months) to see if you're getting any noticeable benefit. If not, stop taking the supplement.

Vitamin D may protect against RA as well. When US researchers at the University of Iowa followed 29,368 women aged 55 to 69 for 11 years, they found that women whose intake of vitamin D from food or supplements was less than 5mcg (or 200IU) were 33 per cent more likely to develop the disease.

While the UK Department of Health guidelines suggest that most people can obtain enough vitamin D from a healthy balanced diet and moderate sun exposure, it does recommend supplements for children aged 6 months to 5 years, pregnant and breastfeeding women, all people aged 65 and over, people with darker skins such as those of African-Caribbean or South Asian origin and people who receive little sun exposure for cultural reasons or because they are housebound. The Department of Health suggests an upper limit of 25mcg per day but some experts believe that higher doses than this would bring more benefit. The safe upper limit is thought to be 80mcg (3,200IU) a day. Taking high doses for long periods of time could weaken your bones.

You'll probably need to take a supplement to get therapeutic benefits. Unless you're eating oily fish such as salmon or sardines every day (100g of either contains about 9mcg, or 350IU, of vitamin D), it's very hard to get enough from food. (A glass of skimmed milk, another good source, has just 2.5mcg, or 98IU.) And while your body makes vitamin D from skin exposure to sunlight, if you can't see your shadow, the amount of sunlight exposure probably isn't enough. To check your vitamin D status, ask your doctor for a blood test at the end of winter, when most people's levels are at their lowest.

Eat colourful foods If it's red, orange, blue or green, chances are it's packed with antioxidants – compounds that neutralise rogue molecules called free radicals, which are thought to interfere with cartilage repair and rebuilding. Mangoes, peaches, oranges and watermelon are all rich in beta-cryptoxanthin, an antioxidant and one of a pair of compounds that lowered the risk of arthritis by an impressive 20 to 40 per cent in a UK study of 25,000 people. The other antioxidant, zeaxanthin, is found in spinach, sweetcorn, peas and orange peppers. People with the highest blood levels of both of these antioxidants cut their arthritis risk by 50 per cent.

Vitamin C is joint friendly too. Eating plenty of citrus fruit, red peppers and broccoli – all good sources – could help slow the development of knee pain if you already have osteoarthritis, according to researchers at Boston University in the USA. In one study, people who got the most vitamin C were three times less likely to have arthritic knee pain than people who got the least.

Latest thinking

If you have a type of arthritis in which the wear and tear is harming the middle of your knee joint – called medial-knee arthritis – special inner soles in your shoes could help. Lateral-wedge inner soles are thinnest at your instep and widest at the outer edge of your foot, realigning your feet and lower legs in a way that can reduce some of the twisting that wears down knee joints. Your doctor can tell you which type of knee arthritis you have.

See also:

Step 2: *Fruit and vegetables*, page 64
Step 3: *Quit smoking*, page 66
Exercises: *Better balance*, page 330
Joint strength, page 334

Asthma

30%
The amount by which you could reduce your risk of asthma by eating oily fish once a week.

Asthma, which is closely linked to allergies, is on the rise in most developed countries. One widely believed reason for this is that children today are not exposed to germs and dirt the way earlier generations were, so their immune systems haven't learned to react appropriately. Studies also find that adults raised on farms are much less likely to have asthma. Still, there's plenty you can do to prevent attacks if you already have asthma.

What causes it

A combination of genes and environment leads to an overly sensitive airway that reacts to triggers such as airborne pollutants, allergens or cold air by releasing inflammatory chemicals. These lead to constriction of the muscles surrounding the bronchial tubes in the lungs, and swelling in the lining of the tubes, often accompanied by extra mucus production.

Symptoms to watch for

Shortness of breath, coughing, chest tightness and wheezing.

Key prevention strategies

Allergy-proof your house More than half of all homes have at least six detectable allergens, and the remainder have at least three. Potential asthma triggers range from dust mites and animal fur and dander, to mould spores and chemical pollutants in the air. The bottom line here is that the higher the allergen levels are in your house, the more likely you or your children are to have asthma. Following are some suggestions for targeting the most common asthma-causing allergens. For dealing with dust mites, see Allergies, page 94.

- **Keep dust down** It's not enough to simply sweep the floor, many allergens can only be removed with washing. It's advisable to choose easy-to-clean hard floors over carpets, and to keep soft furnishings to a minimum. For further advice on keeping your home allergen-free, see page 94.

- **Reconsider your pets** It's hard to face up to the fact that the pet you love may be a cause of health problems. But if a member of the family has a severe asthma problem, you may have to consider finding a new home for the animal. But in all cases, it's sensible to keep some areas of the home pet free, in particular, the living room and bedrooms. Bathing your dog or cat regularly may also help reduce dander. Talk to your vet about the best way to do this.

- **Deal with mice** Mouse droppings and urine can be a source of allergens. To prevent infestation, keep all food in sealed containers Mice can easily gnaw through cardboard boxes. If you know you have a mouse infestation, use mousetraps. There's a wide variety, including humane traps that keep the mouse contained until you find it and are able to set it free away from your home.

- **Dehumidify the air** Damp air can encourage allergy-provoking mould spores as well as dust mites. If you think excess dampness might be a problem in your home, invest in a dehumidifer.

" You're **66%** more likely to have **persistent asthma symptoms** if you're obese. "

Check the scales Gained a few pounds lately? Noticed your asthma is getting harder to control? It's not a coincidence. You're 66 per cent more likely to have persistent asthma symptoms if you're obese than if your weight is healthy. This may have to do with inflammatory chemicals released from fat cells. In one small Italian study, 12 obese women with asthma who had stomach-reduction surgery, and who lost a significant amount of weight, saw a 31 per cent improvement in shortness of breath and an 18 per cent reduction in the use of rescue medication compared to women who didn't have the surgery or lose weight.

Discuss a personal asthma plan A major reason for uncontrolled asthma is the lack of a personalised asthma plan. These plans provide information about how and when to use daily and emergency medications. They also tell you when it's time to seek emergency medical care or call your doctor. Studies find that using these plans significantly reduces asthma attacks and deaths from asthma. It's a good idea to make a list of questions to ask your asthma nurse or GP when you begin treatment, and the following questions are a good start:

- **When should I call you?**
- **When should I seek emergency care?**
- **When is quick-relief medication not enough?**
- **When, if ever, should I increase my use of inhaled steroids?**
- **When, if ever, should I start taking oral steroids?**

Once developed, the plan should be reviewed and updated annually, and given to family members and others who might need to know what to do in the event of an emergency. You can obtain a personal asthma plan pack from Asthma UK (www.asthma.org.uk).

Prevention boosters

Use a peak flow meter If you have trouble recognising the early signs of worsening asthma, this small, inexpensive device may help (available from pharmacies or online). Peak flow meters measure your lung

Got the gene?

Because asthma and allergies, such as hay fever and eczema, tend to run in families, it's been long suspected that certain genes make some people more susceptible. Now we're finding potential culprits for this: a variant in the gene ORMDL3 seems to increase the risk of asthma in children by 60 to 70 per cent.

function, providing an early warning of an impending asthma attack. Using it daily, and adjusting your medication based on the results, can help keep you attack-free.

Learn to use your inhaler properly About a third of people with asthma don't know how to use their inhaler properly. This lack of understanding can increase the risk of asthma attacks, hospitalisation and even death. Ask your pharmacist to show you.

Prevent asthma in children

Believe it or not, asthma prevention actually begins in the womb. Here's what you can do to reduce the risk of your child developing asthma:

1 **Quit smoking** The link between exposure to secondhand smoke in childhood and asthma is strong and undeniable.

2 **Follow the right diet while pregnant** That means one high in foods rich in vitamin E (wheatgerm, sardines, egg yolks and nuts) and zinc (red meat and shellfish). These nutrients influence lung and immune system development. At least two studies find that low levels during pregnancy can increase the risk of allergies and asthma in children. Also include oily fish such as salmon or trout twice a week, or take a daily fish-oil supplement after checking with your doctor, especially if you are taking blood-thinning medication. Studies find that consuming the healthy fats in fish and fish oil during pregnancy reduces the baby's risk of asthma, possibly by leading to healthier immune system development.

3 **Consider allergy treatment** If your child has allergies, ask your GP about treatment with immunotherapy, which may help protect him or her from developing asthma.

4 **Breastfeed for four to six months**

5 **Discuss when to wean** Current advice advocates weaning a baby at six months but some experts believe that earlier weaning may be protective. Talk to your GP.

6 **Avoid acid-blocking medicines while you're pregnant** Research has found that taking medications such as H_2 blockers, including cimetidine (Tagamet), famotidine (Pepcid) and ranitidine (Zantac), or proton-pump inhibitors such as omeprazole (Losec) and esomeprazole (Nexium) during pregnancy increases the risk of asthma in infants by more than 50 per cent.

7 **Limit exposure to dust mites** UK researchers who followed 120 children from birth to eight years found that those who were breastfed and had limited exposure to dust mites due to the use of mattress protectors and pesticides were 76 per cent less likely to have asthma and 87 per cent less likely to have allergies by the age of eight.

Use hypo-allergenic mattress and pillow covers One study found that these covers not only reduced the number of dust mites in beds but also enabled children with asthma to have their dose of inhaled steroids reduced by at least 50 per cent.

See an asthma specialist You may be likely to have fewer problems controlling your asthma and less severe symptoms if your care is provided by a specialist instead of a GP. As you'd expect, a specialist is going to have more in-depth knowledge and will be on top of cutting-edge treatments. Ask your GP for a referral.

Serve oily fish twice a week A study of the dietary habits of 16,000 adults found that those who ate oily fish once a week were 30 per cent less likely to have asthma than those who ate it once a month or less often, and about 36 per cent less likely to have asthma symptoms such as wheezing. One explanation may be the anti-inflammatory benefits of oily fish such as salmon, mackerel and sardines. Asthma is first and foremost an immune system disease, in which immune cells overreact to triggers by pumping out inflammatory chemicals that narrow airways.

Stay away from traffic Diesel exhaust (for example, from lorries and buses) can cause serious problems for people with asthma. Just walking along busy streets can significantly reduce lung capacity and increase inflammation in people with asthma, probably because tiny particles of dust and soot in the exhaust can be inhaled deep into the lungs.

Take an aspirin every other day Research suggests that women who take a small dose (75mg) of aspirin every other day could cut their risk of developing asthma by as much as 10 per cent. Men generally seem to require a higher dose (300mg). Check with your GP before taking aspirin on a regular basis; there are possible risks for some people.

Latest thinking

According to Australian researchers, brief, regular exposure to ultraviolet (UV) light, found in sunlight, can suppress certain immune reactions, including those that trigger asthma symptoms – at least in mice. But don't abandon the usual cautions in respect of exposure to sunlight; too much can lead to skin cancer.

Athlete's foot

An itchy, scaly fungal rash between the toes, in the groin, under the breasts or elsewhere on your skin can be both embarrassing and very uncomfortable. Working up a sweat at the gym or pool, or even just mowing the lawn, is great for whole-body fitness, but if you aren't taking steps to protect sweat-moistened skin, you may end up with a fungal infection commonly known as athlete's foot or tinea.

90%
The odds of staying fungus free if you clear up an existing infection with an antifungal cream.

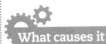

What causes it

The family of fungi called dermatophytes (also known as tinea), which normally live on our skin. Tendrils growing into the top layer of the skin lead to increased cell production with thick, scaly, itchy skin.

Symptoms to watch for

Burning, stinging or itching of your feet; peeling, cracking skin between your toes or on the bottoms of your feet; extremely dry skin on the bottoms or sides of your feet; crumbling, thickened and/or discoloured nails

Key prevention strategies

Keep your feet dry Athlete's foot is a infection caused by a type of fungus that grows in dead skin. The fungus thrives wherever there is moisture and its favourite food – keratin, a substance found in human skin. This means the insides of your trainers and socks are ideal breeding grounds. An important preventive measure you can take is to change your footwear after exercise and when you come home from work or come in from gardening, and change your socks when they're damp. Change your socks every day and try not to wear the same shoes two days in a row, and when you're at home, go barefoot or put on clean socks. In summer, it's a good idea to wear open sandals.

Wear flip flops at the pool and gym Foot protection is the best way to avoid the fungi lurking on the floors of virtually all changing rooms and public showers (they thrive in damp environments such as these). When Japanese researchers swabbed the soles of 140 people taking swimming classes at the University of Tsukuba, they found that 64 per cent carried the tinea fungus.

Stand on a thick towel when in changing rooms It's nearly impossible to keep flip flops on your feet while changing into your clothes, and socks may not offer adequate protection against fungal spores. Researchers have found that foot fungus can easily travel between the fibres of cotton and nylon socks and attach itself to your skin; wool socks and extremely thick cotton socks do keep fungus off your feet, but you'll wind up 'infecting' your shoes. Take an extra towel to use as a floor mat, and when you get home, machine-wash it – and be sure to use a hot setting to kill any spores.

Favourite hosts

Fungi that prefer humans – including those that cause athlete's foot – are generally classed as anthropophile. Other dermatophytes (also known as tinea) prefer soil (geophile) and are known to cause tinea infections in farmers, while fungi preferring animals (zoophile) may live on pets or livestock without causing symptoms, but can transmit skin infections to those who handle them.

Wash or wipe your feet If you forget to wear your shower shoes or flip flops, clean your feet before putting on your socks or shoes. Japanese researchers who studied the spread of athlete's foot in public bathhouses found that washing feet with soap and water or even wiping them thoroughly (don't forget to wipe between your toes) removes a significant amount of the fungus picked up from floors.

Use an antifungal preparation to prevent repeat infections Once your skin is infected, it's hard to get rid of the fungus – and even harder to stay fungus free after the infection seems to clear up. That's because the fungus lies between the skin layers. If you get frequent infections, use an over-the-counter spray, powder or cream containing one of the following antifungal agents: terbinafine, clotrimazole, econazole, ketoconazole, miconazole or tolnaftate.

If you are prone to fungal infections or will be spending a lot of time wearing sweaty shoes or changing in public changing rooms, using an antifungal product every day could help prevent infection.

Prevention boosters

Check your family's feet If anyone in your house has signs of athlete's foot, they could be spreading the fungus to others. Suggest a visit to the GP to rule out other causes. If your doctor confirms athlete's foot, it is important that the person uses an antifungal spray, cream or foot powder until the problem has gone. Disinfect the bath and bathroom floor regularly, avoid sharing towels and wash towels and sheets in hot water to kill the fungus.

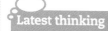

Latest thinking

Toenail fungus? Foot experts now suspect that an ongoing nail infection can be a 'reservoir' of fungus that can infect other parts of the body and that clearing it up could cut your odds of developing athlete's foot. If you have nail fungus, see your doctor; you'll probably need a course of oral antifungal medication to clear up the problem.

Back pain

The reason that back pain is such a common complaint could be because humans were not designed to walk upright. It turns out that the same evolutionary change in our spines that allowed us to walk on two limbs also made it easier for vertebrae (the bones encasing the spinal cord) to crush and strain the soft discs between them. Unfortunately, we can't change our evolutionary heritage, but what we can do is to minimise the effects of this design weakness.

50%
The amount by which you can reduce your risk of back pain by taking regular moderate exercise.

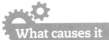

What causes it

Strained muscles or ligaments or the breakdown of the discs between the vertebrae.

Key prevention strategies

Get yourself off the couch or out of the chair If you're sitting around all day (which in itself is bad for the back), you're not getting exercise, a key strategy to prevent back pain. Exercise helps keep extra weight off, strengthens abdominal and back muscles that support the spine, and increases the flow of oxygenated blood to the back muscles, the vertebrae and to other bones that keep your back properly aligned.

Don't worry about what kind of exercise you do; a major review of studies found that no single activity is best, nor is there any clear evidence as to how often and for how long you should work out – it may in fact vary from person to person. Most doctors recommend that you get at least 30 minutes of moderate exercise (walking fast enough so you're slightly out of breath) at least four or five days a week.

Perfect your posture Surprisingly, that doesn't mean sitting up straight. Scottish researchers used specialised scanning (MRI) to evaluate three sitting postures in 22 volunteers. The participants either hunched forward, sat ramrod straight or leaned back slightly. The researchers found the greatest risk of vertebral movement, which can lead to misaligned spinal discs, in people who sat up straight and the least in people who leaned back slightly. So find a chair that provides good back support but also allows you to lean back just a bit. Here are some posture pointers:

- **Sleep on your side or back, not your stomach** Sleeping on your stomach increases the curve of your lower back, pulling it out of alignment.

Mind your mattress

Tempted by a fluffy, pillow-top mattress? Resist. Studies have found that firm mattresses provide the best support for your back, resulting in less back pain. Your mattress shouldn't be as hard as a granite slab, though; one that's medium-firm is best for the health of your back.

> " The **better** your spinal stability, the less likely you are to **develop back pain**. "

- **Stand in front of the mirror and straighten up** Try to memorise how it feels when your entire body – from your ears to your ankles – forms a straight line.
- **Check your workstation** Even when leaning back slightly in your chair, put both feet flat on the floor and keep your eyes level with your computer monitor without bending your neck.
- **Walk with your stomach pulled in** Don't allow your lower back to arch. Hold your head high.
- **Walk lightly** If you literally pound the pavement, you're sending shock waves throughout your body, creating extra stress on your joints, including your pelvic and spinal joints. Ask a friend or family member to watch (and listen) to how you walk. If they observe that you're walking 'too hard', practise walking heel-toe, heel-toe instead of landing on your whole foot. This will cushion each step and distribute your weight more evenly.

Lift like a pro Most physiotherapists and orthopaedic surgeons recommend that you bend and lift in the following ways:
- **Light objects such as a piece of paper** Hold onto a nearby chair or table for support. Then lean over the object, slightly bend one knee and extend the other leg behind you. Push up with your bent leg after you've picked up the object.
- **Heavy objects such as a grocery bag or laundry basket** Stand in front of the object, bend at the knees and lift with your leg muscles. Don't bend at your waist, and don't rely on your arm strength alone for lifting heavy weights.
- **Luggage** Stand right next to the suitcase, bend your knees, grasp the handle and then straighten up.

Treat stress and depression You may think that depression is all in the mind, but in reality it's often all in the back. Chronic pain such as back pain can lead to depression, but it can also work the other way around, according to studies. If you've lost interest in your normal activities, find yourself sleeping significantly more or less than usual,

Symptoms to watch for

Spasms, pain that may or may not radiate down the leg; numbness in your legs and restricted function; pain worsening at night; and bladder or bowel problems.

Bike basics

Cycling is great exercise, but hunching over the handlebars can wreak havoc on your back. Try tilting the front of the bike seat down 10 to 15 degrees. This will relieve pressure on the spine, in turn reducing back pain, according to a British study of 40 recreational cyclists. Also, take your bike into a cycle shop and ask an expert to make sure the seat is at the right height and that the frame itself is the correct size for you. And don't let your shoulders ride up around your neck when leaning on the handlebars; try to draw your shoulders down and back.

have considered self-harm, or have other symptoms of depression, see your doctor immediately. (See also *Depression*, page 152.) If you've ever suddenly found yourself flat on your back and unable to move without excruciating pain after a stressful event, you're not alone. At least 11 studies find a significant relationship between stress, anxiety and back pain. It's not possible to avoid all stressful situations in life, but you can learn better ways to manage your stress. Here are some ideas that work for many people:

- **Take up a new interest** and make it something as exciting and distracting as possible.
- **Learn to meditate** Classes are available in most communities.
- **Volunteer** Helping others in need quite often puts your own issues and problems into better perspective. You'll also make new friends.

Prevention boosters

Try Pilates or see an exercise physiologist There's no evidence that one is better than the other for preventing future episodes of back pain. In both forms of exercise, the practitioner develops a programme of exercises for you that addresses impairments in flexibility and strength, and this may help you enjoy a more active lifestyle. Pilates focuses on strengthening your core muscles – all the muscles that surround your spine and abdomen – that play a role in stabilising your back. But if you already have back problems, make sure you let your Pilates instructor know this before you begin classes.

Work out with an exercise ball Researchers in California tried an experiment on 20 sedentary office workers. Half of them exercised twice a week for 10 weeks with inflatable, oversized balls, also known as stability balls (available online and in sports shops), which are designed to strengthen the core muscles. The other half did nothing. The people who used the ball showed major improvements in spinal stability; the muscles they developed in their abdomen and back acted like a thick belt around the waist to support the spine. The better your spinal stability, the less likely you are to develop back pain. The sizes of stability balls can vary considerably; so be sure to choose the right size for your height. www.exerciseballworkouts.net/exercise-balls.html provides a guide.

Wear flat shoes When you wear high heels, you throw your body weight forwards, which exaggerates the curve of the lower back, making your back muscles work harder.

Set your alarm to get up and move When you're sitting for a long time at the computer, in the car or on a train, set an alarm on your watch or mobile phone to remind you to move every 20 minutes. If you can, get up and walk. If you're stuck in the car, shift your weight from one buttock to the other in a rocking movement and flex your legs as far as possible. On long car journeys, try to stop and walk around for a few minutes at least every hour.

Clean out your briefcase or shoulder bag Large bags may be very useful, but they can cause untold problems for your back, especially if you sling a bag over one shoulder. They make your gait lopsided and pull your neck and shoulder – and hence your back – out of alignment. The best option is a smaller 'bumbag', which puts the weight evenly on your hips. If that's not an option for you, try a backpack or a bag slung across your body, each of which tends to distribute the weight more evenly across your shoulders or chest. And also regularly empty out unnecessary clutter in handbags and backpacks. Regardless of what you're carrying, a bag shouldn't weigh more than 10 per cent of your body weight.

Use a step stool It will keep you from reaching too high, which could pull or strain a back muscle. If the stool has a low step, you can also place one foot on it (occasionally switching feet) to relieve your back a bit while you're washing dishes.

Counteract low kitchen worktops Worktops should be designed at the right height for the people using them, but tall people often end up leaning over to wash dishes or prepare meals. Put a stool or small stepladder in front of your legs and lean the front of your legs against it. A study by Japanese researchers found that this simple change significantly reduced lower-back strain.

Quit smoking Smoking narrows arteries, thereby impeding blood circulation and reducing the amount of oxygen-rich blood that gets to the spine and back muscles, among other areas. An inadequate blood supply interferes with the ability of bone and muscle to repair itself, which spells disaster if you've got back troubles.

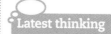

Latest thinking

You may one day be able to blame chronic back pain, in part, on genes. Norwegian researchers believe that there is at least one genetic variant that increases susceptibility to back pain.

See also:

Exercises: *Back strength and flexibility, page 324*
Step 3: *Quit smoking, page 66*

117

Belching

One dictionary definition of burping, 'bringing forth wind noisily from the stomach', has a poetic ring to it. But burping or belching (known medically as eructation) is anything but poetic in real life. Experts say the occasional release of air from your stomach after a large meal is perfectly normal. Sudden, uncontrollable attacks of belching, however, are anything but. These 'attacks' can be embarrassing and even painful. Most of the time, however, the cause is simply air that you've inadvertently swallowed. Here are some tips for avoiding this problem.

50%
The amount of extra air that chronic belchers swallow and release compared to people who don't burp excessively.

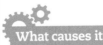

What causes it

Swallowing air, infection with Helicobacter pylori (the bacterium that causes stomach ulcers).

Symptoms to watch for

Expelling air from your stomach, either as a loud belch or a discreet burp.

Key prevention strategies

Put your fork down between bites Gulping down your food or washing down large mouthfuls with a drink are two surefire ways to send more air into your stomach, which is likely to resurface as a belch. Taking small bites, chewing thoroughly and pacing your meal by putting down utensils between bites can all help because they give your body time to move trapped air into your intestines or simply absorb it. Chew especially well if you're eating a plateful of crunchy raw vegetables such as broccoli, cabbage, lettuce and cauliflower. Air becomes trapped easily between the crushed food particles and ends up in your stomach.

More mealtime tips to minimise the amount of air in your stomach include letting hot beverages cool before sipping, not using a straw, cutting out carbonated drinks if they make belching worse for you and taking a few minutes to relax before eating if you're feeling tense. Anxiety has been linked to excess air ingestion in several studies.

Keep cigarettes, gum and boiled sweets out of your mouth Chewing gum or sucking on sweets produces extra saliva, which prompts more swallowing, sending more air into your stomach. Experts say an extra teaspoonful (about 5ml) of air is ingested each time saliva is swallowed. After several swallows, that creates an air bubble in your stomach. When that air is heated by your body to 38°C (98.6°F), the gases expand by about 10 per cent, creating the perfect set-up for a belch.

Conquer nervous air swallowing Dutch researchers who compared 14 'excessive belchers' and 14 'normal burpers' came to a surprising conclusion: While both groups had the occasional 'normal belch', problem

> " Holding a **pencil** between your teeth can help **keep extra air out** of your stomach. "

belchers continually swallowed extra air and immediately let it back out. Digestion experts call this type of nervous belching 'eructio nervosa'. Air swallowing is often an unconscious habit. Experts suggest that approaches such as relaxation exercises, speech therapy, hypnosis, and simply holding a pencil between your teeth (you can't swallow when your jaws are separated in this position) can help keep extra air out.

Prevention boosters

Knock out the ulcer bug Repeated belching can be a sign of infection with the ulcer-causing bacterium *Helicobacter pylori*. This common bug can inflame the lining of your stomach and even trigger a process that burns holes in it. Along the way, it produces bloating and wind. Other signs of an *H. pylori* infection or peptic ulcer include heartburn, indigestion, nausea, chest pain, weight loss and fatigue. If you have unexplained belching, ask your doctor about a blood test or a breath test for *H. pylori*. If the results are positive, you may be treated with an antibiotic.

Fix your dentures and clear your sinuses Poorly fitting dentures and chronic catarrh can lead to excess air swallowing and excessive burping.

Latest thinking

Up to half of all people with gastro-oesophageal reflux disease (GORD) belch excessively. Experts suspect that GORD sufferers may unconsciously swallow air in an attempt to burp and relieve discomfort. If you have GORD and burp a lot, the tips recommended by experts for preventing more belching are the strategies outlined in this chapter: eat more slowly and cut back on air swallowing.

Benign prostatic hyperplasia

As men age, their prostate gland is likely to enlarge, which could lead to symptoms such as difficulty urinating or urinating too often. However, while nearly 80 per cent of men have benign prostatic hyperplasia (BPH) by the time they turn 80, only about a third develop symptoms.

What causes it

Overgrowth of prostate tissue spurred by hormones such as oestrogen and testosterone. Age is the most common risk factor; 40 per cent of men aged 60 and older have it, and 90 per cent of men aged 80 and older.

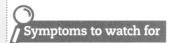

Symptoms to watch for

Increased need to urinate, particularly at night; weaker urine stream; problems starting to urinate and dribbling.

Key prevention strategies

Eat more vegetables When researchers compared the diets of 6,000 men with BPH to 18,000 men without it, they found those who ate about 10 servings of vegetables a day were 21 per cent less likely to have BPH than those who ate less vegetables. Ten servings may sound like a lot, but if you start with a vegetarian omelette for breakfast, snack on a dozen baby carrots with low-fat dip and have a large spinach salad for lunch, you're halfway there.

The best choices, the study found, are vegetables high in vitamin C and the antioxidant lutein, such as Brussels sprouts, peppers and spinach. Also pay special attention to onions. Men who eat several portions of onions a week are far less likely to develop BPH than those who eat less.

Discover flaxseeds and soya Both are sources of hormone-like plant compounds called phyto-oestrogens. These help guard against BPH by blocking an enzyme that converts testosterone into a different form – one that triggers prostate growth. Phyto-oestrogens also counteract the effects of oestrogen (yes, men have oestrogen, too), which also fuels prostate cell growth. Researchers think one reason why men living in Western countries have higher rates of BPH than those living in Asian countries is that they eat lower amounts of phyto-oestrogen-rich foods.

Flaxseeds are easy to add to your diet: buy them ground (store ground seeds in the fridge) and sprinkle them on practically anything, from cereal to yoghurt or salad. You can also add ground flaxseeds to meatballs, bread and cakes.

For soya, you don't have to rely on tofu. Try snacking on soya nuts or soya beans in the pods, known as edamame (available frozen), and using soya milk on your cereal or in smoothies.

50% The amount by which you could reduce your risk by exercising vigorously for 2 hours a week.

Burn off some calories every week A study involving 1,000 men who were followed for nine years found that those who burned the most energy each week through physical activity were half as likely to develop BPH as those who barely moved off the couch. Two hours a week of swimming lengths burns about 1,260kcal – putting you in the 50 per cent risk-reduction zone based on this study. Other good options include running for 2 hours or walking for a minimum of 4 hours each week.

Drugs that prevent disease

Finasteride (Proscar), prazosin (Hypovase), tamsulosin (Flomaxtra) and terazosin (Hytrin) are medications used to treat BPH. Finasteride blocks the enzyme that converts testosterone to dihydrotestosterone (DHT); DHT – three times more potent than testosterone – causes cells in the prostate to grow. Low doses can reduce the risk of BPH worsening over time and also reduce the rate of prostate cancer by 30 per cent. Prazosin, tamsulosin and terazosin belong to a group of drugs called alpha-blockers. They relax the muscles in the prostate gland, bladder neck and urethra, reducing some of the symptoms of BPH. Using finasteride with an alpha-blocker provides more benefit than using a single agent, but they all have side effects.

Check your cholesterol levels
Here's something you possibly didn't know: reproductive hormones such as testosterone are largely made of cholesterol. There is some evidence that men with high levels of LDL ('bad') cholesterol are more likely to have BPH.

Prevention boosters

Forgo unhealthy snacks Cutting out sugary snacks and simple carbohydrates such as doughnuts, white bread and crisps is a good way to lose weight and also guard against high blood glucose levels. Men who are very obese (defined as a body mass index of 35 or higher) are three and a half times more likely to develop BPH than men of normal weight. Men with high blood glucose levels are three times more likely to develop BPH than men with normal levels.

Stop at one beer Cutting back on alcohol intake is a good idea. Men who have two or more drinks a day are 30 per cent more likely to develop BPH than those who have less than one a month.

Reach for low-fat or fat-free options If you're getting more than 38 per cent of your energy from fat, you're about 30 per cent more likely to develop BPH than someone who consumes fewer than 26 per cent of his energy from fat.

Latest thinking

Men with fast-growing BPH may be more likely to develop prostate cancer, particularly if they have metabolic syndrome.

See also:

Cause 2: Intra-abdominal fat, page 24
Cause 5: Bad cholesterol balance, page 30

Bladder cancer

Most men worry about prostate cancer, but few think about bladder cancer – the second most common cancer in middle-aged and elderly men. Women can be affected, too, although less commonly. About one in five cases of bladder cancer occur after exposure to certain chemicals used to make dyes, paints, textiles and other products, most of which people are exposed to 30 to 50 years before the cancer develops. There's not a lot you can do about that if you fall into that category, but there's a surprising amount you can do to prevent bladder cancer from other causes.

30% The amount your bladder cancer risk drops within four years of quitting smoking.

What causes it

Most often, toxins coming into contact with bladder cells. Over time, they can affect the DNA in these cells, leading to cancer. These toxins can come from the food you eat and the water you drink, tobacco by-products, and environmental and occupational chemicals. Other causes include infection with certain parasites (schistosomiasis).

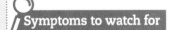

Symptoms to watch for

Blood in the urine, pain during urination, frequent urination or feeling that you need to urinate but can't, and abdominal pain.

Key prevention strategies

Quit smoking If you smoke, your risk of developing bladder cancer is two to four times higher than someone who has never smoked. In fact, researchers estimate that two-thirds of all cases of bladder cancer are related to smoking. The longer you smoke and the more cigarettes you smoke, the greater your risk.

Don't try to give up on your own. Studies prove that you're more than twice as likely to be successful if you combine nicotine replacement products such as gum or nasal spray with some form of organised support, such as a counselling programme or a telephone help line. (See page 66 for more advice on how to quit.)

Munch on raw broccoli and cauliflower Cruciferous vegetables such as broccoli, cauliflower, cabbage, pak choy and Brussels sprouts are filled with isothiocyanates. These antioxidants inhibit enzymes that make certain chemicals in the body more likely to cause cancer. One study found that eating three or more servings a month cut bladder cancer risk by about 40 per cent. Cooking destroys the enzyme needed to produce isothiocyanates, reducing available amounts by 60 to 90 per cent, so eat these vegetables raw as often as possible.

Prevention boosters

Eat foods rich in selenium This trace mineral is a powerful antioxidant linked with lower rates of several cancers, including bladder cancer. In your body, selenium comes into direct contact with bladder cells, where it is thought to prevent damage from free radicals (the

" Brazil nuts *are rich in selenium, which is linked to* **lower rates** *of bladder cancer.* **"**

unstable molecules that wreak havoc on DNA) and reduce levels of cancer-causing toxins. In one 12 year study of nearly 26,000 people, those with the lowest blood levels of selenium were more than twice as likely to develop bladder cancer compared to those with the highest levels. Selenium is found in numerous foods, including brazil nuts (the best source by far), wholemeal flour, barley and fish.

Switch to skimmed milk and low-fat yoghurt High levels of saturated fat (found in full-fat dairy products, not to mention fatty meats and cheese) more than doubled the rate of bladder cancer in a large Spanish study. Other studies find the overall amount of saturated fat in your diet increases your risk, so opt for low-fat dairy foods and trim cuts of red meat; your risk will drop.

Latest thinking

Surgery to remove just the tumour, followed by chemo-therapy and radiation therapy, may be just as effective as removing the entire bladder for most stages of bladder cancer.

See also:

Step 7: Cut back on saturated fat, page 72

Breast cancer

Breast cancer is the most common cancer in women and the most common cause of cancer deaths in women, but it has a good cure rate, especially when caught early. It's also the only cancer with two medications approved to prevent it (for women at high risk). However, most women don't need to take medication to prevent breast cancer.

What causes it

High circulating levels of hormones such as oestrogen are the main disease drivers. After menopause, obesity and weight gain drive up hormone levels and thereby increase risk. The longer you live, the more oestrogen and environmental toxins you've been exposed to and the greater your likelihood of developing the disease. The one-in-eight statistic you may have heard only applies if you live to be 90 or older. Inherited genetic mutations account for only about 5 to 10 per cent of breast cancer cases.

Drugs that prevent disease

If the threat of breast cancer is a real worry for you, talk to your GP A simple quiz can determine your five-year and lifetime risk of breast cancer. If it's at least 60 per cent higher than that of other women your age, you may be a candidate for chemoprevention (taking one of two medications – tamoxifen or raloxifene – for five years). These medications mimic oestrogen in the body, preventing the real thing from affecting breast cells. Studies find that either medication reduces breast cancer risk by a staggering 49 per cent in high-risk women. If you're 35 years or older, you can calculate your own risk of developing breast cancer at www.cancer.gov/bcrisktool.

Key prevention strategies

Limit hormone replacement therapy (HRT) after the menopause Giving breast cells extra oestrogen is like pouring petrol on a fire. It makes the cells divide faster, raising the risk that some will mutate during division, producing a cancerous cell. Your immune system can typically destroy a few cancerous cells, but if you're taking oestrogen, those mutated cells could quickly overwhelm your natural defences. One study suggested that undergoing HRT for just three years quadrupled the risk of developing one of the most dangerous types of breast cancer.

Researchers suspect that the nearly 7 per cent drop in breast cancer diagnoses in the USA between mid-2002 and mid-2003 – after 20 years of increasing rates – was due to the fact that millions of women stopped taking HRT in 2002, the year a major report showed that the most commonly prescribed hormone medication increased the risk of breast cancer, heart disease and stroke, especially if taken in the long term.

Researchers don't think HRT causes the cancer; instead, it may enable microscopic cancers that might have faded away or remained tiny for decades to become destructively active.

Skip the rich chocolate cake Here's another good reason to say no to decadent desserts and over-sized portions: every 11lb (5kg) you gain after menopause increases your breast cancer risk by 1 per cent. The major reason appears to be that fat cells release chemicals that can convert other hormones such as testosterone, which both men and women have, into oestrogen. On the other hand, if you're postmenopausal and you lose 5kg (11lb) or more and keep the weight off – and you don't take HRT – your risk is 57 per cent lower than that of women whose weight stays the same (and is presumably a bit higher than it should be).

Schedule that mammogram Breast cancer screening using mammography is the best way to reduce deaths from breast cancer. It is especially effective in women aged 50 to 69 years, but also in women aged 40 to 49, and those 70 and older. In the 50 to 69 group, for every 10,000 women who are screened, up to 20 deaths from breast cancer will be prevented over a 10 year period. But mammography isn't foolproof. There is a chance that the test will either miss a cancer (false negative) or suggest a cancer where there is none (false positive), leading to extra tests and anxiety. The chance of a misreading is higher in younger women because their breast tissue is denser, making it more difficult to interpret X-ray changes. In the UK all women between the ages of 50 and 70 are invited to have a mammogram every two years.

Prevention boosters

Limit alcohol intake A glass of wine with a meal is good for your heart, but it can very slightly increase your risk of breast cancer – probably not enough to really worry about. If you have more than one drink a day, however, you should worry. About 4 per cent of breast cancers are thought to be linked to this level of alcohol intake, and the more you drink, the higher the risk. Researchers think it's because alcohol increases oestrogen production.

If you tend to drink more than a glass of wine a day (which is not recommended), taking a daily supplement containing at least 400mcg of folic acid could help to reduce your increased risk of breast cancer. This B vitamin can help to repair mistakes that cells make when they divide.

Keep moving Regular physical activity for at least 30 minutes a day, five days a week, can reduce your risk of breast cancer. The reason is that the more physically active you are, the lower your body fat, which in turn lowers breast cancer risk.

Symptoms to watch for

A lump or thickening in or near the breast or in the underarm area; tender nipples; changes in how the breast or nipple looks, including the size or shape; scaly, red or swollen skin on the breast, nipple or areola (the dark area surrounding the nipple); a nipple that turns inward; or nipple discharge.

Latest thinking

Even if you carry mutations in the genes BRCA1 and BRCA2, the 'breast cancer genes', your risk of developing breast cancer by the age of 70 is far less than once thought. Instead of the 80 per cent risk often cited, new research from the USA finds a risk of between 36 and 52 per cent.

See also:

Cause 2: Intra-abdominal fat, page 24
Step 1: Exercise, page 62

Bursitis and tendonitis

Doing the same movements over and over again can end in tendonitis, which is caused by inflammation of a tendon, a tough band of tissue that connects bones to muscles. Unfortunately, tendons lose some of their elasticity with age, making the condition more likely. Overuse of a joint can also cause bursitis, or inflammation of the fluid-filled sacs that cushion pressure points where muscles and tendons move across the bone. You can even get a form of tendonitis by leaning on your elbows too much.

90% Risk reduction by following a balanced exercise programme of aerobics, stretching and strengthening

What causes it

Ageing, repetitive movements and biomechanical problems with joints.

Symptoms to watch for

Pain and tenderness near a joint that gets worse with movement. The skin over the area may become red or warm to the touch. Your doctor can tell whether it's bursitis or tendonitis based on where the problem occurs.

Key prevention strategies

Get moving Exercise is an important part of a healthy, balanced life, but for some conditions, such as bursitis and tendonitis, you'll need to be careful to adopt the right approach.

- **Revamp your exercise routine** Overuse or misuse of joints and muscles causes the majority of tendonitis and bursitis cases. But that doesn't mean you should stop exercising; instead, follow our tips for injury-free movement.
- **Book a session or two with a personal trainer** This way you can evaluate your regular work-out and identify movements that may be putting unnecessary strain on your joints and tendons. Working with a personal trainer is also a great way to stay motivated.
- **Start slowly** It takes a few minutes for your muscles and joints to warm up when you start working out.
- **Be consistent** That means exercising several times a week, not just once or twice a month. It also means you shouldn't throw yourself into a competitive basketball game if you haven't played or exercised for a while. Increase exercise by no more than 5 to 10 per cent each week, in terms of either time spent or weight lifted.
- **Switch activities throughout the week** For instance, if you work out with weights twice a week, spend one day on leg exercises and one day on upper-body exercises. If you run three times a week, cycle on the other days. If you garden intensively one day, just water the garden or take a walk the next day.
- **Rest** Give yourself at least one day off each week. And if you feel any joint soreness after a workout, put an icepack on the joint to ward off inflammation.

126

Stretch and strengthen Range-of-motion exercises and weight-bearing exercises designed to strengthen muscles can reduce strain on joints, helping to prevent overuse injuries. For best results, book a few sessions with a personal trainer or physiotherapist to identify the best exercises for you based on the activities you do most.

Cut your calorie intake As with many conditions related to joints, being overweight increases the pressure on joints, bones and tendons, increasing your risk of injury.

Prevention boosters

Use innersoles or orthotics if you need them A major cause of Achilles tendonitis, an injury to the tendon that attaches the calf muscle to the heel bone, is hyperpronation of the foot – a medical term that simply means your ankles roll in. When you shop for trainers or walking shoes, do it at a specialist sports shop, not a department store, and ask the salesperson to help you find a shoe with the level of support you need.

If your pronation is bad, it may be advisable to consult a podiatrist to be fitted for custom orthotics, or start with a basic pair of shoe inserts from a pharmacy to see if they help. In addition, take advice and wear the right shoes for the sport you're playing.

Pay attention to pain If your joint feels sore, take some ibuprofen or put an icepack on it. Both can relieve inflammation, possibly preventing long-term damage.

Use a band or brace where you need it Supports for elbows and knees help reinforce and protect tendons during activities. There are many different types available, so check with your doctor or personal trainer about which one to choose.

Help for 'housemaid's knee'

If you kneel a lot at work, while cleaning, or when gardening, you're at risk of developing this condition, officially known as prepatellar bursitis. Investing in a thick pair of knee pads, available from DIY stores and garden centres, can save you from the pain.

Latest thinking

The antibiotic ciprofloxacin and others in its family (moxifloxacin and norfloxacin) can cause an inflamed Achilles tendon and even cause tendon rupture. Ask your doctor how you can protect your Achilles tendon if you need one of these antibiotics.

Carpal tunnel syndrome

If your job involves typing for long periods, cutting meat, using sign language or any other repetitive task involving your wrists and hands, you could be at risk of developing carpal tunnel syndrome. Hobbies such as sewing, knitting and guitar playing also put you at risk. Caused by swelling within the carpal tunnel, the channel though which the nerve running through the base of your palm passes, the condition is marked by numbness, tingling and pain in the hand and fingers. Prevent the pain with the following suggestions.

49%
The percentage of people whose carpal tunnel symptoms improved after wearing a wrist splint at night.

What causes it

Repetitive hand movements, particularly if you have to pinch or grip something while your wrist is bent. This inflames the nine tendons in the carpal tunnel, a narrow passageway that runs from the forearm through the wrist. These tendons enable you to flex your fingers. When they become inflamed, they put pressure on the median nerve, which also runs through the tunnel and supplies feeling to several fingers.

Key prevention strategies

Embrace proper ergonomics Good posture can help you avoid carpal tunnel syndrome. That means sitting up straight and not letting your shoulders roll forward, which puts pressure on nerves in the back and arms, and not rounding your lower back or thrusting your chin forwards – common postural mistakes that squeeze the muscles in the neck and in turn can affect muscles and nerves in your hands, wrists and fingers. It's also important to keep your wrists relatively straight – not bent up or down.

Warm up and take breaks Flex your fingers up and down 10 times whenever you've been away from your computer for more than 5 minutes. It's also important to give your wrists a rest. Take a 30 second break every 20 minutes and a 5 minute stretching break every hour.

Carpal tunnel as a symptom

Studies find much higher rates of carpal tunnel syndrome in people with rheumatoid arthritis, Type 1 diabetes, hypothyroidism, fibromyalgia and certain other conditions. It can also be caused by disorders including multiple myeloma, non-Hodgkin's lymphoma and acromegaly – a disease in which the bones grow very long. If you have any of these diseases or conditions, effective management may reduce your risk of carpal tunnel syndrome, or improve symptoms if you already have it. Pregnancy and menopause also increase the risk, suggesting that hormones may also play a role.

Vary your tasks If you have just spent 2 hours typing, switch to a task away from the keyboard – for example, work with pen and paper, do some reading, file your correspondence or meet with colleagues.

Use a wrist splint Wearing a splint that keeps your wrist in a neutral position can help prevent the kind of damage that turns into carpal tunnel syndrome. In one study, 63 people with early signs of carpal tunnel wore

Typing technique

Practise sensible ergonomics at work, and you'll be less likely to end up with carpal tunnel syndrome.

1 **Adjust your chair** so your spine is against the chair back and both feet are flat on the floor or on a footrest.

2 **Keep your wrists flat while typing** and type with your elbows at a 90-degree angle.

3 **Set your keyboard** so you can tap the keys instead of pounding them.

4 **Ensure the keyboard-supporting surface** is at least 75 cm wide and between 70–75 cm off the floor.

5 **Place the monitor directly in front of you** Position the top of the screen at eye level or below and keep materials used for typing at eye level.

custom-fitted wrist–hand splints nightly for six weeks. After six weeks, about half reported that their symptoms improved.

Perform gentle stretching Try the exercises starting on page 332, as they tone and stretch muscles and ligaments in your hands and wrists to help guard against injury.

Prevention boosters

Use the right tools Choose household implements and kitchen tools that distribute the force of your grip across the muscle between the base of your thumb and your little finger, not the centre of your hand. If you use power tools, add shock absorbers to reduce vibration or wrap the vibrating part in a towel.

Check your risk of metabolic syndrome This condition is marked by three of the following factors: low HDL ('good') cholesterol, a waist measurement greater than 88cm (34½in) (for women) or 102cm (40in) (for men), high blood pressure, high triglyceride levels, and insulin resistance. When researchers studied 107 people, they found that 75 per cent of those with metabolic syndrome also had carpal tunnel syndrome.

Lose a few pounds If you're overweight, your risk of carpal tunnel syndrome is twice that of someone of normal weight.

Eat more B vitamins Vitamin B_6 may also be a useful part of your prevention stategy. Brown rice, salmon, macadamia nuts and some breakfast cereals are good food sources.

Symptoms to watch for

Pain, numbness and tingling in the affected hand and/or fingers, especially the thumb and index and middle fingers. The pain and numbness may be worse at night; sometimes it's bad enough to wake you up. You may find you have trouble holding objects tightly and have weakness in your thumb.

Latest thinking

Contrary to popular belief, work may not be the prime cause of carpal tunnel syndrome. One study found that people who used a keyboard for 4 hours or more a day were significantly less likely to have carpal tunnel than those who used it for an hour a day or less. Other risk factors include rheumatoid arthritis, hypothyroidism, Type 1 diabetes and non-Hodgkin's lymphoma. Pregnancy and the menopause also increase risk.

Cataracts

66% The potential drop in your risk if you shield your eyes from sunlight by wearing a broad-brimmed hat and sunglasses.

When the lenses in your eyes grow cloudy, you know you've got cataracts. Your vision becomes blurred, driving at night can become difficult due to headlight glare, and colours become muted. The painter Claude Monet had cataracts and was forced to choose colours by reading the labels on tubes of paint. Cataract surgery can replace clouded lenses with artificial ones, but taking steps to prevent getting cataracts in the first place is a much better option.

What causes it

Sunlight, smoking, a low-antioxidant diet, high blood sugar and other factors seem to deactivate compounds, called alpha-crystallins, that normally prevent proteins in the eye's lens from clumping. Clumped proteins make the lens cloudy, distorting or even blocking the passage of light.

Symptoms to watch for

Cloudy or blurry vision, glare or a halo around lights, poor night vision, double vision, colours that look faded and frequent changes in your prescription for glasses or contact lenses.

Key prevention strategies

Enjoy a spinach salad with hard-boiled eggs, red peppers and sunflower seeds Getting plenty of the antioxidants lutein and zeaxanthin, as well as vitamin E, cuts cataract risk by 16 per cent according to a Harvard School of Public Health study of more than 23,000 women. Other studies show that a high intake of vitamin C also provides protective benefits.

Your body stores lutein and zeaxanthin in high concentrations in the lenses of your eyes, where they seem to work like sunglasses to filter out harmful ultraviolet rays. Antioxidants, including vitamins C and E, also seem to protect proteins in the lens from damage by destructive oxygen molecules known as free radicals.

Eating just seven servings of fruit and vegetables a day plus two servings of nuts is enough to provide your body with plenty of these important nutrients. Top sources of lutein and zeaxanthin include dark green vegetables such as spinach, broccoli and courgettes, as well as eggs and sweetcorn. For vitamin E, try tahini (sesame paste), sunflower seeds, hazelnuts, almonds and whole grains. Good sources of vitamin C include red and green peppers, Brussels sprouts, oranges and strawberries.

Keep your blood glucose low and steady Diabetes raised cataract risk 80 per cent in one study of 6,000 people. Experts suspect that high blood glucose damages proteins in the lens of your eye. Even high to normal blood glucose and prediabetes increase your odds. In a UK study, people with a prediabetic condition called impaired fasting glucose had double the normal risk. If you have diabetes, work with your doctor to keep your blood glucose under control. If you're at risk, follow all the steps in the entry on *Diabetes*, starting on page 156, to keep your blood glucose levels healthy.

Wear sunglasses and a broad-brimmed hat When scientists checked the eyes of nearly 900 US fishermen, they found that those who spent the most time in the sun were three times more likely to have cataracts than those who spent the least. But wearing sunglasses and a broad-brimmed hat reduced the risk by two-thirds. Similarly, French researchers who studied 2,584 residents in Sete, France, discovered that people who were exposed to high levels of sunlight were up to four times more likely to develop cataracts. Experts suspect that solar radiation alters proteins in the eye's lens, causing it to cloud. When buying sunglasses, look for a label that says the lenses protect against 99 per cent of UVB and 95 per cent of UVA rays – or UV absorption up to 400nm.

Quit smoking Smoking cigarettes doubles your risk of cataracts. Quit and your risk begins to drop, say Swedish researchers who tracked the health of 34,595 women. Light smokers (who smoked 6 to 10 cigarettes a day) completely erased their added risk 10 years after quitting; heavier smokers (over 10 cigarettes daily) who quit needed 20 years to reduce their risk to that of nonsmokers.

Prevention boosters

Lose weight Carrying extra weight can raise your risk of getting cataracts by as much as 36 per cent, according to a US study of 133,000 people. If you're overweight you're more likely to have blood glucose problems (even if you're not diabetic). You may also have high blood pressure or high levels of triglycerides.

If you use steroid medications, get your eyes tested soon
Oral steroids increase cataract risk; in one study of 2,446 people taking steroid medication – for example, for rheumatoid arthritis, asthma, emphysema, chronic bronchitis, lupus and inflammatory bowel disease – those who took a dose of 10mg per day for a year increased their cataract risk by 68 per cent. After 18 months, their risk increased to 82 per cent. At higher doses, inhaled steroids, steroid creams and steroid eye-drops may also raise the risk of developing cataracts. If you're taking steroids long term, have an eye examination and ask how often you need repeat checks.

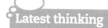
Latest thinking

Cholesterol-lowering statin medications have a surprising vision bonus. In a study of 6,000 people, published in the *Journal of the American Medical Association*, those who took statins cut their risk of cataracts by 60 per cent. Researchers suspect that statins act as antioxidants, protecting proteins in the lens from damage.

See also:

Cause 4: *Insulin resistance,* page 28
Step 2: *Fruit and vegetables,* page 64

Cervical cancer

Advances in the prevention of cervical cancer provide an excellent example of the fast pace of modern medical research. As recently as 20 years ago, experts didn't even know what caused cancer of the cervix. Now they know it's caused by the human papillomavirus (HPV) – and a vaccine has been created to prevent infection with that virus. Someday, possibly in the not-too-distant future, cervical cancer will have gone the way of polio, diphtheria and other viral illnesses prevented by vaccination. Until then, here are some key tips for doing all you can to protect yourself.

70%
The percentage of cervical cancers that could be prevented with the Gardasil vaccine.

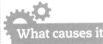

What causes it

The primary cause is the human papillomavirus (HPV), which is spread via sexual contact.

Symptoms to watch for

There are no symptoms with early cervical cancer. In later stages, the most common symptoms are abnormal vaginal bleeding (that is, not during a period) – for example, bleeding after intercourse; or discharge. In the very late stages cervical cancer may cause pelvic pain.

Key prevention strategies

Get vaccinated We prevent tetanus, whooping cough, meningitis and numerous other illnesses with vaccines; now, we can prevent cancer with a series of three shots. The Gardasil vaccine was developed by a team of medical scientists, and protects against infection from four HPV viruses that cause about 70 per cent of all cervical cancers. Ideally, young women should be vaccinated before they become sexually active. In the UK it is given in secondary schools to girls aged 12 to 13. In theory, any woman can be vaccinated as long as she is not pregnant, but there is no evidence of a benefit in women who have already been infected with HPV.

Have regular cervical smears Cervical cancer is one of the few cancers that can be prevented with regular screening. Cervical smears, in which a doctor or nurse takes cells from your cervix for examination under a microscope, can pick up very early cellular changes that could eventually turn into cancer. Burning, cutting or freezing off those cells can prevent the cancer from developing. Such screening is the primary reason cervical cancer rates have plummeted 70 per cent since the 1950s.

In the UK, smear tests are offered to women between the ages of 25 and 49 every three years and from 50 to 64 every five years. If your last test showed any abnormalities, you may need more frequent screening.

Prevention boosters

Choose a non-hormonal contraceptive If you're worried about cervical cancer, avoid taking oral contraceptives that combine oestrogen with progestogen. Research by the International Agency for Research on

Cancer has linked this type of Pill to cervical cancer. A review of 24 international studies found that the longer you use the combination Pill, the greater your risk. Using oral contraceptives for 10 years from around the age of 20 to 30 appeared to almost double the risk of cervical cancer. As soon as they are stopped, the risk appears to drop; after 10 years, it's the same as that of a woman who never used contraceptives.

The risk seems to be linked to evidence that women who use birth control pills are more likely to be infected with HPV – possibly because they are not using condoms, which help to prevent sexually transmitted infections (STIs). But before abandoning this type of contraception, it is worth considering that the Pill reduces the risk of ovarian and endometrial cancer.

Watch your stress levels Being infected with HPV doesn't automatically mean you'll develop cervical cancer; many women, especially those under the age of 30, can shake off the virus as easily as they shake off dozens of other viruses they encounter on a daily basis. But daily stress – from a demanding job, problems with your children or spouse, or money worries – can impair your ability to fight off all viruses, including HPV, increasing your risk of long-term infection that could lead to cervical cancer.

Increase your intake of folate Low levels of the B vitamin folate increase the risk that pre-cancerous cervical cells will turn into actual cancer. Folate is found in green leafy vegetables such as spinach and cabbage. However, don't take a folate supplement before discussing this with your doctor, as it can mask symptoms of vitamin B_{12} deficiency, which is a serious condition.

Latest thinking

An interaction between cigarette smoking and HPV may increase the risk of cervical cancer. Carcinogens in cigarette smoke are thought to enable the virus to persist for longer and replicate, making the cervix more vulnerable to cellular changes that can lead to cancer.

Chronic obstructive pulmonary disease

The best thing you can do to avoid emphysema and chronic bronchitis – two types of chronic obstructive pulmonary disease (COPD) – is avoid tobacco smoke, dust and fumes. Although it sounds rare and obscure, COPD is shockingly common. In some countries, it's the fourth leading cause of death, just behind heart disease, cancer and stroke. Emphysema weakens the air sacs in your lungs so that they can't force out stale air, leaving little room for your next fresh, oxygen-rich inhalation. Chronic bronchitis occurs when damaged bronchial linings produce excess mucus and can't remove it. COPD makes you cough, wheeze and feel incredibly tired; it also raises your risk of lung infections.

What causes it

Smoking and chronic exposure to smoke, other fumes and dust. Occasionally, genes play a role.

Symptoms to watch for

A cough that brings up yellowish, grey or green mucus; chest soreness or tightness, or a tickling feeling when you breathe; infections, chills and a low fever; tiredness; wheezing; sore throat; and sinus congestion.

Key prevention strategies

Quit smoking Smoking cigarettes, cigars and pipes causes an estimated 85 per cent of COPD cases. Over a lifetime, half of all smokers will develop this debilitating lung disease. Giving up is the most effective way for smokers to reduce their risk. To be honest, if you already have COPD quitting won't reverse lung damage that's already occurred, but experts say it's still crucial. By kicking the habit, you may cut future declines in lung function by half.

Avoid second-hand smoke Passive smoking exposes you to chemicals and particles that irritate your lungs. Living with a smoker raises your own odds of developing COPD by 55 per cent. Working in a smoky environment, such as a bar, was shown to raise the risk by 36 per cent in one study. In the UK it is now illegal to smoke in the workplace, in restaurants or in bars, but it's essential that you also insist on smoke-free air in your home and car.

Bad air at work? Ask for a respirator Chemical fumes as well as dust from grain, cotton, wood or mining products can raise your risk of lung damage whether or not you smoke. A face mask fitted with special air filters could save your lungs.

Keep the air at home clean If you already have COPD, you can cut your risk of an attack by avoiding fumes from paint as well as perfumes and the smell of burning candles and incense. Even cooking odours can make you cough or wheeze. Keep the humidity in your home between 40 and 50 per cent (you can buy a hygrometer that measures humidity online or from some DIY or hardware stores) and, if you have them, change air filters on your central heating systems regularly.

Prevention boosters

Skip bacon, sausages, salami and other cured meats Eating cured meats at least once a day raised smokers' risk of emphysema and other progressive lung problems 2.64 times higher than that of those who ate these foods only a few times a year, according to a Harvard School of Public Health study of nearly 43,000 men. Nitrites in these meats generate cell-damaging particles, called free radicals, in the body. People with high levels of free radicals are more susceptible to lung damage.

Eat more fibre Eating about 27g of fibre a day produced a 15 per cent reduction in the risk of developing emphysema and other lung problems compared to eating just 9.5g a day, according to a study of nearly 12,000 people. Those who obtained a lot of their fibre from fruit cut their risk further – by 27 per cent. The reason may be that fibre simply acts as a marker for a diet that includes more fruit and vegetables. It's possible that the real protectors are the antioxidants in fresh fruit and vegetables, which protect lungs from free-radical damage.

How to prevent flare-ups

If you already have COPD, try these strategies to help you avoid wheezing episodes.

Get a yearly flu vaccination Viral and bacterial infections can make COPD worse. This vaccine can cut the risk of flu for those with COPD by up to 81 per cent.

Get a pneumonia vaccine at least once COPD raises your risk of life-threatening forms of pneumonia.

Use an over-the-counter mucus thinner Medications such as guaifenesin and acetylcysteine thin the mucus in yourir lungs and make it easier to cough up, cutting flare-ups by 20 per cent.

Use an inhaler A long-acting bronchodilator or an corticosteroid administered in an inhaler can each cut flare-ups by 20 per cent. Combining the two cuts their likelihood by 25 per cent. Ask your doctor's advice.

Follow an exercise routine Work with your doctor or physiotherapist. Half an hour of exercise most days of the week can ease breathlessness significantly.

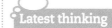

Latest thinking

A new twist on standard breathing exercises has been found to make exhaling easier for people with emphysema. US researchers at the University of Michigan have found that people with emphysema who learned to play the mouth organ improved their breathing significantly.

See also:

Step 3: Quit smoking, page 66

Colds

30% The amount by which you can cut the risk of colds if you use a saline nasal spray every day.

To reduce sniffing, sneezing and sick days by as much as 45 per cent all you need is hand cleanser and water. Together with sound sleep and good nutrition, hand washing is the best defence against cold viruses, which can survive for up to seven days on light switches, ATM keys, doorknobs and other surfaces – and for at least 3 hours on unwashed hands. Cultivating a strong immune system is also your best bet in the fight against viral infection.

What causes it

At least 250 viruses – and possibly hundreds more. The sheer number has made it impossible so far for scientists to develop an effective vaccine. But time's on your side: the human body develops some resistance to each cold virus it encounters, which is one reason we get fewer colds as we age.

Latest thinking

Perhaps your mum was right: being cold can increase your risk of catching a cold, at least according to one study. People exposed to cold temperatures were three times more likely to develop cold symptoms than those who stayed warm, according to a study of 180 people from the Common Cold Centre in Wales. The causal connection is that being chilly constricts blood vessels in the nose, reducing the supply of nutrients to infection-fighting white blood cells. This may allow dormant infections to come to life.

Key prevention strategies

Wash your hands frequently Do this even if your hands don't look or feel dirty. Scrubbing five times a day with soap and water reduced the number of upper respiratory infections among naval recruits by 45 per cent in one two-year study. A brisk, 10 second scrub rinses away 99 per cent of viruses. This cuts your odds of infection substantially, but not completely; a single viral particle can start a cold. For the best results, wet your hands, lather vigorously for a full 20 seconds, rinse, then dry with a clean paper towel. Use the towel to turn off the tap, too. Any hand cleanser will do – washing works by scrubbing viruses off your skin, not by killing them (an anti-bacterial handwash doesn't kill viruses).

Walk five days a week Regular exercise invigorates your immune system's natural killer cells and virus-killing antibodies. American researchers from the University of South Carolina found that adults who exercised moderately to vigorously at least four times a week had 25 per cent fewer colds over one year than those who moved less. A brisk 40 minute walk five days a week should do it; in another study, this amount of exercise halved the number of days during which volunteers suffered from cold symptoms. But don't overdo it: working out for an hour and a half or more could be counter-productive; it may reduce immunity.

Use a saline nasal spray Moist nasal passages are less receptive to cold viruses than dry ones. In one 20 week study of military recruits, those who used a saline nasal spray every day had 30 per cent fewer colds and 42 per cent fewer days with runny noses or congestion. Use the spray during winter, when heated indoor air is dry, and also during plane flights.

Prevention boosters

Tame the stress monster In a year-long Spanish study of 1,149 university staff, colds were twice as likely among people who felt stressed compared to those with the least stress in their lives. And once you catch a cold, stress can also make symptoms worse.

Season or supplement with garlic This ancient remedy may help by boosting the activity of your immune system's virus-killing T cells. When 146 women and men took either a garlic capsule or a placebo daily during the cold season, the garlic group caught 24 colds, compared with 65 in the placebo group. Researchers at the UK's Garlic Centre say that garlic takers who did become ill recovered in just a day and a half, while the placebo group had the cold for an average of five days. (Other research is less positive about garlic.) If you love garlic, use it liberally. Always let chopped, crushed or bruised garlic sit for 10 minutes before you use it to maximise levels of its active healing component.

Use alcohol-based hand sanitisers when you can't wash These gels and sprays kill bacteria and some viruses, but hand washing is preferable. Studies show that brands containing 60 per cent ethyl alcohol are powerless against rhinoviruses (which cause colds). Some researchers report that a 70 per cent ethanol sanitiser can be effective.

Hop into a sauna twice a week In an Austrian study, people who did this twice a week for six months had half as many colds as those who didn't. The link may be air temperature – at over $27°C$, sauna air is too hot for cold viruses to survive.

The new cold fighters

Echinacea may be one of the top-selling herbal supplements, but its cold-battling prowess remains controversial. One authoritative German review of 16 clinical trials concluded that echinacea doesn't prevent colds (though other research says it does). And it seems that vitamin C is even less likely to prevent colds. A definitive analysis of 29 well-designed studies involving over 11,700 people concluded that vitamin C has no power to prevent a cold. Instead, you may want to try one of these alternatives:

Andrographis In one well-designed study, volunteers who took two 100mg tablets a day for three months had half as many colds as volunteers who took placebos.

Probiotics These beneficial bacteria seem to increase production of immune cells where you need them most to fight colds: in the tissues lining your respiratory system. Capsules containing the bacteria *Lactobacillus gasseri*, *Bifidobacterium longum* and *B. bifidum* MF shortened colds by an average of two days in volunteers who took them daily for three months.

Symptoms to watch for

Sore throat, stuffy and/or runny nose, sneezing, coughing and even a mild fever. It may be the flu if you have chills, body aches, significant fatigue and/or a very high fever.

Colorectal cancer

Surprisingly, clinical study reviews have found that high-fibre diets don't protect against cancer of the colon in the way that was once thought. However, while colorectal cancer is among the most common cancers in the UK and the second leading cause of cancer deaths, it's also the most preventable cancer in the world after lung cancer. There are many steps you can take to protect yourself against this type of cancer, many of which, as you might imagine, still involve what you eat.

50%
The risk reduction achieved if you get the vitamin D you need from sunshine, food or supplements.

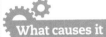

What causes it

Ageing, genetic abnormalities and diseases such as inflammatory bowel disease.

Symptoms to watch for

Blood in your stools; narrowing of stools; a change in bowel habits, including diarrhoea or constipation for more than a couple of weeks; cramping, wind or pain; abdominal pain with a bowel movement; feeling that your bowel doesn't empty completely; weakness or fatigue; and unexplained weight loss.

Key prevention strategies

Get screened The NHS offers bowel cancer screening to all men and women aged 60 and over every two years, using a bowel cancer testing kit. Often, but not always, bowel cancer leads to microscopic amounts of blood in the stool, which can be detected with special kits. The cure rate for patients who have surgery before the cancer has spread is about 90 per cent. As with all tests, there is a risk of missing a cancer or getting a positive result from the kit when no cancer is actually present. To get accurate results from some kits, you mustn't eat red meat, specific fruit and vegetables (for example, raw broccoli), vitamin C supplements, and aspirin or anti-inflammatory medications for three days before taking each test sample, so follow the instructions carefully. If your father, mother or a sibling has had bowel cancer, you have a higher risk and should see your doctor to discuss your individual risk; genetic testing and five-yearly colonoscopies may be recommended.

Get out there and exercise An analysis of 19 studies found that men who are physically active reduce their risk of colon cancer by about 21 per cent; for women, the benefit of brisk walking, heavy gardening, cycling or swimming, etc., yields a 30 per cent risk reduction.

Cut back on red meat The less red meat you eat, the lower your risk of colorectal cancer. Eating 500g a week (the amount in two large steaks) increases your risk by about 30 per cent; every 45g after that increases your risk by another 15 per cent, according to the American Institute for Cancer Research. There are several possible reasons for the link. Firstly, people who eat a lot of meat tend to eat fewer health-protective fruit and vegetables. And a diet high in fatty red meat also contributes to 'oxidative stress'; in other words, it creates harmful free radicals in the body that can damage cells, DNA and other microscopic components of your digestive tract. Some of those interactions are as dangerous as those caused by radiation, which is why eating plenty of fruit and vegetables is so important, because they contain valuable antioxidants that help to combat oxidative damage. So have no more than a hand-sized portion of meat at each meal and eat plenty of fresh vegetables and salad with it.

Should you go 'virtual'?

Many doctors agree that virtual colonoscopy, which involves lying on a table and passing painlessly through a CT or MRI scanner to have detailed 3-D images of your colon taken and examined, isn't ready yet as a tool to replace traditional colonoscopy. So it doesn't excuse you from the pre-test bowel-cleansing ritual that no one enjoys. And if the test finds a polyp, you'll need to follow up with a traditional colonoscopy – and repeat the bowel cleansing – to have the polyp removed.

Skip the cold cuts Eating about 60g of processed meat (about two slices of salami) a day could increase your risk of colorectal cancer by 50 per cent compared to people who eat no processed meat. The culprit may be N-nitroso compounds (NOCs), the result of nitrates used to preserve meat.

Go heavy on fish Feeding fish oil to animals reduces the number of colorectal tumours they develop, along with the overall risk of colorectal cancer. This effect in humans is not yet proven, but it appears that people who eat fish once or twice a week reduce their risk by about 12 per cent compared to those who eat it less often; each additional serving reduces the risk by another 4 per cent. The link between fish and colorectal cancer prevention may be due to the high levels of selenium and vitamin D in fish, both of which are also recognised for their value as colorectal cancer preventives.

Limit yourself to one unit of alcohol a day A unit contains 10ml of alcohol. The volume of liquid making up the drink depends on the concentration of alcohol, so look at the label. One unit of alcohol is defined as 100ml of wine (small glass), half a pint of beer or one small measure of spirits.

As your body breaks down alcohol, cancer-causing acetaldehyde forms. Alcohol also appears to make cells more permeable to other cancer-causing compounds. An analysis of more than 4,600 cases of colorectal cancer among 475,000 participants found that those who drank more than 4.5 units of alcohol a day increased their risk of colorectal cancer by 41 per cent. The risk increased by 16 per cent in those drinking 3-4.4 units daily.

Prevention boosters

Eat more pulses Lentils, beans and peas are excellent sources of folate, a B vitamin also known as folic acid. According to a Harvard study of nearly 89,000 women, those with a family history of colon cancer who consumed more than 400mcg of folate each day lowered their risk by more than 52 per cent compared to women who consumed 200mcg a day. You can get almost 300mcg by eating a cup of chickpeas or cooked spinach, another great source. If you take a multivitamin, you may already be getting enough folate.

Season with garlic About six cloves of garlic a week, whether raw or cooked, can help reduce your risk of colorectal cancer by as much as 31 per cent, according to one University of North Carolina analysis of many studies from the USA. The benefit probably comes from allicin compounds in garlic (its active ingredient), which prevent colorectal tumours from forming, possibly by forcing abnormal cells to commit the equivalent of cellular suicide.

Drink a glass of skimmed milk every day Just 250ml a day reduces women's risk of colorectal cancer by 16 per cent and men's risk by 10 per cent, according to an analysis of studies by US researchers at Brigham and Women's Hospital, and Harvard Medical School. Every two additional glasses reduces the risk by another 12 per cent. Why? It may be the vitamin D that's routinely added to milk in the USA, or its calcium (high calcium consumption is also linked to lower rates of colon cancer). Milk also contains the fatty acid conjugated linoleic acid and the protein lactoferrin, both of which help prevent colon cancer in animals.

Drugs that prevent disease

If you're already taking aspirin or another non-steroidal anti-inflammatory drug (NSAID) such as celecoxib (Celebrex), you may enjoy a happy side benefit: a lower risk of colon cancer. Research suggests that if women take at least 325mg of regular aspirin twice a week for at least 10 years, their risk of colon cancer plummets by a third compared to women who take aspirin less often. And in a study of people who had already had pre-cancerous polyps removed, those who were taking 400mg of celecoxib a day were a third less likely to develop more growths within three years. But it's too soon to recommend taking medications such as these solely to prevent the cancer, as they can have unwanted side effects.

Statins, prescribed to lower cholesterol, may also lower the risk of colon cancer. A study involving 4,000 people found that taking a statin for at least five years reduced the risk of colon cancer by nearly a half. But as with aspirin and NSAIDs, statins have side effects, and doctors aren't ready to prescribe them unless they're necessary to regulate blood cholesterol.

All these medications reduce inflammation, which can contribute to cancer development. They probably work in other ways, too. Researchers around the world are now studying their mechanisms to try to find a way to create a medication with all the cancer-preventing benefits but none of the negatives.

> ❝ *Colorectal cancer is one of only two **cancers** that can be **completely prevented** through screening.* ❞

Use olive oil, not butter, as your fat of choice Animal fats such as butter are associated with an increased risk of colorectal cancer, probably because diets high in fat lead to increased levels of bile acids in the colon which are required to break down that fat. These bile acids can be converted to cancer-causing compounds. This is another reason to get your protein from sources such as fish, soya beans or pulses rather than fatty red meat.

Lose a few pounds Being overweight considerably increases your risk of cancer, including colorectal cancer. An analysis of numerous studies found that men's risk increased 37 per cent if they were overweight or obese; women's risk rose by 7 per cent. Researchers think the higher levels of hormones such as insulin, leptin and insulin-like growth factor in overweight people are to blame. All provide fuel for cancer cells.

Get 15 minutes of sunscreen-free sunshine a day It's your best source of vitamin D, one of the most important vitamins when it comes to preventing colorectal cancer. An analysis of five studies found that getting at least 2,000IU a day from diet, sunlight or supplements could cut the risk of colorectal cancer in half. How? By detoxifying a dangerous form of bile.

Most people in the UK obtain adequate amounts of vitamin D from their diet and exposure to sunlight. However, deficiency is a real risk for elderly people, who may be confined indoors by illness or mobility problems; in people who, for religious or modesty reasons, keep most of their skin covered; or those who spend less than 10 or 15 minutes a day in the sun without sunscreen. About 100g of sardines or salmon has 400IU and 100g of chicken livers has 10IU. If you take vitamin D supplements, aim for 400IU daily.

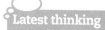

Latest thinking

A simple blood test could provide a warning about pre-cancerous colorectal growths. The test, currently under investigation, detects chemical markers of colorectal cancer that make their way into the bloodstream.

See also:

***Step 7**: Cut back on saturated fat, page 72*

Congestive heart failure

Heart failure is one of the fastest-growing heart conditions in the world, thanks to everything from the obesity epidemic and rising rates of high blood pressure to the fact that more people are surviving heart attacks and facing life with damaged hearts. When your heart is too weak or too stiff to pump enough blood to the organs and tissues in your body, your lungs can fill with fluid, your kidneys may fail and you become very, very tired. This condition kills 80 per cent of men and 65 per cent of women within six years of diagnosis. Here's how you can take steps to try to avoid it.

What causes it

Damage or death of heart muscle due to narrowed arteries or a heart attack; high blood pressure, which makes heart muscle grow large and stiff; malfunctioning heart valves (due to a birth defect, infection or heart disease); and heart-rhythm problems.

Symptoms to watch for

Breathlessness, especially when lying down; coughing and wheezing; swollen feet, ankles, legs or abdomen; fatigue; lack of appetite; nausea; confusion and memory loss; and rapid heartbeat.

Key prevention strategies

Exercise and follow a heart-healthy diet

If you think heart failure happens only to other people, consider this statistic: your odds of developing it after the age of 45 are one in five. The biggest contributors are high blood pressure and heart attack, so the best defence is to stay active, and at your next meal, fill your plate with fruit and vegetables, and whole grains. Small changes can make a big difference. Simply eating a whole-grain breakfast cereal every morning can lower your risk by as much as 30 per cent.

If you already have heart disease or high blood pressure, talk to your GP about the type and amount of exercise that is right for you.

Maintain a healthy weight Each additional point in your body mass index (BMI) – increases a woman's risk of heart failure by 7 per cent and a man's by 5 per cent, according to the landmark Framingham Heart Study from the USA. Having a BMI of 30 or higher, doubles your odds. Extra weight damages your heart by raising your risk of high blood pressure and diabetes. Excess weight also puts a strain on your heart that can lead to muscle damage.

Reduce high blood pressure Ninety per cent of people who have heart failure had pre-existing high blood pressure. This results in your heart having to pump harder to force blood through blood vessels in your body. Over time, enlargement of the heart muscle can reduce the capacity of the chambers of your heart, a condition called left ventricular hypertrophy that interferes with the heart's ability to pump sufficient blood around the body. A 10-point drop in systolic blood pressure (the top number) can cut

30%
The possible reduction in heart failure risk if you ea whole-grain cereal for breakfast every day.

your risk of heart failure by 50 per cent, according to research.

If you need medication for high blood pressure, ask about a diuretic. Studies suggest that these drugs cut heart failure risk more than other drugs such as ACE inhibitors and calcium-channel blockers.

Ask about ACE inhibitors and beta blockers after a heart attack

About one in four men and half of all women who survive a heart attack will be disabled by heart failure within six years. ACE inhibitor and beta blocker drugs reduce that likelihood. In one study, an ACE inhibitor called ramipril (Tritace) cut heart failure risk by 23 per cent in 9,000 high-risk patients, many of whom had had heart attacks. These medications ease the strain on the heart by relaxing blood vessel walls and lowering blood pressure.

Prevention boosters

Maintain good blood glucose control if you have diabetes If you have Type 2 diabetes, your risk of heart failure is five times higher than normal if you're a woman and nearly four times higher than normal if you're a man. Since people with diabetes often have coronary artery disease or high blood pressure, or may have had 'silent' heart attacks, your doctor may prescribe medications to help guard your heart. But don't overlook the power of blood glucose control. In one study, people with diabetes who kept their blood glucose within a healthy range were half as likely to develop heart failure as those whose blood glucose remained high.

Eat fish Researchers at Harvard Medical School tracked the health of 4,738 adults and found that those who ate grilled or baked tuna, or other fish, once or twice a week cut their risk of congestive heart failure by 20 per cent. And more is better: those who had fish five times a week cut their risk by 32 per cent.

Check your weight

If you have any health conditions that put you at increased risk of heart failure, stay alert for early signs. Watch out for unexpected weight gain: an increase of 5lb (2.5kg) or more in a week could mean you're retaining fluid because your heart is losing its ability to pump blood effectively. Another possible sign is if ankles or calves swell enough to make your socks feel tight.

Latest thinking

Depression can make heart muscle stiffer, raising the risk of heart failure. US scientists at the University of Maryland School of Medicine found that depression raised levels of chronic inflammation in the body, which stimulated the production of collagen, a protein that can stiffen heart muscle.

See also:

Cause 1: Hypertension, page 22
Cause 4: Insulin resistance, page 28

Conjunctivitis

55% The chances of avoiding eye itchiness and redness if you use olopatadine for seasonal allergic conjunctivitis.

If you've ever woken up feeling as though someone has thrown a handful of sand into your eyes, you'll know how uncomfortable conjunctivitis can be. Not only is it painful and unsightly but, if caused by infection, it can also spread like wild fire. Conjunctivitis occurs when the conjunctiva, the clear membrane covering the white of the eye and inner eyelid surface, becomes irritated. Irritation may be the result of an infection or allergic reaction, and may also occur if a chemical substance or a foreign body gets into the eye. Conjunctivitis accounts for more than a third of all eye-related visits to the GP and is most common in babies and children, older people and contact lens wearers. It often clears up on its own, but in cases where the infection is bacterial, it needs to be treated with antibiotic eye drops. Meanwhile, here's what you can do to help stop it occurring in the first place.

What causes it

Sometimes known as pink eye, conjunctivitis can be caused by infection (viruses and bacteria), allergy (for example, to pollen or house dust), or irritant chemicals such as substances in cosmetics or chlorine in swimming pools.

Symptoms to watch for

Symptoms may affect one or both eyes. Red or pink whites of the eye; pain, itching or a 'gritty' feeling; discharge from the eye that may be thick and yellowish (bacterial conjunctivitis) or clear and watery (viral, irritant or allergic conjunctivitis).

Key prevention strategies

Avoid allergens If you think your conjunctivitis is caused by an allergy, try to identify the trigger and then avoid it. Common culprits include pollen, animals, make-up and contact lens solutions.

Don't touch your eyes It may be tempting but don't rub itchy eyes with fingers or palms. Touching your eyes is a sure-fire way to spread or introduce infection. If you do inadvertently touch them, wash your hands well and dry them with a disposable towel.

Follow contact lens cleaning instructions to the letter This will prevent the lens becoming contaminated by bacteria, which are likely to irritate the eye. If you wear daily contact lenses always dispose of them after use and never re-use them.

Keep your make-up to yourself To prevent the spread of infection, never share eye liner or mascara. And the same goes for eye drops.

Use your own towel and face flannel These are prime breeding places for viruses and bacteria so never share yours – not even with friends or family. These items should also be washed frequently.

Wear goggles If you are a swimmer, wear protective goggles in swimming pools. Exposure to chlorinated water in pools can trigger irritant conjunctivitis.

Prevention boosters

Teach children to use tissues
Encourage them to use a tissue to cover their mouths and noses when sneezing or coughing and discourage them from rubbing and touching eyes to prevent the spread of bacteria and viruses.

Wash your hands frequently and encourage children to do the same This is a key strategy for preventing the spread of all kinds of infection. Make sure there is always soap available.

Clean surfaces frequently Table tops, door handles, telephone handsets and TV remote controls are ideal breeding places for germs so keep them as clean as possible.

Beware re-infection If you do develop infective conjunctivitis, don't wear eye make-up until it has completely cleared. Throw away any make-up you were using when it developed.

Keep dust down To avoid allergic conjunctivitis, dust and vacuum frequently to get rid of allergens in the home. And keep windows and doors closed on days when the pollen count is high.

Don't wear contact lenses when you have conjunctivitis You could risk extending or worsening symptoms. When infection has cleared, sterilise non-disposable lenses thoroughly before wearing them again. Replace contact lens solutions in which contaminated lenses may have been soaking.

Similar symptoms

Conjunctivitis can sometimes be confused with other conditions such as iritis (in which the coloured part of the eye – the iris – becomes inflamed). If you experience severe pain or intense redness in one or both eyes, sensitivity to light or disturbed vision, contact your GP or go to your nearest A&E department as soon as you can.

Latest thinking

Antibiotic eye drops for bacterial conjunctivitis became available over the counter in 2005, leading to a huge rise in their use. But a study carried out at Oxford University in the same year claims that eye drops do little to speed recovery time in most cases. A more recent study performed in 2009 reiterates this and warns that overuse could lead to antibiotic resistance. 'It's very important that antibiotics aren't used where they are not needed,' says Dr Peter Rose, who led the study. 'Our research shows that selling eye drops over the counter has resulted in greater use at the same time as the evidence shows that they have little benefit.'

Drugs that prevent disease

For seasonal allergic conjunctivitis, the anti-inflammatory olopatadine (Opatanol) appears to be effective at preventing eye itchiness and redness. One 2004 study carried out during the high pollen season showed that people using olopatadine hydrochloride ophthalmic solution 0.2% once daily were 55 per cent less likely to experience symptoms than those using a placebo.

Constipation

Normal bowel movements range from three a day to three a week, so don't automatically assume you're constipated, if you can't seem to open your bowels as often as you expect to: the chances are that you're not eating enough fibre or drinking enough fluid. Anxiety, medications and conditions such as pregnancy and diabetes can also contribute to the problem.

What causes it

Slow movement of waste material along the intestinal tract due to a lack of fibre and fluids, ageing, lack of a regular toilet routine, taking medications or having a health condition (such as diabetes) that slows bowel activity.

Symptoms to watch for

Bloating, abdominal discomfort, having two or fewer bowel movements per week (with hard stools), straining and pushing when you have a bowel movement, and feeling that your bowel movement was incomplete.

Key prevention strategies

Increase the fibre in your diet Including at least 20g of fibre a day in your diet could cut your risk of constipation by 46 per cent, according to Harvard School of Public Health researchers who tracked more than 60,000 women. Those who ate less than 7g a day had the highest constipation rates. Fibre helps by making your stools bulkier and heavier, which allows the muscles in the inner walls of the intestines to move stools towards the rectum with greater ease. Fibre may even make your bowels move faster.

You can get to 20g by starting the day with porridge or a high-fibre cereal such as All Bran. You can get even more fibre if you top your cereal with berries and a sprinkling of wheatgerm or ground flaxseeds (linseeds). At lunch make your sandwich with whole-grain bread, eat a serving of barley or brown rice at dinner and consume a wide variety of fresh fruit and vegetables (including pulses) throughout the day. Remember to keep at it, as it can take a few weeks to see an improvement.

Drink plenty of water If you've just started a higher-fibre diet or have been following one and feel constipated, drink plenty of water. If you're taking a fibre supplement, water is even more important. When researchers gave 117 people with chronic constipation a fibre supplement, those who were also told to drink 2 litres of water a day reported more improvement than those who drank half that amount.

Take a walk When middle-aged Dutch men and women with chronic constipation took a brisk 30 minute walk every day, researchers found that they didn't have to strain as much during bowel movements and had fewer hard stools. Food also passed more quickly through their intestinal tracts. As a result, the number with constipation dropped by a third. And in a study of 62,036 women, those who exercised every day were 44 per cent less likely to be constipated than women who were active less than once a week. In this study, active women who also ate a high-fibre diet were 68 per cent less likely to be constipated than inactive women who ate a low-fibre diet. So adapting your diet as well as getting more exercise seems to be the best strategy.

Prevention boosters

Eat prunes or sip prune juice
Research has confirmed something many of us have experienced first-hand: prunes really get your bowels moving. Studies show that they stimulate contractions of the intestinal wall and seem to make bowel movements wetter, which can make elimination easier. In one US study from Boston University, prunes stimulated the bowels more than any other food tested.

Change your prescription Experts estimate that prescription and over-the-counter medications and remedies are responsible for up to 40 per cent of constipation problems. If you take any of the medications in the following list, and are having trouble with regularity, ask your doctor if you can switch to another medication that is less likely to result in the same problem: antacids containing aluminium or calcium, antidepressants, antihistamines, calcium-channel blockers, diuretics, iron supplements, opioid painkillers and pseudoephedrine (found in many cough and cold preparations).

Try to go half an hour after eating The gastrocolic reflex – a wave of muscle activity along the intestines that leads to a bowel movement – usually happens within half an hour after a meal. Digestion experts often recommend that people prone to constipation make a point of spending some time on the toilet after meals as a form of bowel retraining – getting your body on a schedule that can lead to better regularity. If nothing happens, don't linger, as sitting for a long time won't help.

Trying biofeedback

One in three people with chronic constipation gets little relief from standard approaches, say US researchers from the University of Iowa. In a little-recognised, lifelong constipation problem called dyssynergic defaecation, the muscle contractions that should move stools along are weak and uncoordinated, and it's hard to sense when there's a stool ready to exit the bowels. The solution? In one study, a biofeedback technique that involves using a pencil-thin rectal probe and artificial 'practice stools' helped 80 per cent of people with this problem learn to push at the right time and overcome constipation.

Latest thinking

People with chronic constipation are twice as likely to have frequent headaches as people with regular bowel movements, report researchers from the Norwegian University of Science and Technology. The more frequent the headaches, the worse the constipation. Experts aren't sure why the two are connected, but they warn that prescription painkillers such as codeine and oxycodone could make constipation worse.

See also:

Step 1: *Exercise, page 62*

Coronary artery disease

The stage is set for getting heart disease as early as your teens, or even pre-teens. Taking too little exercise and eating too much saturated fat pads artery walls with plaque. Fast forward 20, 30 or 40 years, and you may have chest pain as narrowed arteries can't deliver enough blood to heart muscle or worse, a heart attack. While genes play a role, your heart's fate is mostly in your hands. Even if your arteries are slightly blocked, changing your ways can change your future.

80% The cases that could be prevented through simple lifestyle changes such as getting more exercise.

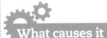

What causes it

Damage to the inner layers of arteries in your heart due to raised blood pressure, smoking and high blood glucose. As your heart tries to heal itself, fatty plaque accumulates in artery walls, especially if you have high levels of 'bad' LDL cholesterol. This build-up narrows arteries and can lead to the formation of heart-threatening blood clots. Infections (e.g. gum disease) and excess belly fat fuel the process by releasing inflammatory compounds into the bloodstream that spur the growth of plaque.

Key prevention strategies

Walk for 30 minutes five times a week
Getting out for a walk at a moderate pace, brisk enough to quicken your breathing a little, five days a week can cut heart disease risk in half, according to one large study of middle-aged and older women. Researchers looking at men found that those who rarely if ever exercised were three times more likely to die from heart disease than men who exercised on at least five days a week.

Exercise helps your heart in many ways. It raises HDL ('good') cholesterol, lowers LDL ('bad') cholesterol and triglycerides, reduces high blood pressure and heart-threatening inflammation, and can even improve the circulation of antioxidants that protect the cells of the heart and the cells lining blood vessels from injury.

One particular study demonstrated the heart-friendly powers of exercise. Researchers looked at 101 men who had surgery to open blocked arteries in their hearts: half of them received stents to keep the arteries open; the other half didn't. Instead, they rode exercise bikes for 20 minutes a day to achieve the same effect. The result? The bike riders had fewer heart attacks, strokes and serious chest pain, which is reason enough to invest in an exercise bike.

Quit smoking Cigarette smoking doubles, triples or even quadruples your risk of developing heart disease, and once you have it, smoking doubles your risk of sudden cardiac death. Smoke damages arteries, giving plaque an easier foothold, and nicotine constricts blood vessels, while the carbon monoxide in cigarette smoke displaces oxygen in the bloodstream, forcing your heart to pump harder to oxygenate cells. Quit smoking, and you'll begin to lower your risk almost immediately.

Within two years after your last cigarette, your risk of heart disease drops by more than 30 per cent, and goes down to normal within 10 to 14 years. (Turn to page 66 for some top strategies for kicking the habit.)

Eat more oily fish If you eat more fish rich in omega-3 fatty acids, you'll eat fewer calories than you would if you were to eat red meat, and you'll not only avoid unhealthy saturated fats that raise cholesterol levels but also increase your intake of 'good' fats that are heart-healthy. In one study of nearly 85,000 women, those who ate oily fish just one to three times a month cut their risk of developing coronary heart disease by 21 per cent; eating fish five times a week or more lowered it by 34 per cent. The oils in fish help prevent blood clots and inflammation of the arteries, and protect against irregular heart rhythms (arrhythmias), that can lead to heart attacks.

The British Heart Foundation recommends that people with heart disease eat one to two portions of oily fish a week – that is up to 300g of fish such as salmon, trout, sardines, mackerel or tuna. However, pregnant women are advised to avoid oily fish such as shark, marlin and swordfish which may contain high levels of mercury.

Consider fish-oil capsules If you don't like fish, consider a daily supplement of 1g of fish oil. In one study, people who took 1.5g of omega-3 fatty acids a day in the form of fish-oil capsules saw plaque regress after two years. Even if you don't have heart disease, ask your doctor about the benefits of taking a 1g supplement of fish oil daily. Vegetarians can look for omega-3 capsules that provide DHA from algae instead of fish.

Eat nuts and heart-healthy oils Walnuts, rapeseed oil, ground flaxseeds (they must be refrigerated), tofu and soya beans are all good sources of alpha linolenic acid (ALA), a type of omega-3 fatty acid that your body converts into DHA and EPA. Eating two slices of soya and flaxseed bread with a rapeseed-based spread will provide 2g of omega-3s. You can get a similar amount from 30g of walnuts (about a small handful). These foods are not a perfect replacement for fish and fish oil, but they're a good add-on.

Eat foods that 'offer best protection' It's a mnemonic device for remembering the foods richest in soluble fibre – oats and oranges; beans and berries; and pears and peas. Soluble fibre forms a gel in your intestines that actually reduces the absorption of the fat you eat, which, in turn, lowers cholesterol. In one study that followed 9,776 women and men for 19 years, those who consumed about 6g of soluble fibre a day (about the amount in a bowl of porridge) had a 15 per cent lower risk of heart disease than those who ate less than a gram a day.

Choose better carbs The key is whole grains. Studies show that people who eat more of them (such as 100 per cent whole-grain bread, whole-grain breakfast cereal and whole grains such as brown rice and bulghur wheat) are less likely to have heart disease, whereas those who eat a lot of refined grains (white bread, white rice and snack foods such as crackers, biscuits and cakes) have more heart attacks. The difference is largely due to the effects of these rapidly absorbed carbohydrates on insulin; they tend to raise insulin more than whole grains do, and high insulin levels raise heart disease risk. A diet that keeps insulin low also helps to lower levels of potentially harmful blood fats called triglycerides.

Cut your salt intake A recent US study from Harvard Medical School shows that cutting back on salt reduces the risk of heart disease by 25 per cent, even if you don't have high blood pressure. Taking the salt cellar off the table is the first step. Infinitely more important is avoiding processed foods, from which we get 70 to 80 per cent of the salt we eat. That means everything from ham, salami and canned soups to microwave meals and salad dressings (make your own or look for low-sodium versions).

Ask your doctor about wine Drinking any form of alcohol in moderation (for healthy men and women, no more than two units with meals, on any day) can lower your risk of heart disease as much as 30 per cent by improving cholesterol ratios and helping to prevent blood clots. But if your triglycerides are high, consume wine only in moderation or not at all. While some studies suggest that just one small glass a day may lower triglycerides, this strategy doesn't work for everyone. Consume in moderation as binge drinking even once a month increases your heart attack risk.

Tackle high blood pressure High blood pressure puts added stress on your heart, making the heart muscle thicker and stiffer. This extra pressure damages artery walls, speeding up plaque formation. It can also diminish your sensitivity to chest pain to the point that you don't notice the warning signs of heart disease, and could even suffer a 'silent' heart attack, according to Canadian researchers who studied 900 people with hypertension. Taking steps to lower your blood pressure can cut heart disease risk by up to 30 per cent, according to current research.

Symptoms to watch for

Chest pain, or angina, which occurs when the heart muscle can't get enough oxygen-rich blood. Angina can feel like pressure or squeezing in your chest, but you may also feel it in your back, jaw, shoulders, neck or arms. It usually gets worse during activity and improves at rest.

> *Getting out for a **walk** five days a week can **cut** **heart disease** risk in half.*

Watch your cholesterol levels If you don't know your cholesterol levels – LDL, HDL and total cholesterol – ask your doctor if you should have them tested. You should have your cholesterol levels checked every five years between the ages of 40 and 75, but more frequently if you have already been diagnosed with raised cholesterol. While many people who have heart attacks don't have elevated blood cholesterol, having high cholesterol does increase risk. If your cholesterol levels are less than ideal, take steps to improve them (see *High cholesterol*, starting on page 216).

Prevention boosters

Brush and floss regularly Using a toothbrush and dental floss are two very basic ways to protect your heart. When used daily (brush at least twice and floss once), good dental hygiene can cut your risk of gum disease, which recent studies suggest doubles your odds of developing heart disease. The link is thought to be inflammation caused by bacteria. People with severe gum disease have four times higher levels of bacterial by-products, called endotoxins, in their bloodstream than people with healthy gums. Battling these toxins involves an immune system response that triggers inflammation, and chronic inflammation contributes to the formation of plaque in artery walls.

Have a guilt-free treat Just one small piece (30g) of dark chocolate a day helps arteries to stay flexible and can help reduce your blood pressure, some studies show. For the most antioxidants it has to be dark chocolate, so look for a minimum of 60 per cent cocoa solids.

Avoid secondhand smoke Living with a smoker raises your own risk of developing heart disease by a significant 25 to 30 per cent.

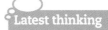
Latest thinking

Marital stress can harm the heart. In a US study of 150 couples, those who unleashed angry, mean-spirited verbal assaults during a 6 minute conversation about a 'touchy' subject had more atherosclerosis (caused by severe plaque build-up). Husbands had a 30 per cent higher risk of atherosclerosis when either spouse was dominant or controlling; wives' risk rose by 30 per cent when either partner was hostile.

See also:

Cause 1: Hypertension, page 22
Cause 5: Bad cholesterol balance, page 30
Cause 6: Inflammation, page 32

151

Depression

When more than 100 doctors were asked which health conditions are most likely to cause chronic disease, depression ranked surprisingly high – not far below high blood pressure. Depression is linked with a higher risk of nearly every major health problem, from diabetes to heart disease, and is the leading cause of physical disability in the world. And it's not the type of thing you just 'snap out of'. The best way forward is to prevent depression in the first place or, failing that, prevent a recurrence (up to 60 per cent of people who have had one major depressive episode go on to have another). Here are strategies that research has found to be helpful.

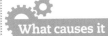

What causes it

Usually a mix of factors that results in an imbalance in mood-regulating chemicals called neurotransmitters (such as serotonin and dopamine). These factors may include a genetic predisposition, a single traumatic event and stress, particularly the kind of stress that comes from feeling a loss of control over your life. Other triggers include specific situations, such as the death of a loved one.

Key prevention strategies

Learn to solve problems Quite often, depression starts with a particular challenge in life that you just don't know how to cope with. Finding ways to manage the issues you're facing now may well help you avoid depression in the future – think of it as a form of preventive health for your mind.

One study looked at older adults who were recently diagnosed with macular degeneration, a leading cause of vision loss. Those who were taught to solve many of the problems they would encounter as their sight failed were 61 per cent less likely to be depressed two months after their diagnosis than those who didn't receive such coaching. They were also less likely to have to give up an activity they enjoyed – the very types of activities that help prevent depression.

Learning to solve problems can be as simple as sitting down with pen and paper, listing the issues that are making you unhappy, and identifying three concrete steps you can take to improve things. Other options include brainstorming solutions with close friends or family, or making arrangements to consult a therapist who is trained in cognitive behavioural therapy.

Try to view the glass as half full Numerous studies find that optimistic people are less likely to develop depression than pessimists. In fact, in one study of 71 older adults, researchers found that people who expected bad things to happen in the coming month experienced more depressive symptoms at the end of the month than those who didn't have negative expectations, regardless of what actually happened.

Not everyone is born hopeful, but anyone can work on adopting a more positive attitude. Being an optimist begins with the belief that bad events are temporary and changeable. For instance, rather than complaining about a bad boss and assuming nothing will change, an optimist would update his or her CV and apply for a new – possibly better – job. It also involves looking on the bright side. If a pessimist were diagnosed with breast cancer, she might immediately assume she's going to have bad side effects from chemotherapy, lose her hair and eventually die from the disease. An optimist might count herself lucky that women today are much less likely to die from breast cancer and that new treatments address many of the negative effects of chemotherapy.

Drugs that prevent disease

If you've had at least two episodes of major depression, or you have a chronic illness such as diabetes, heart disease or cancer, talk to your doctor about continuing your antidepressant medication for longer than the recommended 12 months after the depression recedes. A review of several studies found that about 60 per cent of people are at risk of having another depressive episode within a year of ending treatment, but just 10 to 30 per cent of people who continue their medication will have a recurrence. Another study found that people with a form of depression called seasonal affective disorder (SAD), which occurs in some parts of the world during winter, can prevent an episode by starting antidepressants while they still feel well.

See a therapist once a month If you've ever been diagnosed with major depression, a monthly counselling session may be all that's required to prevent a recurrence. Researchers randomly assigned 99 previously depressed women to interpersonal psychotherapy (a form of counselling that focuses on resolving issues related to grief, role transitions or problems interacting with others) weekly, twice a month or once a month for two years or until they had another depressive episode. The result was that just 26 per cent of the women who completed the maintenance phase saw their depression recur (versus an average 60 per cent recurrence rate), no matter how often they had therapy.

Stay connected Join a football team, a knitting or sewing club, or a committee at your child's school or your local church – anything to bring you into regular contact with others and enhance your social network. According to research, these sorts of connections are highly effective for guarding against depression.

Symptoms to watch for

Changes in your sleeping and/or eating habits; loss of pleasure in things that you used to enjoy; thoughts of hurting yourself; lack of interest in sex; feeling hopeless or worthless; crying for no apparent reason; difficulty concentrating and making decisions; irritability or restlessness; feeling fatigued or weak; unexplained physical problems such as back pain or headaches.

Prevention boosters

Seek treatment for anxiety If you find that you're worrying beyond reason, obsessing over events in your life or pathologically afraid of certain things such as going outside or being around other people, you may have an anxiety disorder and thus an increased risk of depression. The more severe your anxiety, the more likely you are to become depressed. Researchers think that anxiety may alter the way the brain releases and takes up serotonin, a chemical important to mood. Or it may be that anxiety changes your normal interactions and lifestyle so much that it triggers depression. Regardless, your best option is to seek out a therapist trained in cognitive behavioural therapy, which studies suggest is the best way to treat most anxiety disorders.

Get moving regularly Countless studies underscore the emotional boost that exercise provides and its ability to help relieve symptoms of depression. And there is plenty of research that also suggests that people who get regular exercise are less likely to become depressed in the first place. A recent UK study showed that, at least in middle-aged men, more intense exercise (such as running or playing soccer) was most effective.

Ten instant mood boosters

Snapping at your children, spouse or the supermarket check-out person? Feeling out of sorts or just sad for no reason? Here are 10 quick ways to raise your spirits.

1 **Call a friend and chat about anything** Staying in touch and laughing is a great stress buster.

2 **Take a walk in the sunshine** Sunlight has proven mood-boosting properties, as does exercise.

3 **Meet someone for coffee** Good conversation coupled with an energy burst from the caffeine is a quick way to lighten things up.

4 **Give thanks for something** You'll remember how much you have to be grateful for and stop dwelling on your problems for a while.

5 **Plant some brightly coloured flowers** The physical activity of gardening and the bright colours of the flowers are likely to raise your spirits.

6 **Bake a loaf of bread** Nothing spreads contentment like the scent of freshly baked bread filling the house. Even instant-mix bread can do the trick.

7 **Clean out a cupboard** You'll get an instant sense of accomplishment. Give away old clothes and get the added mood benefit of helping someone else.

8 **Soak in a hot bath** Light some scented candles (try lavender or vanilla, which studies find can relieve anxiety and boost mood), listen to music or just drift for 20 minutes. Relaxing helps to improve mood.

9 **Stroke a puppy** Or – equally good – a fully grown dog or a cat. Studies suggest that stroking animals reduces stress and boosts mood.

10 **Enjoy a small piece of dark chocolate** It contains compounds that influence levels of serotonin, a feel-good brain chemical.

> **" Anyone can** *work on adopting a more* **positive** *attitude.* **"**

In another study of older adults with arthritis, taking aerobics classes led to fewer symptoms of depression. The key may be to get your heart rate up; slow walking may not do the trick.

Grill some salmon for dinner Twice-weekly meals of salmon, trout or tuna can help keep depression at bay. Oily fish such as these are great sources of omega-3 fatty acids. In countries where people consume a lot of these healthy fats, depression rates tend to be low. In fact, women who eat oily fish regularly often have half the risk of developing depression than those who don't. If you don't eat fish, ask your doctor about taking a daily fish-oil supplement containing at least 2g of omega-3 fatty acids.

A Spanish study showed that eating Mediterranean-style had significant benefits. Those who ate more fish and white meat than red meat, plenty of fruit, vegetables, pulses and monounsaturated fats, such as olive oil were 30 per cent less likely to develop depression.

It's also worth trying to cut back on corn, safflower and sunflower oils as well as processed foods such as crisps and biscuits. These are high in omega-6 fatty acids, which counteract the beneficial effects of omega-3s.

Get a good night's sleep Researchers used to think that insomnia was a symptom of depression. Now they're finding that it typically precedes depression, with up to 50 per cent of people with insomnia that lasts two weeks or longer later developing a major depressive episode. Of course, the insomnia may be a sign of an underlying problem in your life that may lead to depression, but evidence shows that poor sleep by itself can lead to symptoms of depression. (See *Insomnia*, starting on page 232.)

Include more folate-rich foods in your diet Just a cup of cooked green soya beans contains about 200mcg of folate, a B vitamin in which many people who are depressed are deficient. Many whole-grain breakfast cereals are fortified with folate. Studies find that men who consume 234mcg of folate for every 1,000kcal they eat are half as likely to become depressed as men whose intake is 119mcg. Other great sources of folate include spinach, chickpeas and lentils.

Latest thinking

People who have had depression are more likely to develop Alzheimer's disease than those who were never depressed. Researchers don't know yet whether the depression contributes to the development of Alzheimer's or whether something else is at work to cause both the depression and the Alzheimer's.

See also:

Cause 3: Depression, page 26
Step 1: Exercise, page 62

155

Diabetes

Genes play a role in developing diabetes, but the less exercise you take and the more you weigh, the greater your risk – especially for Type 2. If you aren't part of the 'diabetes epidemic' yet, congratulations. But watch out for pre-diabetes – blood glucose that is elevated but not yet high enough to trigger symptoms – in case you need to address that issue now. Doctors don't always check for pre-diabetes (a fasting blood test can indicate it), so now's the time to prevent it from turning into diabetes.

What causes it

Heredity definitely plays a role, but it usually takes extra weight and a sedentary lifestyle to develop Type 2 diabetes. Excess body fat (especially fat around the abdominal organs) and inactivity conspire to make cells stop obeying signals from insulin to absorb blood glucose. Your body compensates by pumping out more insulin, but if it can't keep pace, your blood glucose will rise, leading to Type 2 diabetes.

Key prevention strategies

Lose a few pounds Excess weight is the number one reason adults and children are at higher risk for Type 2 diabetes now than ever before. Gaining weight can pack excess fat around internal organs at your midsection – especially if you're stressed out on a regular basis (stress hormones can send extra fat to the abdominal area). New research shows that this dangerous abdominal fat sends out chemical signals that desensitise cells throughout your body to insulin, the hormone that enables cells to absorb blood glucose. Insulin resistance is the first step on the path to Type 2 diabetes.

In a landmark clinical trial that followed 3,234 people with pre-diabetes for three years, those who lost just 7 per cent of their body weight (11lb if you now weigh 11 stone) and took 150 minutes' exercise a week reduced their diabetes risk by 58 per cent. In fact, weight loss worked better than insulin-sensitising diabetes medications at cutting the risk of diabetes.

A brisk aerobic work-out three to five times a week can get rid of belly fat better than dieting, say US researchers at Syracuse University. Brisk walking for 30 minutes each day also works.

Aim for at least five servings of fruit and vegetables daily And factor in three servings of whole grains, too. Following a low-glycaemic diet packed with fresh fruit and vegetables and whole grains – and cutting back on white bread, white rice, foods made with white flour, and sweets – helps keep blood glucose low and steady. Research shows it also redresses chronic low-grade inflammation in the body, which interferes with the action of insulin and the absorption of blood glucose by body cells.

58%
The reduction in your risk of developing Type 2 diabetes if you lose 7 per cent of your body weight and take enough exercise.

In a recent study of 486 women, Harvard School of Public Health researchers found that those who ate the most fruit were 34 per cent less likely to have metabolic syndrome, a cluster of risk factors, including insulin resistance, that predispose a person to diabetes. Women who ate the most vegetables cut their risk of metabolic syndrome by 30 per cent. Meanwhile, German researchers who followed 25,067 women and men for seven years recently found that those who got the most fibre from whole grains were 27 per cent less likely to develop diabetes than those who got the least.

Give up sugary drinks Quench your thirst with plain water, sparkling water (with a squeeze of lemon or lime), unsweetened tea or skimmed milk instead of sweetened soft drinks, fruit juices, coffee or tea.

A single sweetened soft drink a day raised the risk of developing metabolic syndrome (described above) by a staggering 44 per cent in a headline-grabbing study from Boston University School of Medicine in the USA. Experts have many theories as to why this is. It could simply be the result of all those extra calories in sugary drinks or in the high-fat, high-calorie foods we tend to pair them with (for example, chips and pizza). What's more, experts are also finding that drinking even a single soft drink a day is associated with being overweight – perhaps because the calories in drinks don't reduce appetite, so we don't compensate for them by eating less food.

Another possible culprit is high-fructose corn syrup. It's essentially sugar in liquid form, which for technical chemical reasons, some experts believe is more likely to lead to insulin resistance.

For a healthier thirst quencher, drop several tea bags (black, green or herbal) into a jug filled with water and refrigerate overnight before drinking. Or drink a glass of skimmed milk. The calcium, vitamin D and other minerals in dairy products may be the reason that having at

Ten low-glycaemic snacks

Low-glycaemic foods are those that have a slower effect on blood glucose. Studies show that people who eat more of these foods and fewer high-glycaemic foods are less likely to develop insulin resistance, a core problem underlying Type 2 diabetes. Low-glycaemic foods are often rich in fibre, protein or fat, though it's not a good idea to eat fatty foods just for the sake of your blood glucose unless they're healthy (unsaturated) fats.

1 An apple with skin

2 Whole-grain bread with peanut butter

3 Carrot sticks dipped in low-fat sour cream

4 A small handful of walnuts or almonds

5 Low-fat yoghurt sprinkled with fresh fruit or untoasted muesli

6 Toasted wholemeal pitta with white bean dip

7 Edamame (fresh soya beans)

8 Lentil soup (with no added salt)

9 A small handful of dried apricots

10 A hard-boiled egg

least one serving of low-fat or skimmed milk (or yoghurt or cheese) a day lowered metabolic syndrome risk by up to 62 per cent in one particular UK study.

Turn off the TV and go for a walk Exercise helps protect against diabetes by transporting blood glucose into fuel-hungry muscle cells and making cells more sensitive to insulin. A Harvard study of 40,000 women found that 30 minutes a day of brisk walking, plus a TV limit of 10 hours per week, cut diabetes risk by 43 per cent. If you get bored walking, sign up for an aerobics class, take up swimming, gather your children or grandchildren for a country walk, or just put on some music and dance.

Eat less fast food Do regular take-away meals lead to diabetes? When US researchers at the University of Minnesota tracked the eating habits and health of 9,514 people aged between 45 and 64 for up to 10 years, they discovered that those who ate two portions of red meat (beef in hamburgers) a week were 26 per cent more likely to develop metabolic syndrome. A daily helping of fried foods raised the risk still further. These foods are high in saturated and trans fats, which have been linked to diabetes.

Swap burgers and butter for fish and olive oil Each bite of a burger and each smear of butter you consume is full of saturated fat. These fats not only clog arteries, they also increase insulin resistance, which propels you down the path to full-blown diabetes. Saturated fats also trigger inflammation, which is toxic to cells, including those that handle blood glucose. Fish and olive oil have the exact opposite effect and could actually lower your diabetes risk. The same goes for nuts (including peanuts) and rapeseed oil.

Of course, you don't want to overdo even these good fats, which are high in calories. Cutting total fat intake as well as saturated fat helped participants in the US Diabetes Prevention Program study reduced their diabetes risk. Participants limited their intake of saturated fat to 7 per cent of total calories a day, which is about the amount in 60g of cheese plus 5g of butter if you eat 2,000kcal a day.

Get out the tape measure

Women whose waists measure 32in (80cm) or more and men whose waists measure 37in (94cm) or more are more likely to have fat deep in their abdomens, which can triple the risk of diabetes. While you're probably overweight if your waist is big, researchers report that they're seeing more people at a normal weight who also have larger waistline measurements, so don't think it's enough to simply watch the numbers on the scale.

Prevention boosters

Eat breakfast In one study, people who ate breakfast were 35 to 50 per cent less likely to be overweight or have insulin resistance than those who skip their morning meal. Why? An overnight fast puts your body into 'starvation mode'. If you don't eat breakfast, your liver churns out stored glucose to keep your blood glucose levels up.

At the same time, skipping breakfast flips biochemical switches that reduce the body's response to insulin. And it raises levels of an appetite-stimulating hormone called ghrelin so you want to eat more all day long. Do this often enough, and you gain weight, say scientists from Children's Hospital Boston in the USA.

Avoid eating fried foods or shop-bought pastries (too many calories and unhealthy fats) for breakfast. Instead, pour yourself a bowl of muesli or high-fibre cereal with skimmed milk and sprinkle some berries over it. One Canadian study from the University of Toronto looked at people with pre-diabetes and found that high-fibre cereals made their cells 'listen' better to insulin than lower-fibre ones. Low-fat yoghurt with fresh berries is also a good breakfast choice.

If you're depressed, get help If you're depressed, you're much less likely to exercise and eat well. But the health dangers don't end there. US scientists from Stanford University think that depression itself alters body chemistry in profound ways that spell trouble for anyone at risk of diabetes. Rates of insulin resistance were 23 per cent higher among depressed women than among women who weren't depressed, regardless of body weight, exercise habits or age. (See *Depression*, page 152.)

Get better sleep A chronic lack of sleep leads to weight gain and reduces your body's sensitivity to insulin. In one US study of 1,709 men, those who got an average of 5 to 6 hours of sleep per night had double the risk of diabetes of those who slept for longer. Studies of women have found similar results.

Symptoms to watch for

Often, there are none. You can have Type 2 diabetes for years without noticing anything's amiss. But as it progresses, symptoms include thirst, frequent urination, intense hunger, weight changes, tiredness, blurry vision, sores that are slow to heal and more frequent bladder and vaginal infections for women.

Latest thinking

Diet soft drinks aren't safe, either. Sipping just one can of diet soft drink per day raised the risk of metabolic syndrome by 34 per cent in one recent study and 48 per cent in another, although experts aren't sure why.

See also:

Cause 2: Intra-abdominal fat, page 24
Cause 4: Insulin resistance, page 28
Step 1: Exercise, page 62
Step 2: Fruit and vegetables, page 64

Diarrhoea

When you're in the midst of an attack, diarrhoea can seem more like an uncomfortable inconvenience than one of nature's most ingeniously simple health-protection strategies. It's designed to flush out invaders as quickly as possible, but it can have serious consequences such as dehydration and loss of electrolytes – sodium, calcium, potassium, magnesium and other important minerals. You can side-step bouts of diarrhoea by tackling the germs, the medication and the foods that trigger it. If your problem is irritable bowel syndrome, see the advice on page 236.

59%
The amount by which you can lower your risk if you wash your hands regularly and use hand sanitiser when you can't wash.

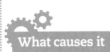

What causes it

Bacteria, viruses, parasites, antibiotics, some artificial sweeteners, stress.

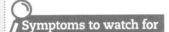

Symptoms to watch for

Frequent, loose, fluid-filled stools, perhaps accompanied by abdominal pain, cramps and bloating.

Key prevention strategies

Wash your hands frequently It's the best defence against the viral and bacterial infections that cause most cases of diarrhoea, say researchers who reviewed 14 studies of hand washing and diarrhoea risk. They conclude that hand hygiene can cut risk by at least 30 per cent. Wash for 20 seconds. There is no need to use an antibacterial soap; washing works by rinsing viruses and bacteria off your skin. University of Michigan researchers found that plain soap was just as effective at preventing diarrhoea.

Rub on an alcohol-based hand sanitiser when you can't wash. Using a hand-sanitising product regularly in addition to ordinary hand washing cut the risk of diarrhoea and vomiting by an impressive 59 per cent in a study of nearly 300 households. Families in the study all had at least one child aged 5 or younger enrolled in a nursery, where the germs that cause gastrointestinal illnesses sometimes run rampant. Participants kept sanitiser gel in the bathroom and kitchen and near nappy-changing tables and rubbed it on their hands after using the toilet, before preparing food and after changing nappies.

Practise good food safety Food poisoning – from undercooked meat, food left out of the fridge for too long or contaminated by contact with cutlery and chopping boards used for raw meat – cause millions of cases of mild to severe diarrhoea every year. Just a few of the rules: don't let other foods touch raw poultry or other raw meats; don't put cooked meat, fish or poultry back on the plate that held the raw product; wash chopping boards and knives in hot, soapy water after using them for raw meat (wash the sink, too); wash your hands frequently during and after handling raw meat; don't eat or serve food that's been out of the refrigerator, off the stove, or out of the oven for more than two hours; and if food looks or smells bad, throw it out. Be careful to cook meat properly. Although it's safe to eat rare beef or lamb as long as it's seared on the outside, chicken and pork should always be cooked so that the meat and the juices are no longer pink or red. (See also *Food poisoning*, starting on page 182.)

Prevention boosters

Cut back on sugar-free and low-carb treats Many 'sugar-free' and low-carbohydrate chewing gums, boiled sweets, chocolates, biscuits and cake mixes are sweetened with sugar alcohols such as sorbitol and mannitol. Your body can't absorb most of the sugars (and calories) in these sweeteners, making them seem like the perfect choice for dieters. But the unabsorbed sugars draw water into your intestines and encourage the growth of bacteria, leading to bloating, wind and sometimes severe diarrhoea.

Eat more 'good bacteria' Antibiotics can trigger diarrhoea by killing beneficial bacteria in your intestines. Studies show that increasing the levels of these helpful germs in your gut by eating yoghurt with live, active cultures or taking a probiotic supplement can help. When British researchers studied 135 people taking antibiotics, those who also drank a yoghurt drink every day cut their risk of diarrhoea by 21 per cent compared to those who had a placebo drink without beneficial bacteria. The yoghurt drink contained the bacteria strains *Lactobacillus casei*, *L. bulgaricus* and *Streptococcus thermophilus*, commonly found in commercial yoghurts and in a variety of probiotic supplements available in health food shops or pharmacies.

Prevent traveller's diarrhoea

Planning a trip to an out-of-the-way foreign destination?
Be prepared. Your odds of getting traveller's diarrhoea in a developing country are one in three. These infections are usually bacterial and can put you out of action for three to five days – waylaying your plans to explore museums, ruins, markets and other exotic wonders. Experts say that observing the five 'P's below can cut your risk of getting diarrhoea dramatically.

○ **Take Pepto-Bismol** four times a day. Take two 262mg tablets at each meal and at bedtime. Studies show it can cut your risk by 65 per cent. You can do this daily for up to three weeks.

○ **Peelable, packaged, purified or piping-hot food** is safest. Stick with bottled water (don't drink water from the tap in your hotel bathroom); skip ice cubes in drinks (even alcoholic ones); and avoid salads and other raw vegetables, fruit you can't peel, mayonnaise, iced cakes or pastries, unpasteurised dairy products and undercooked shellfish.

Latest thinking

Love tortoises, snakes or lizards? If you keep a reptile as a pet or can't resist touching or picking one up at a pet shop, zoo or a friend's house, be sure to wash afterwards. Reptiles can be carriers of salmonella bacteria, which cause bloody diarrhoea, fever and vomiting.

Diverticular disease

Years of constipation, straining during bowel movements and eating a low-fibre diet can take an invisible toll on the walls of your intestinal tract. Hard stools and repeated high-pressure straining can create tiny, pea-sized pouches that balloon outwards. These sacs, called diverticula, can number in the hundreds – and usually don't cause any trouble. But if faeces get trapped in a pouch, the sac can become inflamed and even infected, and you have diverticulitis, which can cause intense abdominal pain, fever, nausea and constipation or diarrhoea, putting you at risk of intestinal blockages or tears, and bleeding if a blood vessel bursts.

37%
The possible reduction in your risk of diverticulitis if you eat 30g of fibre a day.

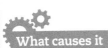

What causes it

Increased intestinal wall tension from hard stools plus straining to have a bowel movement can make tiny sections of the wall bulge outwards. If these pouches become infected or inflamed, you may experience pain, bleeding or even perforations in the intestinal wall.

Key prevention strategies

Eat more fibre Incorporating about 30g of fibre into your diet each day could cut your risk of developing diverticulitis by 37 per cent, say Harvard School of Public Health researchers who tracked the health and diets of nearly 44,000 men for four years. And if you've already had a painful episode, boosting the fibre in your meals could help prevent a repeat attack. In one UK study of people who had been hospitalised once for diverticulitis, 90 per cent of those who switched to a high-fibre diet were symptom free and stayed that way when researchers checked up on them seven years later.

Provided you drink plenty of fluids together with the fibre you eat, fibre will protect intestinal walls by making stools soft and therefore easier to pass, and by reducing tension within the bowel. Researchers now suspect that it also promotes a healthier environment in the intestines by providing a haven for beneficial bacteria and by maintaining the layer of protective mucus that lines the inner walls. This healthy 'inner landscape' seems to prevent the immune system from overreacting and causing inflammation in diverticula.

If you're planning to increase your fibre intake, take it slowly. Add a few high-fibre foods to your diet each week over the course of a month or two so you and your body grow accustomed to the changes. And be sure to drink several large glasses of water a day to avoid discomfort.

Add a fibre supplement If you can't get 30g of fibre every day from the food you eat, experts say it's OK to use a fibre supplement to make up the difference. (However, you should avoid taking fibre supplements during flare-ups of diverticulitis as this can sometimes increase discomfort.)

Snack on fruit instead of crisps, biscuits and chips Eating chips, biscuits or a small bag of crisps five or six times a week raised the risk of diverticular disease by as much as 69 per cent in one study of 48,000 men. In contrast, those who snacked regularly on peaches, blueberries, apricots, apples or oranges lowered their risk by as much as 80 per cent. However, it's important to avoid eating too many fruits that might give you diarrhoea.

Have chicken or fish instead of fatty or processed red meat Greek researchers have found that a diet packed with red meat can raise your odds of diverticulitis an incredible 50 times more than a vegetarian diet. Eating even a medium (110g to 170g) serving of beef, pork or lamb five or six nights a week tripled the risk of diverticular disease in the Harvard study noted earlier. Having a weekly hot dog raised the odds by 86 per cent; a serving of processed meat (such as sausage or ham) five or six times a week nearly doubled the risk. In contrast, fish and chicken eaters barely increased their risk at all.

Some experts speculate that red meat may prompt bacteria in your colon to produce substances that weaken the intestinal wall, so it's easier for pouches to form.

Don't worry about coffee or tea In the past, people at risk of diverticulitis have been warned to avoid these popular beverages. But newer research suggests that they actually have little effect on diverticulitis. (Of course, if a food or drink makes your symptoms worse, you should eliminate it from your daily diet.)

Eating the right foods

Fruit, vegetables and whole grains packed with a type of insoluble fibre called cellulose seem to be particularly helpful for protecting intestinal walls from damage that leads to bowel problems. The foods listed below contain the most cellulose.

Food	Serving	Total fibre	Cellulose
Beans and lentils (cooked or canned)	75g	6.7g	2.8g
Potato, with skin	1 medium	4.2g	1.6g
Peas	80g	4.8g	1g
Apple	1 medium	3.3g	0.9g
Tomato pasta sauce	125ml	2.3g	0.7g
Whole-grain cereal	40g	6.0g	0.7g
Carrots	80g	2.6g	0.5g
Banana	1 medium	1.5g	0.3g
Whole-grain bread	1 slice	1.1g	0.3g
Orange	1 medium	3.0g	0.3g

Symptoms to watch for

You may have severe, sharp pain in your abdomen (often on the lower left side) or milder pain that lasts for several days and may occasionally get worse. Other symptoms include fever, nausea, bouts of diarrhoea or constipation, and bloating. If you have severe pain or bleeding, call your doctor immediately.

Start exercising Perhaps because it can prompt stools to move more swiftly through the intestinal tract, physical activity lowered the risk of diverticular disease by as much as 48 per cent in one study. People who jogged got the most benefit, but any kind of exercise may help, especially if you also eat a high-fibre diet.

Schedule in some 'toilet time' Straining to have a bowel movement puts extra pressure on the intestinal walls, setting the stage for the formation of pouches. If you're prone to constipation, be sure to take advantage of a key, after-meal opportunity for a bowel movement. During the half hour or so after eating, your gastrointestinal system makes room for the new food by moving everything else further down the line. This wave of muscle activity, called the gastrocolic reflex, often results in a bowel movement if you give it a chance by spending a few minutes on the toilet about 30 minutes after a meal.

Ask about your medications Ask your doctor if constipation is a common side effect of any prescription or over-the-counter medication you're taking. Common culprits include antacids that contain aluminium or calcium, antidepressants, antihistamines, calcium-channel blockers, diuretics, iron supplements, opioid painkillers, and pseudoephedrine (found in many over-the-counter cough and cold preparations). You may be able to substitute a different medication.

Prevention boosters

Consume more healthy fats Getting plenty of omega-3 fatty acids from fish, flaxseeds (linseeds), which also act as a laxative, and flaxseed oil, walnuts, or fish-oil capsules may reduce levels of inflammation in your colon – a big plus because inflammation can trigger serious diverticulitis symptoms. Taking 1g of fish oil once or twice a day could help, according to digestive disease experts from the University of Maryland in the USA. However, you should always check with your doctor before taking any supplement.

Take probiotics Diverticular disease can destroy beneficial bacteria in the gut. These 'good' bacteria, available in supplements known as probiotics, play a role in the speedy movement of stools, in protecting the lining of intestinal walls and even in reducing inflammation. Studies from Italy and Germany are beginning to suggest that bolstering their levels may cut the risk of repeat attacks of

> " People who snacked regularly on **peaches**, blueberries, apricots, apples or oranges **lowered their risk** by as much as 80%. "

diverticulitis. Look for *Lactobacillus acidophilus*, *L. gasseri* and *Bifidobacterium bifidum*. Many probiotic products include a combination of these. And the yeast *Saccharomyces boulardii* may help to prevent diarrhoea caused by infections.

If you've had an attack of diverticulitis, probiotic supplements alone may not be enough to prevent a recurrence. Make an appointment to see your doctor and follow his or her advice about medication and any lifestyle steps you should take.

Lose weight Traditionally, diverticular disease has been a problem for people over the age of 50, brought on by decades of low-fibre intake and constipation, but that may be changing. As more and more people become obese, doctors are beginning to notice that people as young as 20 have the thin-walled, bulging pouches along their intestines – which suggests that poor diet linked to overweight at any age puts you at risk.

Latest thinking

You can eat nuts, seeds and popcorn. In the past, doctors have told people with diverticular disease to avoid these foods, fearing that they could get stuck in the intestinal pouches. But when researchers tracked more than 47,000 men for 18 years, they found that those who ate these healthy, high-fibre foods had no extra risk of problems. In fact, those who ate popcorn twice a week had a 28 per cent lower risk of flare-ups than those who indulged less than once a month, possibly because popcorn is a good source of fibre.

Dry eyes

Tears are your eyes' first line of defence against infection and damage from dust and airborne debris. Each time you blink, a new layer of moisture rolls across the surface of your eyes. Or at least it should. If tears evaporate too quickly (perhaps due to age-related changes in tear production) or aren't renewed often enough (perhaps because you've been staring at a computer screen for too long), your eyes begin to dry out. Try the following steps to keep your eyes comfortably moist.

68% The reduction in your risk of having dry eyes if you eat foods high in omega-3 fatty acids five or six times a week.

What causes it

Ageing; eye problems that interfere with blinking or tear production; medications such as antihistamines, diuretics, sleeping pills, oral contraceptives and tricyclic antidepressants; exposure to dry air; for women, hormonal changes around the menopause; and, for both sexes, medical conditions such as diabetes, rheumatoid arthritis, lupus, scleroderma and Sjögren's syndrome.

Symptoms to watch for

A stinging, burning or scratchy sensation in your eyes; sensitivity to light, wind and/or smoke; stringy mucus in or around your eyes; and blurry vision at the end of the day or after focusing intently on a close-range task.

Key prevention strategies

Remind yourself to blink Your 'blink rate' drops from a normal 17 to 22 blinks per minute to as few as four when you're doing anything that requires intense visual focus. In one study, people playing computer games blinked just once every 2 to 3 minutes! Keeping your eyes wide open increases the rate of evaporation of the protective film of tears. To protect your eyes, try to blink whenever you turn the page of a book or check your rear-view mirror while driving (which should be several times each minute). If you're working at a computer, try the 20-20 rule: give your eyes a 20 second rest every 20 minutes. Look out of a window or at something across the room and be sure to blink.

Lower your computer monitor Shifting your eyes upwards to read the top lines on your screen could double your risk of dry eyes. The reason is that looking up exposes more of the surface of your eyes to the air. (This is one reason computer use dries out eyes more than reading a book does – when you read, you tend to look down, which partially closes your eyes.) Raise your chair or lower your monitor so you can see the top third of the screen while looking straight ahead.

Eat healthy fats When researchers from Brigham and Women's Hospital in the USA checked the diets and eye health of nearly 32,500 women, they found that those who ate the most omega-3 fats had the lowest risk of dry eyes. In fact, those who ate five or six servings of oily fish a week were 68 per cent less likely to have dry eyes than those who had less than one. Try to get your omega-3s from a variety of sources, including herring, sardines, salmon and trout, as well as flaxseed

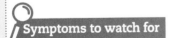

(linseed) oil, walnuts, freshly ground flaxseeds, rapeseed oil, walnut oil and pumpkin seeds.

Eye experts think supplements of fish oil or flaxseed oil may also promote eye health, but they're still debating the best dosage. Follow the package directions on one of the dry-eye prevention supplements available in pharmacies, such as TheraTears Nutrition, or take fish-oil capsules with a total of 1g of DHA and EPA per day. It may take up to three months to notice a difference, so stay with this treatment to see some results.

Stop smoking Research that checked lifestyle habits against the eye health of several thousand people found that smokers had an 82 per cent higher risk of dry eyes than non-smokers.

Medical help for dry eyes

If self-care steps aren't keeping your eyes moist, see your doctor. He or she may suggest one of these treatments:

Ocular lubricants Artificial tears, gels and lubricating ointments are the main treatment. They may need to be applied as often as every hour. If you need to use eye drops more than six times a day, it's important to use preservative-free products (frequent exposure to preservatives can irritate the eye). Ask your pharmacist or GP for advice.

Punctal plugs for more tears These tiny silicone stoppers, inserted by an ophthalmologist, close off your eyes' drain holes for tears. Sometimes temporary plugs are inserted first so you can see if they'll help. They are usually recommended for people with moderate to severe dry eyes who haven't been helped by other treatments.

Prevention boosters

Treat rosacea, blepharitis and eyelid problems All can cause dry eyes. People with rosacea have a 50 per cent chance of developing ocular rosacea, which can cause dry eyes, frequent styes and the feeling that there's something in your eyes. Tell your eye doctor that you have rosacea and ask about a check for related eye problems, too. Your doctor can also help treat blepharitis, or inflammation of the eyelids, as well as eyelids that curl outwards or inwards with age. Both conditions can change the way you blink, resulting in tears not spreading across the entire eye.

Use artificial tears Keep artificial tears, also called lubricating drops, on hand for times when you'll be in air-conditioned or heated buildings, or in a car, aeroplane, desert or any other place with extremely dry air. Eye experts recommend choosing preservative-free drops if you'll be using them more than four to six times a day for more than two or three days; otherwise, your eyes may become sensitised to preservatives and become inflamed.

Latest thinking

Before having laser eye surgery, have a dry-eye check-up. In the USA, 50 per cent of people who opt for laser surgery to improve their vision develop dry eyes for at least a few months after surgery – and 10 per cent develop ongoing, severe problems. If your eyes are dry, ask your doctor about starting treatment with artificial tears and/or punctal plugs before considering surgery.

Ear infections

As anyone who has had earache knows only too well, ear infections can be excruciatingly painful. There are two types: outer ear infection (otitis externa), also known as 'swimmer's' or 'tropical' ear, affects the outer ear, while middle ear infection (otitis media or OM), affects the middle ear, the space between the eardrum and the inner ear. It can be acute or chronic. Middle ear infection with effusion (fluid accumulation) – known as 'glue ear' – is very common in young children; around 80 per cent of children in developed countries have had a bout of glue ear by the age of four.

What causes it

Infection by bacteria, viruses or fungal spores. You are more likely to develop an outer ear infection if liquids get into the ear canal or if the lining is irritated. Some soaps, shampoos or other personal hygiene products can irritate the ear as can hearing aids or earplugs or damage to the ear canal from a cotton bud or fingernail. The risk of a middle ear infection is increased by blocked Eustachian tubes, enlarged tonsils or adenoids, and a weak immune system.

Symptoms to watch for

Outer ear infections may cause pain, itching, discharge from the ear and temporarily dulled hearing. A middle ear infection may cause severe pain, slight deafness, a temperature of 38°C (100.5°F) or above, and in children, vomiting and lethargy. Pus or fluid may also be present.

Key prevention strategies

Outer ear infections

- **Protect against water** Take measures to keep the water out of your ears while bathing or swimming – for example, wear a bathing cap that covers the ears, or use earplugs (kept clean to prevent reinfection).
- **Empty it out** After swimming or bathing make sure your ears are clear of water by tilting your head and pulling on the ear to help water escape. You can 'wick out' any water left in your ear canals by gently inserting the corner of a soft towel into the ears after swimming or bathing. Alternatively, dry your ears with a hairdryer on the lowest heat.
- **Rinse well** After swimming in the sea or swimming pool, rinse your ears with fresh water. This will wash out bacteria, foreign debris or plankton, all of which can trigger infection.
- **Drop it** Use astringent and acidifying eardrops or spray to keep your ears clean and prevent recurring outer ear infection. These are available over-the-counter; ask your pharmacist for a suitable product.
- **Treat underlying skin conditions** If you suffer from dermatitis, psoriasis or eczema, keep them under control; an outbreak can increase susceptibility to infection.

Middle ear infections

- **Practise good hygiene** Middle ear infections are usually caused by the common cold. Wash your hands frequently, encourage children to do the same, and don't share towels or flannels with other members of the family – especially if they have a cold.
- **Breastfeed if possible** Studies suggest that children who were breastfed for three months are less likely to suffer from middle ear infections.

- **Limit your baby's dummy use** Sucking on a dummy can increase the chance of an infection travelling from the mouth into the Eustachian tube, the passage connecting the middle ear with the back of the throat.
- **Don't smoke** Spending time in a smoke-filled atmosphere is a major risk factor for ear infections in children, according to a major review.
- **Chew gum** A study carried out in Finland showed that children who chewed two pieces of sugar-free gum containing the sweetener xylitol five times a day for two months or who took this sweetener as syrup had fewer ear infections. It is thought xylitol may help to reduce the growth of bacteria that cause infection.

Prevention boosters

Go easy on the cleaning A little earwax is healthy because it protects the lining of your outer ear from moisture, so only use cotton buds to sweep around the visible, outer part of the ear. If you think excess earwax has become a problem, ask your GP or practice nurse to syringe your ears.

Gently does it If you have a cold, blowing your nose too hard can push bacteria back into your middle ear, via the Eustachian tube, causing an infection there.

Try food elimination Frequent middle ear infections could be a sign of a food allergy. Common trigger foods include dairy products, wheat, peanuts and oranges. Try removing these for several weeks then add them back one at a time. If your ears start aching exclude that particular food from your diet.

Ask your doctor about vaccinations The pneumococcal vaccine, part of the standard childhood immunisation schedule, may help prevent middle ear infections in children over two. In a study, which followed up children to the age of three and a half years, vaccination reduced visits to the doctor for treatment of middle ear infection by 8 per cent, antibiotic prescriptions by 6 per cent, recurrent acute middle ear infections by 10–26 per cent and the use of grommets (part of the treatment for glue ear) by 24 per cent. A new vaccination specifically against ear infections is currently under trial in the USA.

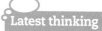

Latest thinking

The arguments for and against the use of grommets (ventilation tubes) in the treatment of glue ear have raged for years. But a 2010 Cochrane Review concludes that the effect of grommets on hearing is only small and diminishes after six to nine months. Most grommets come out over this time and by then the condition will have resolved in most children. Watchful waiting seems to be the best way to manage glue ear in children, as it will usually get better on its own without surgical intervention.

Eczema

Could itchy skin be worse than a life-threatening health condition such as diabetes or high blood pressure? When scientists asked 92 adults with severe eczema about the quality of their daily lives, they reported that having a serious medical problem might be easier than dealing with itchy, bumpy, scaly skin all the time. Half said they would trade up to 2 hours a day of their lives for normal skin, and 74 vowed they'd spend whatever it took for a cure. The following strategies may help avoid flare-ups, and beat the 'itch, scratch, itch' cycle that makes skin so much worse.

20% The reduction in itching, dryness and skin crusting if you keep eczema-prone skin moisturised.

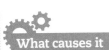

What causes it

Experts are still trying to identify the culprits behind eczema. While the causes aren't fully understood, allergies, dry skin and low levels of a skin-protecting protein may play a role.

Key prevention strategies

Avoid hidden triggers Among the everyday things that can cause an outbreak are: perfumes and dyes in laundry and personal-care products, dust, cigarette smoke, walking barefoot on sand (or letting it rub the creases of your legs or arms at the beach), and chlorine or bromine left on the skin after swimming in a pool or soaking in a hot bath. Avoid them or shower them off your skin as soon as possible. Sunburn is another possible trigger.

Bathe less often Long hot baths or showers can take the natural oils out of skin, making it drier and more easily irritated. While some experts recommend a long soak in a tepid bath to soothe skin, many others say it's better to go a day or two between washing. When you do bathe, keep it short and use warm – not hot – water. Avoid using harsh soaps, including antibacterial or deodorant soaps, that may strip more moisture from your skin. In fact, use a mild soap only where you really need it: on your underarms, genitals, hands and feet. Try using just water, or emulsifying ointment and water, everywhere else. When you've finished, pat yourself dry, then apply plenty of unperfumed moisturiser.

Keep your skin super-moist If you have eczema, you know first-hand how dry, itchy and sensitive your skin is, and that dryness makes itching and rashes even worse. That's why it's important to apply a thick layer of moisturiser once or twice a day to seal the water in the top layer of skin. Keeping your skin moist may mean you'll need less steroid cream to control rashes. In a Spanish study of 173 children with eczema, those who applied moisturisers daily needed 42 per cent less high-potency steroid cream.

Always apply moisturiser generously. In one German study of 30 adults with eczema, those who applied the amount their doctors recommended saw their itching, dryness and skin crusting improve about 20 per cent more than those who skimped. If you're using moisturiser and a steroid cream, apply the steroid first.

Keep a steroid cream handy just in case Steroid creams, ointments, gels and lotions can't cure eczema, but when it flares up, they're the number-one choice for controlling it. The catch is that overuse (more than four continuous weeks) can lead to thinning of the skin, reduced bone density in adults and growth problems in children, but these side effects are rare. In fact, some researchers say fear of steroid creams can have worse side effects than the creams themselves. In one UK study of 200 people with eczema, 73 per cent admitted to being worried about using a steroid cream, and 24 per cent said that they had skimped or skipped the treatment as a result. But studies show that sensible use brings relief, usually without adverse effects. If you're worried about high-dose steroid creams prescribed by your doctor, remember that they're safe and very effective when used as directed. When UK researchers followed 174 children and teenagers with mild to moderate eczema for 18 weeks, they found that when treating flare-ups, three days of a high-dose cream worked as well as seven days of a low-dose cream. Both groups had the same number of itch-free days and neither showed signs of skin thinning.

Get tested for allergies Pet dander, pollen and dust mites can all trigger eczema flare-ups. In fact, one Scandinavian study of 45 people with eczema found that everyone with severe skin problems was allergic to at least one of these airborne allergens. So it's sensible to ask your doctor for an allergy test.

Experts have conflicting opinions about the effectiveness of strategies for avoiding allergens at home (such as removing carpets, keeping pets out of the bedroom and covering mattresses and pillows with allergen-proof covers). While some recommend it, studies tend to show that these steps often don't reduce eczema flare-ups, simply because it's difficult to

Sunlight or a sunlamp?

Use a sunlamp. Stubborn, severe eczema that isn't healed by creams or even steroid medication may respond to exposure to ultraviolet (UV) light. In one study of 73 people with moderate to severe eczema, those who got twice-weekly narrow-band UVB treatments with sunlamps for 12 weeks saw a 28 per cent reduction in itching, oozing and crusting of their skin rashes. In contrast, those who were exposed to regular sunlight saw a 1.3 per cent improvement. See a dermatologist about UV therapy – and don't go to a tanning salon; any potential benefit has to be balanced against the risk of skin cancer.

Symptoms to watch for

Small, itchy bumps that may leak fluid when scratched; dry, itchy, red to brownish grey patches of skin or areas of thick, scaly skin, especially on the hands, feet, arms, neck, face and chest, and behind the knees.

keep the air completely allergen free. Immunotherapy (anti-allergy injections) may help. In one German study of 89 people with eczema who were allergic to dust mites, those who got immunotherapy found it easier to keep their eczema under control than those who didn't have the injections. Ask your GP if these might be suitable in your case.

Consider food allergies Intolerance to milk, wheat and other foods can cause flare-ups in children with eczema. While food allergies are usually rare among adults with eczema, don't rule them out. In one Danish study, 25 per cent of adults with severe eczema were allergic to at least one food. Before you start cutting whole food groups out of your diet on your own, though, talk to an allergy specialist or a registered dietitian about the best way to test yourself. Often this involves keeping a detailed food diary, removing one suspect food from your diet for several weeks and then reintroducing it again to see what happens.

Try an immunomodulator cream For severe eczema, an immunomodulator cream may help. Pimecrolimus (Elidel) reduces eczema symptoms by 50 per cent or more, according to UK researchers who reviewed 31 well-designed studies.

Pimecrolimus cream doesn't have the skin thinning and other side effects of steroid creams, so it is often used for sensitive areas such as the face or body folds. It can also be used for long-term control of eczema. However, because there are reports of serious side effects, it should only be used under the supervision of an eczema specialist.

Cut the risk of eczema

Most eczema begins in early childhood. Now it appears that what the mother eats during pregnancy can lower her child's risk of the condition. Scientists from the University of Aberdeen in Scotland tracked the eating habits of mothers as well as allergies and asthma in 1,212 children from birth to the age of five and found that the babies of women who ate fish once a week or more often during pregnancy were significantly less likely to develop eczema. They also concluded that a woman's diet during gestation may have a bigger impact on a child's risk of developing eczema than the child's own diet in the first few years of life. Fish is a rich source of inflammation-soothing omega-3 fatty acids, but scientists aren't yet sure how this healthy food may bolster protection in a child. For toddlers who are eating solid foods and can have dairy products, adding probiotic-rich foods such as yoghurt with active, live cultures may help, too.

Prevention boosters

Soothe your emotions Several studies have linked stress and anxiety to eczema outbreaks. If anger, frustration or stress seems to trigger a rash, consider adding a little 'emotional therapy' to your skin-care routine. Studies show that relaxation therapy, cognitive behavioural therapy and biofeedback can all help. For best results, ask your doctor for a referral to a psychologist or to a programme specifically designed for people with skin conditions.

Dress for comfort Rough, scratchy fabrics and clothing that's too tight can irritate sensitive skin. Instead, choose smooth cotton weaves and knits to avoid irritation and to allow skin to breathe. And avoid itchy wool next to the skin and synthetic fabrics that tend to trap sweat.

Wash all new clothes before you wear them to remove irritant chemicals used to make them look smooth and wrinkle free in the shop. If you suspect that your laundry detergent or fabric softener is irritating your skin, switch to products without perfumes or dyes and rinse clothes twice in the washing machine.

Keep the temperature and humidity levels comfortable Too much humidity in the air can make you sweat; too little can leave skin parched and flaky. Both situations can prompt an eczema flare-up. Keep your home's humidity level comfortable by using a humidifier in winter if your heating system dries out the air too much. Research suggests that large temperature swings can also trigger flare-ups, so try to keep the room temperature constant.

Keep using your medications A recent study showed that people's use of medication recommended for eczema dropped by 60 per cent within three days of starting treatment – perhaps because their skin improved quickly or because they were afraid of side effects. Discuss with your doctor any concerns you may have about your treatment, and how often you actually use the medication so he or she can plan the treatment that's best for you.

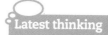

Latest thinking

While many experts have traditionally believed that allergies trigger eczema, there's evidence that a genetic quirk that makes skin fragile could be behind many eczema cases. Researchers in Ireland and Scotland have found a lack of filaggrin, a compound that normally makes the skin's outer layer watertight, in up to half of adults and children with eczema. The result is that the skin dries out, and particles of dust or pollen from the outside can penetrate the skin causing irritation. While investigations continue into this intriguing clue, experts say it underscores the importance of protecting eczema-prone skin by the generous use of moisturisers.

See also:

Step 8: *Reduce chronic stress,* page 74

Erectile dysfunction

Before 1998, it was quite rare to hear anyone speak openly about erectile dysfunction (ED) or impotence. Then Viagra arrived on the scene, and suddenly everything changed. Overnight, conversations about the ability to have and maintain an erection became commonplace. Although there are now five medications approved to treat ED, including two injectable agents, simple lifestyle changes are still the best way to try to prevent it occurring in the first place.

70%
The amount by which you can reduce your risk if you stay physically active in middle age and beyond.

What causes it

Anything that affects the health of blood vessels – heart disease, diabetes, high blood pressure or smoking – can affect a man's ability to have an erection. Stress and relationship problems are other causes.

Key prevention strategies

Eat like the ancients The Mediterranean diet is rich in healthy monounsaturated fats from foods such as olive oil. It's also packed with fruit, vegetables, nuts, pulses, whole grains and fish and is relatively low in red meat. When Italian researchers compared 100 men with ED to 100 men without it, they found that those whose diets closely matched a Mediterranean diet were significantly less likely to be impotent. The reason, researchers speculate, is probably the anti-inflammatory effect of the diet. Inflammation contributes to plaque build-up, narrowing blood vessels, and narrow vessels mean less blood gets through to the penis, making an erection less likely.

Get into sport Exercise isn't just good for your muscles; it's also good for an erection. Men who become more physically active in middle age drastically reduce their risk of ED by 70 per cent compared with men who stay on the couch. In fact, physical activity – no matter what kind – reduced the risk of impotence even more than giving up smoking, losing weight or drinking less alcohol.

Stop smoking If the idea of protecting your heart and lungs isn't enough to make you stop smoking, perhaps the threat of sexual embarrassment is. One study of 7,684 Chinese men found that smoking

Drugs that prevent disease

Although medications such as sildenafil (Viagra) are designed to be used on an as-needed basis, preliminary studies suggest that taking them every night for a year could actually prevent impotence once you stop using the medication. In one German study, 112 impotent men took either 50mg of sildenafil every night for a year or 50–100mg only as required. Following the research, after six months without treatment, 58.3 per cent of the men who had taken nightly sildenafil had normal erections without medication, compared to only 8.2 per cent of those who had used the tablet only as needed.

" Even **one day**
without a cigarette can
improve erections. "

probably accounted for about one in five cases of ED. The more you smoke, the more likely you are to have problems. The study found that smoking 20 cigarettes a day increased the risk by 60 per cent compared to not smoking at all. The reason could be that smoking constricts blood vessels and contributes to the build-up of plaque, both of which reduce blood flow – which obviously results in trouble getting and maintaining an erection. Smoking also reduces levels of nitric oxide, a chemical compound that keeps blood vessels, including those in the penis, dilated. Even one day without a cigarette can improve erections.

Take care of your heart A study published in the *Journal of the American College of Cardiology* found that men who could not achieve an erection were 40 per cent more likely to develop cardiovascular disease. It may be that erectile dysfunction is an early warning sign of heart trouble, so it makes sense to pay special attention to the advice given for preventing coronary artery disease, starting on page 148. And this finding also underlines the importance of discussing this problem with your doctor, who may decide to carry out further tests.

Prevention boosters

Maintain normal blood glucose levels Half of all men with diabetes have erection problems – twice the rate of men without the disease. (See *Diabetes*, page 156, to find out how to prevent Type 2 diabetes.)

Take medication The three most popular choices include: sildenafil (Viagra), tadalafil (Cialis) and vardenafil (Levitra). All work by increasing levels of nitric oxide, the chemical that helps dilate blood vessels in the penis and keep them dilated so you can have and maintain an erection. The major difference between the three is how long they take to begin working. Vardenafil works the fastest, with one study finding it began working within as little as 10 minutes and remained effective for up to 12 hours. However, if you're away for a romantic weekend, consider tadalafil: studies find that one dose continues working for up to 36 hours.

Symptoms to watch for

The inability to have or maintain an erection.

Latest thinking

Men with erectile dysfunction have an increased risk of Parkinson's disease. Researchers evaluating the medical records of 32,616 medical professionals found those with a history of ED were nearly three times more likely to develop Parkinson's than those who didn't have erection problems. The link seems to be related to damage in the autonomic nervous system, which regulates functions such as breathing and digestion. Identifying the underlying reasons for the link could theoretically lead to ways to prevent Parkinson's disease.

See also:
Cause 6: *Inflammation*, page 32
Step 3: *Quit smoking*, page 66

Fatigue

Fatigue is classically characterised by a chronic lack of energy. When you're fatigued, you may not need to sleep, but you don't feel like doing much else. Your brain feels muddy and your muscles feel like lead. Fatigue can be the result of a condition such as depression, cancer, diabetes, fibromyalgia or congestive heart failure, but about one in four people experience fatigue that's not related to any medical problem.

65%
The amount by which walking for 20 minutes a day three times a week can reduce fatigue.

What causes it

The most common reason for fatigue is lack of sleep, but it can also be a side effect of illness, cancer treatment or medical conditions such as fibromyalgia, chronic fatigue syndrome, diabetes, lupus, multiple sclerosis, low iron levels or hypothyroidism. Depression and boredom may also contribute. Fatigue is also a side effect of certain medications, both prescription and over-the-counter.

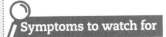

Symptoms to watch for

Lack of energy and the inability to concentrate.

Key prevention strategies

Get a good night's sleep It's the most obvious way to keep your natural energy up. If you're tossing and turning, waking up in the middle of the night or waking up too early, see *Insomnia*, starting on page 232. If you snore, also read *Snoring*, starting on page 296. Obstructive sleep apnoea, which is associated with severe snoring, is a common cause of daytime tiredness.

Step out As little as 10 minutes of brisk walking helps to raise energy levels more effectively – and for much longer – than eating a chocolate bar. Just 20 minutes of walking three times a week can increase energy levels by 20 per cent and reduce fatigue by 65 per cent.

Get your blood tested Common causes of fatigue that a blood test can reveal are low iron levels (you don't have to be anaemic to be low on iron) and hypothyroidism, which occurs when the thyroid gland doesn't make enough thyroid hormone. Both are common in women and often go undetected. One US study found that about 16 per cent of women had low iron levels.

Eat a high-fibre breakfast One study found that people who started their mornings with a high-fibre meal, such as muesli or baked beans on whole-grain toast, were more alert throughout the morning, probably because these meals take longer to digest than, say, a bowl of cornflakes or a muffin, so blood glucose levels remain steadier. It also helps to include some protein with breakfast – and every other meal, too.

Good breakfast options, then, are whole-grain toast with a slice of cheese or a teaspoon of peanut butter and a piece of fruit, a bowl of high-fibre cereal (aim for at least 5g of fibre per serving) with skimmed milk, or a bowl of porridge sprinkled with freshly ground flaxseeds (linseeds).

For an afternoon snack, instead of a chocolate bar or crisps, choose a small handful of almonds or a couple of whole-grain crackers spread with peanut butter.

Prevention boosters

Enjoy the sun Bright light – whether from the sun or a full-spectrum fluorescent light designed to mimic the sun's rays – pumps up alertness levels like a shot of adrenaline. You don't have to sunbathe; in one Japanese study, women who sat near a sunny window for 30 minutes reported feeling more alert than when they sat in a darkened room for the same amount of time. Sunlight boosts activity in brain regions associated with alertness and dampens levels of the so-called 'sleep hormone', melatonin.

Sip small coffees Too much caffeine can backfire by keeping you up at night, but sipping just 60ml of coffee every hour from about 10am to 2pm boosts alertness levels, thanks to caffeine's ability to block a sleep-inducing brain chemical called adenosine.

Use the power of peppermint If you need a quick pick-me-up, the smell of peppermint may do the trick. Purchase peppermint essential oil from a health-food shop or pharmacy and rub a drop between your hands once every hour, or place a few drops on a tissue and breathe in the scent for an instant boost.

Find a new hobby Boredom and loneliness are twin contributors to depression, which is a major cause of fatigue. Join a book group, a tennis or golf club, a knitting or sewing circle –anything that gets you out of the house, helps you meet new people and gives you something interesting to do.

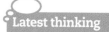

Latest thinking

In women with breast cancer, fatigue from chemotherapy can last up to six months or more after the treatment ends. But a recent review of studies shows that moderate exercise is effective at relieving even cancer-related fatigue.

See also:

Cause 3: Depression, page 26
Step 1: Exercise, page 62
Step 5: Sleep, page 70

177

Flatulence

Flatulence is hardly a disease. In fact, everyone passes wind from 14 to 23 times a day (women emit as much as men), but most of the time it's odourless. However, knowing that doesn't make passing wind in company any less embarrassing. If smelly emissions are worrying you, here's some advice.

75%
The reduction in wind experienced by people with IBS after taking a peppermint oil preparation.

What causes it

Gas is produced when bacteria in your bowel ferment indigestible carbohydrates in high-fibre foods and fibre supplements. Lactose intolerance, gluten intolerance, irritable bowel syndrome, ulcerative colitis and Crohn's disease can also cause wind. So can antibiotics, some diabetes medications, laxatives, weight-loss drugs, medications to help you stop smoking and gastric bypass surgery. Eating foods sweetened with sugar alcohols such as sorbitol and mannitol can also cause cramps and excess wind.

Symptoms to watch for

Passing wind, sharp abdominal cramps and bloating.

Key prevention strategies

Go easy on beans and 'windy' vegetables Dried beans are very good for you, but an increase in wind is often the downside. The culprit is an indigestible sugar called raffinose, also found in cabbage, Brussels sprouts, broccoli and asparagus. Humans lack an enzyme needed to break down raffinose, so beneficial bacteria in the intestinal tract do the work of consuming this sugar. The bacteria emit gas, so within a few hours, you do the same. US experts say that by gradually increasing the amount of beans and similar foods in your diet, you can minimise this side effect.

Reduce bean gas Draining and rinsing canned beans before use gets rid of some of the gas-causing raffinose. If you're cooking dried beans, always soak them first. Add 1/8 teaspoon of bicarbonate of soda to the soaking water to leach out more raffinose, and rinse soaked beans well. Never cook beans in their rinsing water.

Eat slowly It's normal to swallow some air when you're eating – accounting for half the wind you pass – but gulping down food or drinking through a straw adds to this considerably. So slow down and cut back on chewing gum, which also increases the amount of air you swallow.

Check your reaction to the major wind producers Many foods contain tough-to-digest sugars that often become food for gassy bacteria in your gut. Everyone reacts differently, so don't write off a nutritious fruit or vegetable unless you're sure it's causing a reaction. Prime culprits include foods high in the sugar fructose, such as dates, grapes, apples and pears, as well as foods that contain sorbitol, such as apples, pears, peaches and plums.

Prevention boosters

Opt for still water over fizzy water All those bubbles in soda or sparkling water and soft drinks contain gas, and you swallow a lot of it when you sip a carbonated drink. Switching from fizzy drinks (including beer and champagne) to still ones helps.

Have rice instead Starchy side dishes such as potatoes, noodles made from wheat flour (including most pasta) and other grains produce gas when they're digested in your large intestine. Rice won't – it's just about the only starch that is completely absorbed in the small intestine, making it a more comfortable choice if you're bothered by excessive wind.

Skip low-carbohydrate sweets Many 'sugar-free' and low-carb chewing gums, sweets, chocolates, biscuits and cake mixes are sweetened with sugar alcohols such as sorbitol and mannitol. When bacteria in your intestinal tract break them down, the result can be tummy rumbling and windy emissions.

Switch antacids Using bicarbonate of soda or an antacid containing sodium bicarbonate to ease heartburn and acid indigestion could backfire, loudly. Experts caution that while it's busy neutralising stomach acid, bicarb produces plenty of carbon dioxide – some of which may exit through your intestinal tract. As little as ½ teaspoon of bicarb could produce enough gas to give you wind. Look for another type of antacid, such as one that contains calcium carbonate, which neutralises acid, or ask your doctor or pharmacist about H2 blockers, which reduce acid production.

Season beans to get rid of gas Researchers from India report that adding garlic and ginger (either fresh or dried) to beans while they cook can reduce gas when you eat them.

When wind is a symptom

Sometimes intestinal gas is a sign of a food intolerance or digestive condition. Among the most common are:

Lactose intolerance If you have wind and abdominal pain after eating dairy products or drinking milk, you may lack the enzyme lactase, needed to break down the sugar, called lactose, in these foods. A simple breath test can diagnose this problem. The solution is lactase supplements, lactase drops to add to milk and lactose-reduced dairy products.

Gluten intolerance If your body can't digest gluten, a protein found in wheat and some other grains, you may experience flatulence, bloating, weight loss, oily and foul-smelling stools, and other symptoms. The solution is to avoid gluten, but get a diagnosis from your GP first.

Irritable bowel syndrome (IBS) If you emit normal amounts of wind but regularly feel bloated and have bouts of abdominal pain, diarrhoea and/or constipation, you may have IBS. Dietary changes, stress reduction and medications may help; discuss options with your doctor.

Latest thinking

If you have irritable bowel syndrome (IBS) and flatulence, meditation may help. In a small study of 16 people, twice-daily relaxation-response meditation for 15 minutes over a two-week period reduced flatulence and belching.

Flu

The odds of catching flu range from 5 to 20 per cent each winter, depending on the virulence of the circulating virus. That sounds low, but once you've had a miserable case of the flu, you'll be motivated to tilt those odds a little more in your favour. Start by doing all you can to keep your immunity strong: eat a healthy diet and get plenty of sleep and physical activity. Beyond that, the following suggestions may help to stack the deck in your favour.

81%
The reduction in your risk if you take Tamiflu as soon as someone in your household shows signs of the flu.

What causes it

Dozens of strains of the influenza virus. These viruses are extremely infectious because they're always mutating. This means that even though you develop antibodies to the flu if you're infected, your immune system won't recognise and fight off a new strain.

Symptoms to watch for

A sudden high fever, severe headache, aches and pains, fatigue, chest discomfort, coughing and sometimes a sore throat, stuffy nose and sneezing.

Key prevention strategies

Get vaccinated Having flu isn't just miserable; it can be dangerous, especially in older people. In a 10 year study of thousands of elderly men and women, having a flu vaccine cut the risk of being hospitalised with flu-like illnesses by 27 per cent and reduced the risk of dying from flu by 48 per cent.

Flu vaccines are not perfect, and they work better some years than others. At best, vaccination protects against 70 to 90 per cent of the flu viruses being passed around. But at worst, it may provide only 40 to 50 per cent immunity. However, those are still far better odds than you'd have with no flu jab.

Definitely ask your doctor's advice about getting vaccinated if you're over the age of 65, if you have long-term medical condition, if you are responsible for the care of an elderly or disabled person (to protect yourself and them), or if you are pregnant.

Take an antiviral drug asap People who took the prescription drug oseltamivir (Tamiflu) or zanamivir (Relenza) after someone in their household caught the flu significantly reduced their risk of getting it themselves in one major study. Among people who took oseltamivir, 81 per cent didn't become ill; among those who took zanamivir, 75 per cent stayed well. People who received a placebo were five to seven times more likely to develop flu symptoms than those who took the antiviral drugs. The potential downside is an upset stomach. Ask your GP for advice if you have been exposed to the flu virus.

Wash your hands often The flu virus can survive for hours on hard surfaces such as metal, glass and plastic – and even on cloth, paper and tissues. Your best defence is washing your hands, and the more you do it the better. Lather vigorously for at least 20 seconds to get rid of all the germs. Choose hand washing over antibacterial hand wipes and gels when you have the option; relying on rubs and wipes could allow bugs to build up on your hands if you don't alternate their use with regular washing.

Carry the right alcohol-based hand sanitiser Viruses are hard to kill; even some alcohol-based hand sanitisers won't kill them if the alcohol concentration isn't high enough. (Hand washing doesn't kill viruses; it simply washes them away. That's why you don't need antibacterial soap.) Buy a sanitiser that contains 60 to 95 per cent ethyl alcohol. Rub the gel or foam on all sides of your hands, then rub your hands together vigorously until they're dry.

Vaccination know-how

The flu vaccine works by introducing a tiny dose of several dead flu viruses into your body. The antibodies you develop in response help to protect you if you're exposed to the real thing. The more antibodies, the better the protection. The following four factors can affect the flu vaccine's effectiveness:

Stress Feeling stressed in the 8 to 10 days after having a flu injection could suppress your immune response to the vaccine by 12 to 17 per cent.

A fever If you have a fever on the day of your injection, reschedule. Fever is a sign that your immune system is already fighting an infection, so don't overload it.

Sleep Getting a few good nights' sleep before the vaccine could boost your antibody production by 50 per cent.

Tai chi or qigong US researchers found that people who performed one of these two activities for an hour three times a week for 20 weeks produced significantly more antibodies after getting a flu vaccine.

Prevention boosters

Sneeze technique Alcohol-impregnated wipes aren't a substitute for hand washing, but they could cut the number of virus particles on your children's hands and may even reduce the number lurking on surfaces in your home. Also, teach your children to sneeze into the crook of their elbow, not their hand.

Move your exercise routine indoors In a small Canadian study, people who exercised most days of the week for three months had fewer flu symptoms and higher levels of flu-fighting immunoglobulin A in their bloodstreams compared to people who didn't exercise. We know that exercising can be a challenge when the weather is cold and wet. If that's the case, try following an exercise DVD at home, or do old-fashioned calisthenics such as sit-ups and star-jumps, or get that exercise bike back into action.

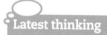
Latest thinking

To avoid flu over the holidays, don't fly. In 2002, the flu season started several weeks later than usual and peaked in March instead of January or February. US researchers at Harvard University suspect the cause was the 27 per cent drop in air travel after the terrorist attacks of 11 September. Exposure to airport crowds and hours spent in close proximity to people who may be carrying the virus can raise your risk of catching flu.

181

Food poisoning

85% The percentage of cases of food-borne illness that could be prevented by safe food-handling in the home.

Most of the foods we eat naturally contain tiny amounts of bacteria and viruses that are harmless for most of us. But if foods are poorly handled or improperly cooked, these germs can grow to threatening levels, causing anything from mild discomfort to serious illness. Don't just rely on the 'sniff' test to tell if a food is okay; while you can smell if food is rotten, you can't smell bacteria that may be multiplying on or in it. In fact, food safety experts say the most dangerous disease-causing bugs don't alter the look, smell, or taste of food. Instead of using your senses, practise safe shopping, cooking and storage. And use good judgement when eating out or when abroad. (For more on traveller's diarrhoea, see *Diarrhoea*, starting on page 160.)

What causes it

Bacteria such as *Campylobacter jejuni, Escherichia coli, Giardi intestinalis, Listeria monocytogenes, Salmonella,* and *Staphylococcus aureus,* as well as viruses such as norovirus, *Vibrio vulnificus,* and *V. parahaemolyticus.*

Key prevention strategies

Separate meat, chicken and seafood from the rest of your groceries Put them in plastic bags to contain any juices. Pack them into separate bags at the supermarket check-out, too. At home, store raw meat, poultry and seafood in containers or sealable plastic bags on the bottom shelf of the fridge to make certain the juices can't leak out and contaminate other foods.

Buy perishables last and refrigerate them fast Place all meat, poultry and seafood in the fridge as soon as possible. Freeze poultry and minced meat that won't be used within one or two days; freeze other meats within four or five days.

Don't defrost on the kitchen worktop Germs can grow quickly on fish, chicken, turkey and other meat products left at room temperature even while defrosting. Use these techniques instead.

- **Plan ahead and defrost in the fridge** Put the frozen item in a sealable storage bag or wrap it well to contain juices. Place the package on a plate or in a bowl in the refrigerator until defrosted.
- **Use the microwave** Set your microwave to 'defrost' or use a low power setting (such as 50 per cent) so the thinner edges of the meat won't cook while the middle thaws. Cook immediately after defrosting.
- **Dunk in cold water** Seal food in a plastic storage bag and place in a large bowl of cold water, or under cold running water, until just thawed. Cook immediately.

Leftover safety

Leftovers can provide an easy meal the next day – but make sure they're safe.

- **Refrigerate or freeze foods promptly** Discard perishable food left at room temperature longer than 2 hours, or 1 hour in temperatures above 32°C (90°F).

- **Divide and conquer** Split large amounts of leftovers into small shallow containers for quick cooling in the fridge. Remove the stuffing from poultry and other meat immediately and refrigerate it in a separate container.

- **In doubt? Throw it out** If you suspect food may have been sitting out for too long, don't take any chances. Bin it.

Marinate safely Keep marinating foods in the fridge. Don't use the marinade from raw seafood, poultry or meat for cooking or on cooked food unless you've brought it to a full boil first to kill any bacteria. Throw away the rest after use.

Wash before you cook and again as needed Scrub your hands vigorously with soap and water for 10 to 15 seconds immediately before handling food. Dry with a clean paper towel. Wash your hands after handling raw food and again before eating. Surveys show that 25 per cent of cooks do not wash their hands after touching raw meat and fish, and 66 per cent don't wash after handling raw eggs.

Guard against cross-contamination Keep raw meat, poultry, seafood and their juices away from ready-to-eat foods. Always wash knives, utensils, chopping boards or other kitchen equipment immediately after contact with raw meat. Serve the food on a clean plate, platter or board – don't reuse the one that held raw food.

Clean up carefully Be sure to clean worktops and other kitchen surfaces (including fridge doors) adequately after contact with raw meat. An antibacterial cleaning product or a solution of one teaspoon of bleach to one litre of hot water will do the trick; dry with a clean paper towel.

Cook it through Kansas State University research reveals that colour isn't a good indicator that meat or poultry is fully cooked; minced beef may look fully browned when the internal temperature is just 55°C (130°F) – well below the 75°C (170°F) that scientists estimate is

Symptoms to watch for

Abdominal cramps, diarrhoea and vomiting 12 to 24 hours after eating contaminated food. You may also have a headache, fever and chills. If vomiting and diarrhoea continue for more than two days or, if you have signs of dehydration, call your doctor. Young children, older people and those with reduced immunity need prompt medical care if affected by food poisoning.

Latest thinking

Should you rewash prepacked salad leaves? Some experts say yes. While studies show that prewashed leaves sold in sealed bags are safe, some food safety experts say rewashing can't hurt. The truth is, you can't always remove all germs from leafy green vegetables; researchers say they're sometimes inside the leaves or cling tightly to them. But washing helps.

necessary to destroy all disease-causing bacteria. To add to the confusion, some lean minced beef and some poultry may look pink even after it's reached a safe temperature. To get it right, use a food thermometer for roasts or poultry. Wash the probe end in warm soapy water and dry with a paper towel after each use.

For seafood, look for these signs that it's done Fish flesh should be completely opaque and flake easily with a fork. Cook lobster or crab until the shells turn red; their flesh – and that of shrimps and prawns should be pearly and opaque. Cook clams, mussels and oysters until the shells open; don't eat any that remain shut after cooking.

Keep fresh produce safe It's not widely recognised that fresh fruit and vegetables also have the potential to cause food poisoning. Although most produce is safe, follow these strategies to keep it even safer.

- Buy fresh-cut produce such as half a watermelon or bagged salad leaves only if they're refrigerated or surrounded by ice. Store perishable produce (such as strawberries, lettuce, herbs and mushrooms), pre-cut produce and peeled produce in the fridge.
- Wash fruit and vegetables under running water before eating, cutting or cooking, even if you're going to peel them. Use a clean vegetable brush on potato skins and the rinds of melons and squash. There is no need to use washing-up liquid or hand soap. Dry with a clean paper towel when possible to remove even more germs.
- Discard the outer leaves of vegetables such as cabbage, pak choy and lettuce.

When is it done?

Cook until food reaches these recommended internal temperatures.

Whole chicken, duck, goose, turkey or dark meat: 85°C/185°F

Poultry breast: 71°C/160°F

Minced beef, lamb, pork or veal: 70°C/160°F

Rare beef: 60°C/140°F

Medium-rare beef: 70°C/160°F

Well-done beef: 80°C/175°F

Roast pork: 80°C/175°F

Fresh ham: 71°C/160°F

All leftovers: heat to 74°C/165°F

○ Make sure that any sprouting vegetables, such as bean sprouts, alfalfa and cress, are really fresh; it's easy for bacteria to flourish in the warm, moist conditions they're grown in.

Keep hot foods hot and cold foods cold If food isn't going to be served and eaten immediately – for example, at a picnic, party or buffet – keep hot food at or above 63°C (145°F) in chafing dishes, a food-warming trolley, oven and/or slow cooker. To keep cold foods at or below 5°C (41°F) put food in containers on ice.

Keep your refrigerator cold One in three refrigerators is set too warm to keep foods cold and safe, researchers say. Be sure yours is set at 0°-5°C (32°-41°F) and the freezer at -18°C (-1°F). If your fridge doesn't have a temperature indicator, buy a fridge thermometer. And don't overload the fridge – air needs to circulate in order to chill food effectively.

Prevention boosters

Keep meat hot – safely Once meat reaches the right internal temperature on the barbecue, keep it hot if you aren't going to serve it right away by moving it to the side of the grill, away from the flames or coals. If you've cooked food in the oven or on the stove, you can keep meat hot in an oven at 90°C (lowest setting) until you serve.

Keep your fridge clean Clean up food spills promptly with a solution of baking soda and water. If meat juices leak, use a weak solution of one teaspoon bleach in one litre of warm water to kill any germs, then wipe with baking soda and water to remove the bleach.

If you're transporting food to a picnic or party, use a cool box Use enough ice or ice packs to keep food at 5°C (41°F) or below. Keep cool boxes out of the sun and try to keep the lid shut as much as possible. Put meat in a separate box from other foods.

See also:

Safeguarding your health: *Keep your food safe, page 82*

Foot problems

Each of us takes an average of 4,000 to 6,000 steps a day, which puts our feet under enormous stress. So it is hardly surprising that three out of four of us experience foot problems at some time in our lives. Some conditions are inherited, some develop from illnesses in middle age, while others are a direct result of pressure from ill-fitting shoes. Here's what you can do to prevent problems and keep your feet in good walking order.

What causes it

Foot pain can be caused by bunions, hammer toes, calluses and corns, veruccas, fallen arches, poorly fitting shoes and strain resulting from carrying too much weight. Other causes include broken bones, arthritis (page 104), gout (page 194), plantar fascitis (inflammation of the band of fibrous tissue that runs from the heel bones to the base of the toes), bone spurs, sprains, bursitis of the heel, tendonitis, ingrown toenails, chilblains, and Morton's neuroma (pain typically between the third and fourth toes caused by thickening of tissue around a nerve in the area).

Symptoms to watch for

Swelling, redness and heat may be a sign of gout or an infection. Cold, painful feet that are white or very pale can be a sign of poor circulation. Sharp pain around the third and fourth toe, which gets better if you take your shoes off, suggests the possibility of Morton's neuroma.

Key prevention strategies

Buy shoes carefully A well-fitting pair of shoes is fundamental to healthy feet. Go for leather uppers that allow your feet to breathe and choose a shoe with a firm heel counter (the rear section of the sole to which the heel is attached). For women, a laced or strapped style with a small heel (ideally no more than 2.5cm) is best. Always try on both shoes and walk a few steps to check that they don't pinch or rub. Remember, feet swell during the day so go shoe shopping in the afternoon when feet are at their largest.

Get the right shoe for the sport If you play more than one sport be sure to buy the correct type of shoe to provide the support you need for each activity. For example, tennis shoes are designed to provide stability for side-to-side motion while running shoes are designed to support toe-to-heel motion. If you walk a lot, choose shoes with laces to keep feet firmly in place. This will help prevent blisters and keep toes from slipping forward.

Maintain good foot hygiene Wash your feet every day in warm soapy water, dry them thoroughly, especially between the toes, and moisturise with a special foot cream – an all-purpose body lotion won't be nearly as effective, as the skin on your feet is considerably thicker than that on the rest of your body.

Avoid high heels A 5cm heel puts 57 per cent more pressure on the ball of the foot than the pressure you experience when wearing no shoes. If you can't resist high heeled shoes, make sure that they fit well and are not too small, and don't wear them for long periods.

64% The number of women who could avoid foot problems in the future by wearing well-fitting, low-heeled shoes.

Take the weight off your feet

With every step you take, all your weight goes through one foot, and one third of that goes through the ball of the foot (first metacarpophalangeal joint). If you weigh more than 16st (101kg) then the pressure under that joint during walking can be greater than under an elephant's foot (75lb per sq in/34kg per 6.5 sq cm) when walking on two feet. Losing those extra pounds will help reduce pain in your feet.

Protect your feet in public Wear flip flops in public showers and around swimming pools to avoid picking up verrucas and other infections. (See also *Athlete's foot*, starting on page 112.)

Lose weight if you need to Being overweight can place added strain on the muscles, tendons and ligaments, which support the arches of the foot leading to pain.

Prevention boosters

Cut across Always cut toenails straight across to reduce the risk of ingrown toenails.

File it Use a foot file or pumice stone on dry skin (such as on the heels or the sides of the big toes) once a week to minimise the build-up of hard skin at key points. Never do this on wet or damp skin or in the shower, as the skin will crack. Always file in one direction: from the heel downwards towards the sole of your foot.

Move them Extend and flex your toes whenever you can and circle your feet when sitting down.

Keep them warm If you suffer from cold feet, wear an extra pair of socks or insulated soles. Try to keep the temperature of your feet constant as suddenly going from cold to hot may cause chilblains.

Latest thinking

You may want to think twice before buying your next pair of high heels to avoid painful problems later in life, according to researchers at the Institute for Aging Research of Hebrew Seniorlife. A study of 3,300 men and women showed that nearly 64 per cent of older women who reported heel and ankle pain had regularly worn high-heeled shoes or sandals at some point in their lives.

The reason? With each step you take your foot gets a shock as it hits the ground. Trainers and sports shoes often have special soles and other features that soften the impact and protect the foot. But in high heels, the heel and the ankle take the brunt of the shock, which is why women who wear them often report pain in this part of the foot. The advice from the Society of Podiatrists is keep high heels for special occasions, and wear them only for short periods.

See also:

Exercises: *Joint strength*, page 26

Fungal skin infections

An itchy, scaly fungal rash in the groin, under the breasts or elsewhere on your skin can be both embarrassing and very uncomfortable. Working up a sweat at the gym or pool, or even just mowing the lawn helps to build whole-body fitness, but if you don't take steps to protect sweat-moistened skin, you may end up with an infection caused by the tinea fungus – the same organism responsible for Athlete's foot (page 112).

90%
The odds of staying fungus free if you clear up an existing infection with an antifungal cream.

What causes it

Tinea, a fungus from the family called dermatophytes. Tendrils growing into the top layer of the skin lead to increased cell production with thick, scaly, itchy skin.

Key prevention strategies

Stay clean and dry Take a shower or bath every day. After a workout, change out of sweaty clothes (including underwear) and shower as soon as you can. Carefully dry your genital area, buttocks, inner thighs and skin folds under the breasts or between rolls of fat with a clean towel. Leaving skin damp gives fungus a foothold, not only because moisture encourages the fungus to multiply, but also because sweat and water dilute your natural oils, which contain fungus-fighting compounds.

Wash all sports clothing, supports and underwear after each use These items will not only be smelly but may also carry fungus. They will have absorbed sweat and the chances are they've been in contact with the changing room floor at some point. Take them out of your gym bag as soon as you get home; fungus can breed in the bag's damp, dark interior. In fact, if your bag is wet, spray it with disinfectant spray, dry with a paper towel, and leave it to air in the sun for extra protection.

Check your pets, too

Dogs and cats can harbour hard-to-see fungal infections on their skin and you may pick up an infection when you touch them. For instance, ringworm (tinea corporis), which produces scaly red patches on the skin, is usually transmitted through contact with furry pets or livestock. In one study of 211 dogs, researchers found 89 fungal strains that can also infect humans – and 11 dog owners who had fungal infections of their feet or groin area. Look for areas of skin where fur is missing or ask your vet to check your dog or cat.

Wear boxers, not briefs Close-fitting underwear traps moisture, so go loose with boxers and roomy shorts or pants. Choose smooth, breathable fabrics such as cotton and wool instead of synthetics. Avoid scratchy material that irritates your skin; fungus thrives on broken skin.

Dust yourself with an antifungal powder Using an antifungal powder, such as Daktarin or Tinactin, in skin folds on clean, dry skin can help discourage itchy fungal growth and keep you dry. Using them during hot weather and when you know you'll be hot and sweaty, such as while doing gardening or exercising, can stop a fungal infection before it has a chance to get started.

Already itchy? Use an antifungal product Unless your rash is severe, start with an over-the-counter antifungal cream, gel, powder or spray. There are plenty of over-the-counter brands to choose from. Products containing terbinafine (Lamisil), clotrimazole (Canesten) or miconazole (Daktarin) are effective. Continue to use these for 10 days after the rash has disappeared to prevent a recurrence.

Safe sex If your partner has a fungal infection in the groin area ('jock itch'), skin-to-skin contact could transmit the fungus to you during sex. Women are much less likely to develop jock itch than men, but it can happen. Ask him to use an antifungal cream until the infection is gone or use an antifungal cream yourself to prevent infection.

Prevention boosters

Enlist your washer and dryer Washing clothes and towels in hot water, then drying them on high heat in the dryer, kills fungus.

In the changing room Don't sit naked on benches. Always use your towel to create a barrier between your skin and any fungal spores that may be lurking on surfaces in the changing room.

Symptoms to watch for

Burning, stinging or itching on your feet, groin, buttocks, inner thighs, below the breasts or underneath rolls of fat. Infection in the groin can extend to the lower abdomen in severe cases.

Latest thinking

The fungus that causes groin infections could be living on the seats of stationary bikes, weight machines and free-weight benches, warn experts from the Institute for Fungal Illness in Berlin, Germany. Most gyms clean down equipment several times a day. If you're concerned, ask the manager about the gym's cleaning policy and before you sit down, clean the seat with wipes or a disinfectant spray.

Gallstones

Built from layers of cholesterol or calcium salts, gallstones grow slowly and silently in your gall bladder or bile ducts in much the same ways as a pearl grows inside an oyster. While most gallstones never cause a problem, some trigger attacks of severe abdominal pain and ultimately have to be treated with surgery or medication. Fortunately, there's a lot you can do to reduce your chances of developing these painful stones and to prevent a recurrence if you've already had them.

What causes it

An imbalance of the 'ingredients' in bile acids (the digestive juices that break down dietary fat) or partial emptying of your gall bladder, allowing cholesterol particles from bile acids to clump together to form stones.

Symptoms to watch for

Indigestion, which may be worse after you eat a high-fat meal. Also wind, bloating, sudden steady pain in your right upper abdomen, nausea and vomiting.

Key prevention strategies

Aim for a healthy weight and a trim waist Being overweight or obese more than triples your odds of developing gallstones; carrying extra fat around your middle is especially dangerous. In a Harvard School of Public Health study of more than 42,000 women, those whose waistlines measured 92cm (36in) or more were twice as likely to have gallstones that required surgery compared to women whose waists measured less than 66cm (26in). If you're overweight, losing extra pounds slowly and steadily is the best way to protect yourself. Don't crash diet; losing more than 3lbs (1.5kg) a week appears to raise gallstone risk; losing a more gradual 1-1½lbs (0.5-0.7kg) a week doesn't.

Avoid yo-yo dieting at all costs The more weight you gain and lose repeatedly, the higher your risk of gallstones becomes. US researchers found that men who lost and regained as little as 4½lbs (2kg) in five years had a 21 per cent higher risk of gallstones than those who maintained the same weight. Men whose weight fluctuated by 11-17lbs (5-8kg) raised their odds by 38 per cent. Fluctuations of 20lbs (9kg) or more increased the risk of gallstones by 78 per cent.

Why is yo-yo dieting so risky? While dieting, you may not be eating enough fat to keep your gall bladder active; this may allow cholesterol to sit long enough to begin forming stones. What's more, when you regain weight, you may develop insulin resistance because most of the weight regained after a diet consists of body fat (not muscle), which increases the risk of this condition. Changes in body chemistry that lead to insulin resistance also increase gallstone risk, according to researchers.

Exercise more Taking 2 to 3 hours of physical exercise per week can lower your risk of gallstones by 20 per cent.

Focus on good fats Cutting out too much fat could cause problems, but regularly eating a little fat helps prevent gallstones by prompting the gall bladder to empty, pumping bile acids into your digestive system to help digest your meal. It's the type of fat that matters. In studies from Denmark and France, people who ate more saturated fat were more likely to develop gallstones, so opt for 'healthy' fats, such as those found in olive and rapeseed oils, nuts and oily fish.

Cut back on sugar and add fibre
Eating 40g of sugar a day, the amount in 8 teaspoons of sugar or a serving of sweetened breakfast cereal plus a couple of biscuits after lunch, doubles gallstone risk, according to research. This may be because of an increase in cholesterol in the bloodstream, which is triggered by the surge of insulin that occurs when blood glucose rises. But eat a high-fibre diet and you'll protect against gallstones by removing cholesterol from your body.

Foods that fight gallstones

A diet rich in magnesium can lower gallstone risk by 30 per cent, according to one US study from the University of Kentucky. Men with the lowest risk had an average intake of 454mg a day from supplements plus food. The richest sources of magnesium are green leafy vegetables and nuts. The eight foods below all contribute a healthy dose of the mineral:

Food	Serving	Total magnesium
Almonds, unblanched	25g	68mg
Wholemeal bread	1 slice	24mg
Bran flakes	30g	36mg
Dried figs	50g	40mg
Pumpkin seeds	25g	68mg
Pearl barley, uncooked	100g	65mg
Brazil nuts	25g	103mg
Spinach, steamed	80g	27mg

Prevention boosters

Enjoy coffee A cup or two of coffee in the morning could cut your risk of gallstones by 40 per cent, according to researchers who tracked the gall-bladder health of more than 46,000 men for a decade. Components in coffee stimulate the release of bile acids, and lower levels of stone-forming cholesterol in bile fluid.

Toast your gall bladder's health One drink a day can lower gallstone risk by 27 per cent. Alcohol may help by raising 'good' HDL cholesterol, which transports 'bad' LDL (found in gallstones) out of your body. Beer, wine and spirits are equally protective.

Latest thinking

Research suggests that people of European ancestry have a 10 per cent chance of having a gene that increases gallstone risk. Carrying the gene doubles or even triples the risk by causing the liver to pump extra cholesterol (a major component of gallstones) into the gall bladder. But eating well and exercising can prevent gallstones from ever causing trouble.

Glaucoma

Glaucoma slowly destroys the delicate fibres of the optic nerve, making it impossible for your eyes to tell your brain what they're seeing. The result is a loss of sight. The damage usually begins decades before you realise something's wrong, as pressure within your eyes builds up and begins erasing peripheral vision. Untreated, glaucoma leaves you with tunnel vision – and then darkness. Regular eye checks can pick up dangerously high pressure in the eyes early and, if it does develop, prescription eye drops and surgery can help bring it under control.

60% The reduction in your risk of vision damage if you treat high pressure in your eyes with prescription eye drops.

What causes it

Untreated raised pressure from fluid within the eye. Pressure can build if your eyes' drainage system doesn't work efficiently. Some people with apparently normal pressure also develop glaucoma.

Key prevention strategies

Make sure you get your eyes tested regularly The NHS recommends that all adults should have an eye examination every two years. People over the age of 60 and those with a family history of glaucoma or other risk factors (see *Know your risk*, below) should be checked for the condition every year. Your optometrist will check for signs of optic nerve damage, measure pressure levels in your eyes and check the thickness of your cornea (a thin cornea is associated with higher glaucoma risk). You should also have a visual field test to check for tiny blind spots in your field of vision.

Know your risk While anyone can develop glaucoma, your risk is significantly higher if other people in your family have it, if you're over the age of 60 or if you're of African or Asian descent and over the age of 40. Diabetes, high blood pressure, shortsightedness, severe eye injuries and long-term use of steroid drugs may also raise your risk. If you're at increased risk, catching early signs of trouble should be a top priority.

Use prescription eye drops If the pressure inside your eyes is elevated, using the pressure-lowering eye drops prescribed by your doctor could save your vision. In a landmark study of 1,686 people with high eye pressure

The coffee controversy

Glaucoma specialists don't all agree, but several studies suggest that a serious coffee habit could raise eye pressure and your risk of optic nerve damage. Harvard researchers found that drinking five cups a day increased glaucoma risk by 61 per cent in a long-term study of more than 76,000 women. Meanwhile, Australian researchers who studied the eye health of more than 3,600 people found that the more coffee they drank, the higher their eye pressure. Some studies suggest that caffeine is the culprit, but in other research, tea and caffeinated soft drinks seemed to have little effect compared with coffee.

but no signs of effects on the optic nerve, those who used drops cut their risk of damage over the next five years by more than half. If eye drops don't work in your case, or if optic nerve damage is progressing despite the use of drops, your doctor may suggest surgery to help lower your eye pressure.

Control diabetes Researchers from the Harvard School of Public Health found that having Type 2 diabetes raises the risk of developing glaucoma by 70 per cent. Experts suspect that diabetes may somehow raise eye pressure or make the optic nerve more vulnerable to damage. If you have diabetes, keep your blood glucose under control and have your eyes checked once a year for glaucoma and other diabetes-related vision problems.

Prevention boosters

Get moving It's no substitute for eye tests and eye drops, but physical activity is a great add-on strategy for lowering glaucoma risk. Studies show that exercise that raises your heart rate – walking, swimming or even vigorous housework – for about 20 minutes can lower your eye pressure by four points immediately afterwards. Exercising four times a week can keep your pressure lower throughout the day. But if you have been prescribed eye drops, keep using them unless your doctor advises otherwise. Avoid movements that involve lowering your head below heart level (such as the downward-facing dog position in yoga or any exercise involving bending over) as they raise eye pressure.

Quit smoking When Greek researchers reviewed seven glaucoma studies, they found that smokers were 37 per cent more likely to develop glaucoma than non-smokers. Not all studies have found an association, but if you've been told you're at risk for glaucoma or already have it, it's just another good reason to kick the habit.

Relax and refresh There's some evidence that emotional stress raises pressure inside the eyes and that relaxation techniques can reverse that trend. In one German study of people with glaucoma, the eye pressure of those who did guided imagery exercises to relax was significantly reduced. Again, it's no substitute for drops if you need them, but it could help.

Symptoms to watch for

Usually, none. In advanced glaucoma, you will develop tunnel vision. A less common form of glaucoma, called acute angle-closure glaucoma, causes very sudden blurred vision, halos around lights, red eyes, severe eye pain and nausea and vomiting, all due to a rapid, dramatic increase in eye pressure. This is a medical emergency.

Latest thinking

Glaucoma may be a warning sign of heart trouble. When researchers followed the health of 4,092 residents of Barbados for five years, they found that those with glaucoma were 38 per cent more likely to have potentially fatal heart disease. The connection could be underlying health problems that lead to both. If you have glaucoma, it makes sense to keep an especially careful watch on your blood pressure and cholesterol levels, too.

Gout

40%
The reduction in your gout risk (if you're overweight) when you lose just 11lbs (5kg).

Gout is an increasingly common condition thanks to the developed world's obesity problem – and to the fact that more people are consuming food, drinks and medications that raise levels of uric acid in the blood. Too much leads to the development of crystals that collect in joints and cause excruciating joint pain. Here's how to cope with this condition, or to simply avoid it.

What causes it

High blood levels of uric acid, which crystallises in joints, causing inflammation and pain. Certain foods and beverages raise uric acid levels, and some medications may make it more difficult for your body to excrete it or may increase production.

Key prevention strategies

Maintain a healthy weight Gaining 33lbs (15kg) could more than double your risk of developing gout, according to researchers from Massachusetts General Hospital in the USA. Losing just 11lbs (5kg)was found to lower the odds by 40 per cent.

Sweat a little In a California study of 228 men, those who were leaner and fitter were less likely to develop gout than men who had only one of those healthy attributes. In the study, men who ran around four miles a day lowered their risk by 50 per cent, but doing any form of aerobic exercise for any amount of time will help to some extent.

Limit red meat or seafood A daily serving of red meat raised the likelihood of developing gout by 45 per cent in a study of 228 men conducted by US researchers. Meanwhile, men who ate the most seafood (including oily fish) increased their risk by 51 per cent in another study. Why? The answer is that these foods contain purines (game and offal, and seafood, including anchovies, sardines and scallops, have especially high levels). When purines break down, blood levels of uric acid – and therefore the risk of gout – rise.

Limit your consumption of meat and seafood to less than three 100g servings a week – try chicken or pulses instead. But if you don't have problems with gout, it's a good idea to keep eating oily fish.

Eat dark red cherries Cherries are a traditional remedy for gout, and now science reveals why they work. When 10 volunteers breakfasted on 45 dark red cherries for two days, researchers at the University of California discovered that levels of uric acid in their blood fell by an impressive 30 points. Black, yellow and red sour cherries are effective, too. Around 200g a day is all you need.

Include soya beans in your daily diet People with gout may benefit from limiting animal protein in their diet, which contains purines, but foods derived from soya beans can be beneficial. Several studies show that soya reduces uric acid, making soya products a helpful way to combat gout, as well as being a source of healthy protein. Try to have soya products such as tofu or soya milk at least twice a week instead of red meat.

Check your hypertension medication Studies suggest that blood pressure-lowering diuretics can increase gout risk three and a half times above normal. Some thiazide diuretics may raise risk the most. If you develop gout and you already take one of these medications, ask your doctor about an alternative.

Drink wine instead of beer A little alcohol may protect your heart, but it also raises gout risk. In one study, men who drank 1½ pints of beer a day or more increased their odds of developing gout 2.6 times more than those who abstained. But two small glasses of wine did not raise the risk. Beer contains higher levels of purines than most wines.

Skip sweetened fruit drinks Sugary soft drinks and beverages raise gout risk by just as much as alcohol. Fructose in fruit-based drinks seems particularly to increase uric acid levels.

Prevention boosters

Enjoy your coffee In one US study of 228 men, those who drank four or five small cups of coffee a day reduced their gout risk by 40 per cent compared to those who drank none. Decaffeinated coffee was also found to lower the risk, but tea had no effect.

Have low-fat milk and yoghurt Two daily servings of milk products can reduce gout risk by about 45 per cent – as long as they are low fat. Proteins in milk called casein and lactalbumin may protect against gout by promoting the excretion of uric acid in urine.

Symptoms to watch for

Sudden, severe pain; redness and tenderness in joints. Gout often begins in the joint of a big toe or in the knee.

Latest thinking

People with gout have a 20 per cent higher risk of heart attack than people who are gout free, according to new research. The connection may be inflammation: gout can trigger ongoing inflammation in the body, and inflammatory compounds may also trigger blood clots that can lead to a heart attack. If you have gout, be extra vigilant about your blood pressure, cholesterol and blood glucose levels. People with gout also have an increased risk of kidney failure.

See also:
Cause 6: *Inflammation*, page 32

Gum disease

Gum disease can affect more than just your mouth. Heart disease, diabetes, pneumonia and chronic obstructive pulmonary disease are all linked to gum disease, probably because of the low-level inflammation created as bacteria from your gums travel throughout your bloodstream.

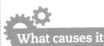
What causes it

Bacteria in plaque (a sticky, colourless film that forms on teeth) inflames gums. Over time, the inflammation can spread beneath the gum line.

Symptoms to watch for

Gums that become reddened (healthy gums are pink), swell or bleed easily; later, you may have loose teeth, bad breath and visibly receding gums.

41%
The reduction in the likelihood of bleeding gums after two weeks of brushing and flossing twice a day.

Key prevention strategies

Brush twice a day To prevent the plaque which causes gum disease from ever forming, the British Dental Association recommends using a fluoride toothpaste and brushing twice a day with a small brush that removes food debris from the gaps between your teeth. You should brush in a circular motion over the surface of each tooth with your brush at an angle of 45 degrees to the gum line.

Try an electric toothbrush After six months of brushing – but not flossing – with an electric toothbrush, people who already had gum disease showed significantly less plaque in the morning and immediately after brushing than those using a regular toothbrush.

Visit your dentist regularly You should have a dental check-up at least once a year and preferably every six months. Your dentist or dental hygienist will also be able to give your teeth a thorough clean, possibly doing a scale and polish to remove plaque.

Floss frequently Flossing takes less than a minute, and it's one of the best ways to prevent gum disease as it helps to remove the plaque and bacteria from between your teeth and from under your gum line. Here's how to make flossing easier.
- **Keep floss everywhere** At your desk, in your handbag, in the bathroom (of course) and in the glove compartment of your car.
- **Use a battery-operated flosser** A 10 week study found that these flossers (available online) got rid of more plaque on molars, premolars and hard-to-reach back teeth than regular floss.
- **Ask for a demonstration** Although the process may seem obvious, there is a right and wrong way to floss. Ask your dentist or dental hygienist for a demonstration.

Rinse with an antibacterial mouthwash daily A study of 156 volunteers found those who brushed their teeth and used either mouthwash containing antimicrobial chlorhexidine or cetylpyridinium chloride had less plaque than those who brushed and flossed or only brushed.

Quit smoking Not only is cigarette smoking a major risk factor for gum disease, but exposure to second-hand smoke can also increase your risk by up to 70 per cent.

Prevention boosters

Watch your blood glucose If you have diabetes, your risk of gum disease is already higher than it is for someone who doesn't have it. But if your diabetes isn't well controlled, you're in the danger zone: researchers find that people with poorly controlled diabetes have more inflammatory chemicals such as cytokines in their gums, which contribute to the development of gum disease.

Eat foods high in vitamin C When researchers evaluated the link between diet and gum disease in 12,400 adults, they found that those who didn't get the recommended daily amount of vitamin C (45mg, or about the amount in one orange) were nearly 20 per cent more likely to have gum disease than those who consumed more. Aim to eat more vitamin C-rich foods, such as citrus fruit, red peppers and broccoli.

Increase your calcium intake People whose intake of calcium was less than 500mg a day (240ml of low-fat milk has about 350mg) are nearly twice as likely to have gum disease as those who consume at least three servings a day of calcium-rich foods (a serving is 240ml of milk or a 150g tub of yoghurt or 100g of sardines with bones). Aim for an intake of around 1,000mg of calcium a day from food. Calcium helps build density in the jaw bone, which supports the teeth.

Don't overdo the alcohol Researchers have found a direct correlation between the amount of alcohol people drink and their risk of gum disease. Ten drinks a week increased the risk by 10 per cent, 20 drinks increased it by 20 per cent and so on.

If you have a dry mouth, see your doctor Many medications, including some antidepressants and cold remedies, contain ingredients that dry up saliva production. Saliva hinders the growth of bacteria, so if your mouth is dry, you may be courting gum disease.

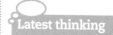

Latest thinking

New research suggests that obesity and gum disease may be related. When you're very overweight, fat cells release inflammatory chemicals that can contribute to numerous health problems, including gum disease.

See also:

Cause 6: *Inflammation*, page 32

Haemorrhoids

Haemorrhoids (piles) are very common in middle age, and also in pregnancy. Over-the-counter treatments can help some people, but if the problem becomes too bad, you may need professional help. In fact, the treatment of haemorrhoids – marked by swollen and inflamed veins around the lower rectum – form a large portion of any colorectal surgeon's workload. They're also probably much more common than we know, since many people are, understandably, too embarrassed to admit they have them. Try to avoid pain, itching and the operating table by following the suggestions outlined below.

75%
The amount your risk of haemorrhoids and tears in the skin of the anus could drop if you eat breakfast every day.

What causes it

Straining during bowel movements due to constipation, obesity and sitting for prolonged periods. Haemorrhoids commonly occur in pregnancy because of abdominal pressure and the effect of hormonal changes on blood vessels.

Symptoms to watch for

Bright red blood covering the stool, on toilet paper or in the toilet bowl. An internal haemorrhoid may protrude through the anus outside the body, becoming irritated and painful. Other symptoms include painful swelling or a hard lump around the anus.

Key prevention strategies

Don't strain If you have to bear down to have a bowel movement, something's wrong. And if you've been sitting on the toilet for more than 5 minutes without a result, get off. Straining is the primary cause of haemorrhoids, and a longer time spent on the toilet doesn't guarantee success. Instead, try again an hour or so later.

Avoid constipation If you're straining, the problem could well be constipation. Keep things moving along by eating a high-fibre diet, and drink plenty of clear fluids to help the fibre through the bowel. See also *Constipation*, starting on page 146.

Focus on fibre When asked what he recommends to his patients to prevent haemorrhoids, one leading gastroenterologist answered with one word: flaxseeds. It's one of the best sources of fibre you'll find, with nearly 3g in 1 tablespoon. Add a couple of teaspoons of ground flaxseeds (linseeds) to your breakfast cereal or and sprinkle it over yoghurt. Try adding freshly ground seeds to salads for added crunch, to pasta sauce for added bulk and even to a bowl of ice-cream. Fibre acts like a sponge in your intestinal tract, soaking up liquid and creating softer, bulkier stools that are easier to move out of your body.

Get out of the chair A good way to get your bowels moving is to get yourself moving with regular exercise. It can be dancing, swimming, walking, golf – anything that gets the blood flowing. One study of 43 people with constipation found that those who walked every day for

Stop the burning

Once you have haemorrhoids, it can make going to the toilet difficult: you may be afraid something might burst, not to mention the discomfort. Try these suggestions:

- **Use moist wipes** These are gentler and much more effective than dry, scratchy toilet paper for wiping after a bowel motion.
- **Use over-the-counter haemorrhoid cream or pads** They usually contain topical anti-inflammatories to reduce inflammation and a local anaesthetic to kill pain.
- **Try a sitz bath** Sit in a bowl containing about 15cm of warm water for about 20 minutes. Dry carefully with a soft towel. Do this several times a day.

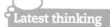

Latest thinking

To treat severe haemorrhoids, instead of surgery or cutting off the blood supply to haemorrhoids with a tight band, doctors can now zap them with infrared light to cut off the blood flow.

30 minutes and did 11 minutes a day of weight-based exercises at home improved their rankings on a scale designed to evaluate constipation by nearly 35 per cent.

Drink up A major reason people get constipated and find it hard to move their bowels is that their stools don't absorb enough water. Often it's because their fluid intake is low, so make sure you are drink enough.

Go on a schedule Believe it or not, there's actually an ideal time for a bowel movement: about 30 minutes after you wake up, just after a cup of hot coffee or tea, and about 30 to 60 minutes after meals. So factor in toilet time, even if nothing happens. What you're doing is training your bowels to 'let go' on time. But at whatever time of day, be sure to go when you feel the urge. Putting it off can lead to hardening of the stools and a greater likelihood of straining and pain.

Prevention boosters

Change your position Modern toilets work against you when it comes to haemorrhoids, since they require you to sit instead of squat (squatting facilitates bowel movements). To get around this, try propping up your feet on a small footstool and pulling your knees up towards your chest.

Eat plenty of berries Not only will the extra fibre help with constipation, but these fruits are also high in flavonoids, natural plant compounds that help reduce inflammation and strengthen blood vessel walls. Try eating a cup of your favourite berries every day.

Headaches

Whether you get a tension headache once in a while or experience excruciating 'cluster' headaches, the best headache is the one you don't get at all. Experts say most headaches can be avoided with the following steps, but if you get a sudden, intense headache which is unlike any previous headache, call your doctor immediately. If you suffer from recurrent severe headaches with other symptoms such as visual disturbances or nausea, it may be migraine (see page 258).

50%
The decrease in the number and severity of headaches if you exercise for 30 minutes most days of the week.

What causes it

We don't know exactly what causes tension headaches, but researchers now suspect that fluctuating levels of serotonin – feel-good endorphins – and other brain chemicals play an important role. Anaemia, anxiety, arthritis of the neck or spine, depression, menopause, muscle tension, severe high blood pressure and sinus infections can cause headaches. So can prescription and over-the-counter medications, including oral contraceptives, some antihistamines and decongestants.

Key prevention strategies

Stick to your schedule Sleeping-in on weekends or not drinking your regular tea or coffee could trigger a headache. One survey found that 79 per cent of sufferers have a headache if they sleep longer than 8 hours. And if you're used to a cup of coffee at 7am, delaying it could restrict blood vessels, leaving you with a pounding headache.

Don't skip meals If you get 'hunger headaches', the culprit could be low blood glucose. Keeping your blood glucose on an even keel with low GI (glycaemic index) foods could help. Try to include whole grains, fruit and vegetables, and protein to keep levels steadier for longer. Avoid filling up on white rice, white bread, white potatoes and sugary foods, which make blood glucose levels rise rapidly and then crash again.

Move your muscles Getting half an hour of exercise on most days of the week can cut headache frequency and severity by an impressive 50 per cent, according to research. Physical activity works in two ways: by boosting feel-good brain chemicals called endorphins and by easing the physiological effects of stress.

Practise relaxation You don't have to meditate – any kind of relaxation that eases stress could help you escape from frequent tension headaches. Italian office workers who took brief relaxation breaks every 2 to 3 hours cut their monthly headaches by 41 per

Drugs that prevent disease

Cluster headaches are excruciating and can be a major problem for weeks, months or years on end. The heart drug verapamil is sometimes prescribed as a preventive treatment, but carries risks. In one study of 30 people, 12 of 15 participants who took this drug had fewer attacks in just two weeks. But verapamil significantly raises the risk of irregular heart rhythm. If you are prescribed this medication, your heart will be monitored regularly.

cent, report researchers from the University of Turin. And when US researchers tracked 203 adults with chronic daily tension headaches, 35 per cent of those who were given five sessions of stress management advice saw headache frequency fall by more than 50 per cent. Ask your GP about stress-reduction training. Meanwhile, try a few minutes of slow, deep breathing on a regular basis.

Check your workstation Reposition your chair, desk and computer screen so you can sit up straight with your feet on the floor. The centre of your screen should be just below your gaze when you look straight ahead. Have your eyesight checked and, if you need a new pair of glasses, it's worth paying extra for the anti-glare coating. Finally, get up and take frequent breaks from the screen.

Give up pain relievers If you take medicine for headaches more than 15 times each month, you may have 'rebound headaches'. These happen when painkillers wear off and blood vessels swell, then pain returns, you take medication to relieve it and the cycle begins again.

Studies show that rebound headaches can happen with over-the-counter remedies such as ibuprofen and aspirin, and as well as with prescription drugs for headaches and migraines. The best remedy is to stop taking your pain reliever (and understand that it'll hurt). But once the rebound effect wears off, your doctor will be able to treat the underlying cause of your headaches.

Prevention boosters

Stay hydrated That nagging pain could be your brain's way of asking for a glass of water. Mild headaches can be a sign of dehydration, so drink up.

Let go of tension in your jaw, face, shoulders and/or neck It's easy to unconsciously clench muscles in these areas when you're tense; this is a frequent cause of chronic tension headaches. So if these muscles are tight, take a few slow, deep breaths and imagine the stress flowing out until you feel relaxed. Repeat several times a day.

Symptoms to watch for

Head pain, of course, as well as trouble sleeping, tiredness, irritability, loss of appetite and difficulty concentrating. If you have cluster headaches, you will have intense pain plus weeping, swollen eyes, a stuffy nose and sweaty skin.

Latest thinking

Chronic headaches and depression are linked. In a study, one in four women and men with chronic headaches also had major depression, report researchers from the University of Tsukuba in Japan. The researchers suggest that if you have had chronic headaches for longer than six months, it's a good reason to ask your doctor to evaluate you for depression.

See also:

Step 8: *Reduce chronic stress,* page 74
Exercises: *Neck strength and flexibility, page 338*

Hearing loss

Hearing tends to worsen with age, partly as a result of some health conditions and years of noise exposure. Thanks to the high-volume sound produced by rock bands, personal music systems and electronic children's toys, noise-related hearing loss is also now more common in younger adults and in children as young as six.

51%
The amount by which you could reduce your risk if you quit smoking.

What causes it

Noise damages minuscule hair cells in your inner ear that transmit sounds to your brain. When these cells die, they can't be replaced.

Symptoms to watch for

Ringing in the ears, dizziness, difficulty perceiving and differentiating consonants, feeling that words often 'run together', and the inability to hear high-pitched sounds such as a ringing phone.

Latest thinking

One reason why noise damages ears may be that it stimulates the production of free radicals, dangerous molecules that can damage cells. In animals, certain antioxidants such as n-acetyl-l-cysteine and acetyl-l-carnitine reduce the risk of hearing damage from excess free radicals, which may point the way to future strategies to protect hearing.

Key prevention strategies

Protect yourself against major disease Diabetes, heart disease and high blood pressure can increase the risk of age-related hearing loss, probably by impeding blood flow to the inner ear. Find tips for preventing them in the entries for those conditions in this book.

Use the lawnmower test If something sounds as loud as a powered lawnmower (about 90 decibels), it's too loud. For prolonged exposure, you need to cover your ears with ear defenders or at least use earplugs. Here's another way to gauge whether your tasks or hobbies are hurting your hearing: before mowing the lawn or listening to the stereo, turn on the television and set the volume on low. Notice how well you hear what's said. Afterwards, try the test again. If you don't hear as well, you're experiencing some temporary hearing loss. With continued exposure, it could become permanent.

Turn down the volume When you're listening to music through headphones, you may not realise how loud it really is. When in doubt, turn down the volume. If you keep the volume control no higher than 50 per cent of its maximum (for an MP3 player that may be 100 decibels or more), you can listen as long as you like. But if you often turn it up much higher, limit yourself to 5 minutes when using earbuds that sit inside your ear and 18 minutes for conventional headphones. Any longer could put your hearing at risk, according to current research.

Quit smoking Add hearing to the list of body functions that can be damaged by cigarette smoke. After analysing eight major studies, researchers concluded that smoking increases your risk of hearing loss by up to 51 per cent. This is probably because it reduces the flow of blood and oxygen to your inner ear, weakening the hair cells that transmit sound to your brain.

Get plenty of B vitamins A growing body of evidence suggests that people who consume low levels of the B vitamins folic acid and B_{12} tend to have poorer hearing. When Dutch researchers gave 728 older men and women 800mcg of folic acid or a placebo daily for three years, those who were given this vitamin had less hearing loss than those who took the placebo. In another study, researchers injected 20 young volunteers daily with either a placebo or vitamin B_{12} for seven days, then exposed each group to a loud noise. The vitamin-taking group's hearing recovered better than the placebo group's.

B vitamins reduce levels of the amino acid homocysteine, which damages blood vessels. When homocysteine is cleared out, blood flow is improved, leading to healthier inner-ear hair cells. That's important, given that loud noises can reduce blood flow to the inner ear by up to 70 per cent. Good sources of B vitamins include soya beans, leafy green vegetables, lentils, beans, mussels (for vitamin B_{12}) and fortified cereals.

Prevention boosters

Hop on a bike, go jogging or take a walk After cycling twice a week for 30 minutes a day over two months, 17 moderately fit young adults suffered less hearing loss after a loud noise than before they started cycling. Researchers suspect this is related to the cyclists' stronger hearts. The better the circulation, which is improved by exercise, the more oxygenated blood gets to the fragile hair cells of the inner ear, helping them resist noise-related damage.

Snack on almonds They're packed with magnesium, which studies find can help prevent hearing-related damage. When researchers gave 20 men a juice drink containing 122mg of magnesium or a placebo for ten days, then exposed them to white noise designed to exhaust the hair cells of the inner ear, they found the men recovered more hearing more rapidly after the magnesium-laced juice than after the placebo drink. Researchers think this is because magnesium helps cells make better use of the energy you need to repair noise-induced damage energy. Oat bran, pumpkin seeds, barley and spinach are good dietary sources.

Got the gene?

While most hearing loss results from noise, everyone's hearing reacts differently. Two people exposed to the same noise level could experience it differently in each ear, even at different times of the day. That makes researchers suspect there's some genetic component to hearing loss. Another clue to your risk may come from your blood type. In one study, researchers found noise-induced hearing loss much more common among people with blood group O. So if your parents or grandparents wear hearing aids, or you have type O blood, you may have a higher risk of noise-related hearing loss, so should be extra careful about prevention.

See also:
Cause 1: Hypertension, page 22

Heartburn and GORD

30% The amount by which you could reduce your risk of acid reflux if you lose excess weight.

A muscular valve at the bottom of your oesophagus normally keeps corrosive digestive juices in your stomach. But if this valve opens at the wrong time – for example, after a big meal – stomach acid can back up into the oesophagus, causing the pain known as heartburn, which can be mild or so strong you could mistake it for a heart attack. Over time, recurrent heartburn becomes gastro-oesophageal reflux disease (GORD), a more serious condition that may raise your risk of oesophageal cancer. Take it seriously – and try to discourage acid reflux.

What causes it

Weakening or relaxation of the lower oesophageal sphincter (LOS), the muscular valve at the bottom of your oesophagus. Normally, this valve keeps digestive juices and food in your stomach. But smoking, alcohol, lying down too soon after a meal, some foods and medications can weaken or partially open the LOS, letting stomach acid back up into the oesophagus.

Key prevention strategies

Lose excess weight Losing 26lbs (12kg) cut reflux episodes 40 per cent in one study reviewed by researchers from Stanford University in the USA. Weight reduction helps because it may lower pressure at the valve, known as the lower oesophageal sphincter (LOS), that normally keeps stomach acid in its place. Losing weight also reduces the body's output of acidic digestive enzymes.

Don't go to bed on a full stomach When Japanese researchers tracked the bedtimes and GORD symptoms of 441 women and men, they found that those who went to bed within 3 hours of finishing their evening meal were seven and a half times more likely to have acid indigestion than those who turned in four or more hours later. If you go to bed at 10pm, aim to finish dinner no later than 6pm.

Prop up the head of your bed Raising the head of your bed about 30cm with bricks or books could cut the number of reflux episodes dramatically and also their duration.

Favour your left side In one study, people who slept on their left sides had only half as much reflux as right-side sleepers. The location of your stomach and oesophagus means that lying on your right side puts increased pressure on the LOS.

When to call the doctor

Chronic or severe heartburn can be a sign of more serious reflux disease or other digestive problems. Call your doctor if you have heartburn for more than two weeks or if it's making you wheeze or giving you a sore throat; preventing you from sleeping; interfering with daytime activities; causing pain in your neck, chest or back; creating discomfort or difficulty when you swallow; making you vomit; or if you have black stools (from digested blood) or unintended weight loss.

Take the pepperoni pizza test There's plenty of controversy about which foods trigger heartburn. The truth is, what bothers you may be no problem at all for the person sitting next to you.

When US researchers from Stanford University reviewed more than 100 studies of lifestyle remedies for acid reflux, they found that avoiding chocolate, mint, spices, greasy foods and late-night eating doesn't help most people. But plenty of other research, and the experience of digestive disease specialists, suggests that, for some people, these are exactly the things they should avoid.

The challenge is to work out what your personal trigger foods are, then steer clear of them. Common culprits include citrus fruit, chocolate, coffee and tea, alcohol, fatty and fried foods, garlic and onions, mint flavourings, spicy foods and tomato-based foods such as pasta sauce and pizza.

Avoid sleeping pills According to a large survey, people who took benzodiazepine sleeping pills such as nitrazepam and temazepam in order to fall asleep were 50 per cent more likely to have GORD at night than those who didn't take them. Other research has shown that these medications relax the LOS, thereby increasing the likelihood of reflux.

Quit smoking A Swedish study of more than 43,300 people found that long-time smokers had a 70 per cent higher risk of heartburn and GORD than non-smokers. Smoking raises risk four ways: it may make you cough more, which puts pressure on the LOS; it can weaken the LOS; it reduces production of saliva, which normally neutralises stomach acids that find their way into your oesophagus; and it boosts production of corrosive digestive acids.

Prevention boosters

Try chewing gum For times when you don't have any antacid handy, you might be able to head off heartburn with some chewing gum. A small UK study found that chewing gum for 30 minutes after a large, fatty meal doubled saliva production and saliva swallowing. It is estimated that 10 extra swallows could cool mild heartburn by pushing acids back into the stomach. Other research shows that gum chewing neutralises the acid in stomach reflux for up to 3 hours after a meal.

Take a relaxation break Science has yet to uncover the link between stress and acid indigestion, but plenty of heartburn sufferers know it exists. In one survey conducted by the US National Heartburn

Symptoms to watch for

A burning pain in your throat or chest, under your breastbone. It may become worse after a meal, at night or when you lie down. Less obvious symptoms include a persistent cough and chronic laryngitis.

Latest thinking

New research shows that nearly 40 per cent of heartburn/GORD sufferers who use an acid-reducing PPI medication once a day still get heartburn symptoms two to four times a week. Many end up taking antacids, which can stop pain but may not protect the oesophagus from damage. If you're taking medication for heartburn or GORD and are still in pain, ask your doctor about changing your treatment.

Alliance, 58 per cent of people who had frequent heartburn said hectic lifestyles made their pain worse. Stress may prompt you to smoke more, drink more alcohol, eat the foods that trigger acid reflux or simply to feel discomfort more intensely. Pay attention to your own stress levels, and when they get too high, look for ways to relax, such as deep breathing.

Control asthma Three out of every four people with asthma also have acid reflux. Coughing and difficulty exhaling may trigger the reflux of stomach acid into the oesophagus. Asthma medications that widen airways in the lungs may also relax the LOS. Keeping your asthma under control can help, but if you still have acid reflux, tell your doctor.

Keep blood glucose at healthy levels Over time, the high blood glucose levels that come with uncontrolled Type 1 and Type 2 diabetes can damage nerves throughout your body, including those that regulate the emptying of your stomach. If food sits in your stomach, it can be regurgitated more readily into your oesophagus. Some research studies suggest that better blood glucose control can help this problem, but it's still important to use the other lifestyle strategies mentioned here.

Find out if any medications are the culprits Many prescription and over-the-counter medications and supplements can keep the LOS from staying tightly shut. These include some antibiotics, antidepressants, calcium-channel blockers, opioid pain relievers such as codeine and oxycodone, osteoporosis medications, sedatives and tranquillisers, as well as over-the-counter pain relievers and supplements such as iron, potassium and vitamin C. If you have heartburn or GORD, ask your doctor if any of these could be contributing to the problem, and whether you should switch to another medication or remedy.

Up your fibre intake People who ate high-fibre bread (whole grain and multigrain) had half the risk of GORD compared to people who ate low-fibre bread (white) in one large Scandinavian study. Fibre may help by soaking up excess nitric oxide, a compound that relaxes digestive-tract muscles. When US researchers scanned the oesophaguses of 164 people, they found that those who ate more fruit, vegetables, whole grains and pulses were 20 per cent less likely to show reflux damage. Those who ate more fat, protein and other high-calorie foods were at higher risk.

Avoid cola drinks When US researchers from the University of Arizona College of Medicine polled more than 15,000 people about their lifestyle habits and history of GORD, they found that those who drank more than

Drugs that prevent disease

If you already have GORD, acid-reducing medications known as proton-pump inhibitors (PPIs) and H2 blockers can help you accomplish two important health goals: halting the searing pain of heartburn and healing damaged tissue in your oesophagus. (It's important to note that there is also non-acid reflux that does not respond to PPIs.)

Proton-pump inhibitors (PPIs) Medications such as esomeprazole (Nexium), lansoprazole (Zoton), omeprazole (Losec), pantoprazole (Protium) and rabeprazole (Pariet) work by blocking production of about 90 per cent of stomach acid. In one study of people with GORD, 78 per cent of those who took a PPI saw their damaged oesophageal tissue heal in four to eight weeks. After about eight weeks, your doctor should check to see if your oesophagus is healing and may cut back on your dosage.

H2 blockers Drugs such as cimetidine (Tagamet), famotidine (Pepcid), nizatidine (Axid) and ranitidine (Zantac) reduce acid levels in your stomach. Your doctor may suggest H2 blockers if you cannot tolerate PPIs. Studies show that H2 blockers work best for people with mild to moderate reflux problems but are less effective if your oesophagus is inflamed or has already been damaged by exposure to stomach acid. If you know which foods or situations are most likely to make your heartburn flare up, taking an H2 blocker in advance may help you avoid discomfort more effectively than if you take an antacid afterwards.

one carbonated, caffeinated drink per day were 24 per cent more likely to have sleep-disturbing night-time reflux than those who drank fewer of these soft drinks. Many carbonated drinks are highly acidic, which may explain the connection.

Try acupuncture if prescription medication isn't working When 30 people with persistent heartburn received either a double dose of proton-pump inhibitors or twice-weekly acupuncture plus their regular dose for four weeks, the acupuncture group enjoyed a significant reduction in GORD symptoms. The group that were given only increased medication didn't see much improvement at all, according to researchers at the University of Arizona.

See also:

Step 3: *Quit smoking,* page 66
Step 8: *Avoid chronic stress,* page 74

Hepatitis

Hepatitis is inflammation of the liver. There are five types of viral hepatitis: A, B, C, D and E. If hepatitis A, B or C gains control, liver cells are infiltrated and turned into virus-producing factories. Sometimes hepatitis heals on its own or it can last a lifetime. Cirrhosis, liver failure and liver cancer are all life-threatening conditions that may result from years of infection.

80-95%
How much you'll reduce your risk of hepatitis B by being vaccinated.

What causes it

Hepatitis A and E Ingesting food or water contaminated by stools from an infected person or through some other contact with an infected person's stool, such as nappy changing or shaking hands with someone who hasn't washed after using the toilet.

Hepatitis B and D Unprotected sexual contact with an infected person, sharing needles or drugs, or a needle-stick injury from an infected person. These viruses can also be passed from mother to infant during childbirth.

Hepatitis C Exposure to infected blood products or sharing needles. It can also be passed from mother to infant during childbirth.

Key prevention strategies

Get vaccinated The number-one way to prevent hepatitis A, B and D is with a vaccine. This is particularly important if you are in a high-risk group – for example, if you have liver or kidney disease. Unfortunately, there are no vaccines yet for hepatitis C or E, though researchers are working on them.

- **Hepatitis A vaccine** The NHS recommends that you should get vaccinated against this form of hepatitis if you are travelling to countries where the virus is common, such as the Indian subcontinent, Africa, Central and South America, the Far East and eastern Europe. You will need one injection four to six weeks before you travel and a booster dose six to twelve months later. If you do not have time for the vaccination to be effective before you travel, an injection of antibodies called immunoglobulin will give you some measure of protection for three to six months (see also *Drugs that prevent disease*, below).

- **Hepatitis B vaccine** This vaccination is recommended for anyone who is at increased risk of being infected with the hepatitis B virus, including those travelling to high-risk countries, those who have many sexual partners or who inject drugs, and people who work

Drugs that prevent disease

If you may have been exposed to the hepatitis A or B virus, see your doctor as soon as possible. He or she may give you a shot of immunoglobulin, which contains antibodies that destroy the virus. The sooner you receive this injection after being exposed to the virus – within two weeks for hepatitis A and 72 hours for hepatitis B – the more likely it is to work.

in high-risk jobs (for example, nurses and doctors). A full list of those for whom this vaccine is advised is given on the NHS website (www.nhs.uk/conditions/hepatitis-b/pages/prevention.aspx). It's typically given in three doses over six months. The protection lasts for at least five years, but can be lifelong. However, if you're over the age of 40 or obese, have kidney failure, are on dialysis, or have a suppressed immune system, it's not quite as effective. This vaccine also protects against hepatitis D.

- **Combined vaccine** There are also combination vaccines that protect against both hepatitis A and B.

Prevention boosters

Wash your hands regularly Not everyone washes their hands properly, so when you shake a person's hand and then touch your mouth, eyes or nose, you could easily end up with a hepatitis A infection. Always wash with soap and water whenever you can (especially when travelling), and for times when you can't, carry hand wipes or hand-sanitising gel. Always wash thoroughly after using the toilet or changing a nappy, and before preparing food.

Use condoms Practising safe sex is one of the best ways to prevent transmission of the hepatitis B virus.

Stay away from injectable drugs In this case the problem is recreational drug use, not insulin injections. This is the most common cause of infection with hepatitis B and C viruses.

Don't share personal items Using razors, toothbrushes or any other personal item that could have come in contact with an infected person's blood can lead to hepatitis B or C infection.

Choose your tattoo parlour carefully It's possible, though unlikely, that you could get hepatitis C when you get a tattoo. Make sure the tattoo parlour you choose complies with health regulations, looks clean and tidy, and uses an autoclave to sterilise all equipment properly. The tattoo artist should remove the needles and tubes from a sealed package and wear gloves while working.

Symptoms to watch for

Infection may initially go unnoticed or it may feel like a mild case of flu. With serious infection, you may experience jaundice, fatigue, abdominal pain, loss of appetite, nausea, diarrhoea, fever and dark urine. Hepatitis B infection may also cause rashes and joint pain and inflammation.

Latest thinking

People infected with the hepatitis B virus should be started on treatment as soon as possible. This may help prevent permanent damage to the liver.

Herpes simplex

Herpes – whether it's cold sores on your lips or blisters on your genitals – is painful in many ways. The blisters sting and burn for days. And while an attack is under way, herpes can be both embarrassing and risky because it's so contagious. Once you've been infected by the herpes virus, it lives dormant in your skin cells or nerve cells until it's reactivated by stress, sun exposure, trauma, surgery, illness or even the hormonal fluctuations of the menstrual cycle. The following strategies can keep it under control and help you to stay safe.

77%
The percentage of genital herpes outbreaks that could be prevented if you take antiviral medication daily.

What causes it

The herpes simplex virus. Type 1 usually causes oral herpes and Type 2, genital herpes. But either type can develop in either area.

Key prevention strategies

Not infected? Practise safe sex – and safe kissing If your partner has herpes blisters around the mouth or genitals, you should avoid skin-to-skin contact. Over 50 per cent of adults in the UK harbour the herpes virus – and at least one in four of those infected have no symptoms, but nevertheless could be contagious. The reason for this is that tiny viral particles can migrate to the skin's surface without causing an outbreak. This is known as viral shedding, and it's dangerous because it makes it possible to pass the virus around even when no one can see it.

That's why it's so important to practise safe sex. This includes using a condom during intercourse, though condoms won't always prevent spread of the virus simply because they don't cover all the areas that are infected or could become infected. The surest way to avoid genital herpes is to abstain from sexual contact or to stay in a mutually monogamous relationship with a partner who has been tested (testing for herpes antibodies is available, although the results may be difficult to interpret) and is known to be uninfected.

Drugs that prevent disease

Those who know they are harbouring the herpes simplex virus can reduce the frequency of outbreaks by taking antiviral drugs. The specific medications are aciclovir (Zovirax), famciclovir (Famvir) and valaciclovir (Valtrex). In one international study of 384 women and men with genital herpes, 71 per cent of those who took valaciclovir every day for six months had no more outbreaks, compared to just 43 per cent of those who took a placebo. Daily use can also reduce viral shedding by 94 per cent, helping to keep partners infection free.

Keep antiviral drugs on hand If you suffer from regular outbreaks of herpes symptoms, ask your doctor to prescribe medication that can short-circuit a cold sore and dramatically reduce genital herpes outbreaks and viral shedding (see *Drugs that prevent disease*, left). In cold-sore studies, antivirals healed outbreaks in three days, compared to just over four days for placebos, and reduced the number of blisters by 50 per cent. You can take these medications in advance to prevent cold sores, too, such as when you'll be outdoors in bright sunlight all day. Your doctor will tell you what dosing schedule to use.

What about antiviral creams? The truth is, many doctors don't recommend them any more. In some studies, they've proven no more effective than a placebo cream for clearing up blisters. Having a supply of oral antiviral medication on hand, and even carrying some for sudden outbreaks away from home, is a much better herpes-control strategy.

Always wear sunscreen The sun's ultraviolet rays may reactivate the herpes virus. In one US National Institutes of Health study of 38 people prone to cold sores, 71 per cent developed blisters after exposure to UV rays. The number dropped to zero when they all wore lip balm with built-in sunblock.

Prevention boosters

Breathe, and try to release the tension In one survey of nearly 500 Canadian doctors, dentists and pharmacists, 60 per cent said their patients and customers complained that emotional upheaval was certain to bring on a herpes outbreak. The best way of preventing stress-related cold sores is to use your favourite stress-busting technique. In one study, men who made time for daily relaxation had lower levels of antibodies associated with herpes.

Keep clean, don't touch If you have an outbreak of herpes sores, you can reduce the risk of the spread of infection by avoiding hand contact with the affected skin as much as possible. Always wash your hands if you have touched the area. Be especially careful not to touch your eyes after contact with herpes sores.

Eat well, sleep well Experts aren't sure why, but letting yourself become run down increases blister risk, perhaps due to stress, lowered immunity or both. When your life is tense, make an extra effort to go to bed earlier and opt for healthier food choices – simply to pamper yourself so you don't feel worn out.

Symptoms to watch for

Open sores or small, painful blisters surrounded by swollen, painful skin. Often there's pain or tingling for a day or two before the blisters appear. They typically occur around the lips or on the genitals, but they can also appear in your nose, mouth or eyes; on your chin or fingers; or on your buttocks or the upper part of your inner thighs. Outbreaks may be accompanied by flu-like symptoms, such as fever.

Latest thinking

A Canadian survey found that 75 per cent of people with herpes say they were never told about antiviral medications that can control this virus, although doctors claimed they were telling 60 per cent of their patients about them. The same situation may be true in the UK as patient information about oral antivirals does not appear to be widely available. Ask your GP if they are a treatment option in your case.

See also:

Step 5: *Sleep*, page 70
Step 8: *Reduce chronic stress*, page 74

211

High blood pressure

If avoiding a single health problem could cut your odds of having a stroke by 30 per cent, reduce your chance of a heart attack by 23 per cent and cut your risk of heart failure and dementia by half, you wouldn't need to think twice about tackling it. These health dividends – and more – all involve keeping blood pressure at a healthy level. After the age of 55, your odds of developing high blood pressure jump to 90 per cent – unless you take action. So have your blood pressure checked and if it's creeping over 120/80mmHg, start tackling it now.

11.4 points
The possible drop in your systolic blood pressure if you eat a healthy, low-salt diet.

What causes it

Stiff arteries and excess salt play a role. Too much salt in the blood prompts your body to pump extra water into your bloodstream in an effort to dilute high sodium levels. Meanwhile, everything from smoking to being overweight to eating a diet low in fruit and vegetables, dairy foods and whole grains can stiffen arteries, leaving them unable to flex, stretch and make room for fast-flowing blood.

Key prevention strategies

Lose those extra pounds Carrying excess weight, especially around your waist, raises your risk of high blood pressure by an astonishing 60 per cent. The reason is that fat around the waistline pumps inflammatory compounds into your bloodstream where they, in turn, stiffen artery walls. Stiff arteries mean higher blood pressure. Excess abdominal fat can also interfere with your kidneys' ability to filter pressure-raising sodium out of your bloodstream.

Being overweight seems to be the cause of half of all cases of high blood pressure, according to research. Losing a modest amount can protect you from this silent killer. When researchers followed 1,191 overweight women and men with high to normal blood pressure for more than two years, 65 per cent of those who lost 11lbs (5kg) and kept it off reduced their blood pressure to healthy levels.

The lesson is to start tackling excess weight sooner rather than later. Researchers suspect that, over time, chemicals produced by body fat can make artery stiffness hard to reverse.

Cut back on sodium A little sodium – a major component of common salt – is essential for human survival; too much is a problem. When sodium levels in your blood rise, your body pumps more water into your bloodstream to dilute it. This results in an increase in blood volume and in the force with which your blood pumps through your body. Too much sodium, research suggests, can also stiffen arteries, further raising your blood pressure.

If you make just one dietary change to lower blood pressure, eat less sodium. In one US study from Duke University, 71 per cent of people with high blood pressure who cut back on salt but made no other dietary changes brought their readings down to normal. If your blood pressure is at a healthy level, the British Heart Foundation recommends a maximum intake for adults of 2,500mg of sodium a day – that's 6g (about a teaspoon) of salt. But, better still, aim for much less. If your pressure is beginning to rise, you should aim to consume less than 500mg of salt or about a quarter of a teaspoon. Remember that most of the salt we eat is found in foods that may not even taste salty, such as packaged and processed foods, some cereals, and processed meats, such as ham, bacon and sausages. When you cook, add salt at the end (if at all); long cooking dulls salt's flavour, so you're more likely to be tempted to add more at the table.

Eat plenty of fresh fruit and vegetables A low-fat diet packed with fruit and vegetables can work wonders for your blood pressure. In one remarkable study, people with high blood pressure who followed a low-fat diet rich in fruit and vegetables and low-fat dairy foods for just eight weeks lowered their systolic pressure (the top number) by 11.4 points and their diastolic pressure (the bottom number) by 5.5 points – an improvement similar to that achieved by some blood pressure medications. Blood pressure began to fall after just two weeks. Other studies show that eating this way daily can lower your odds of developing high blood pressure in the first place.

The key ingredients here are calcium, magnesium and potassium. These three minerals help lower pressure in several ways: potassium helps the body excrete excess sodium, while calcium and magnesium work together to keep artery walls flexible.

The landmark US study of nutrition and blood pressure known as Dietary Approaches to Stop Hypertension, or DASH, found that people who increased their fruit and vegetable intake were able to lower their blood pressure, which lowers the risk of heart attack and stroke. The recommendation is seven to ten servings of fruit and vegetables daily, which is easier to achieve than you might think. Here are the best food sources of the three essential minerals:

- **Calcium** Low-fat dairy foods, sardines (with bones), tofu (firm), tinned salmon (with bones and liquid), almonds, cooked soyabeans and cooked spinach.
- **Magnesium** Almonds (unblanched), buckwheat flour, oat bran, tahini, pumpkin seeds, pearl barley, brazil nuts, cooked spinach, bulghur wheat, tofu and kidney beans.
- **Potassium** Raisins, cooked spinach, potatoes (baked, with skin on), avocados, cooked pumpkin, baked beans in tomato sauce, broccoli, tinned tomatoes (whole, chopped or puréed) and bananas.

Symptoms to watch for

Usually, none. To keep tabs on your pressure, have it checked at least every two years and ask your doctor to tell you your reading. If it's 120/80mmHg or higher, it's time to take action – even if your doctor doesn't suggest it at first.

213

Latest thinking

There's nothing normal about 'high normal' blood pressure. Until recently, experts thought blood pressure readings between 120/80 and 140/90mmHg were perfectly healthy. Now those levels are considered 'prehypertensive' or 'high normal' – and they can raise your risk of dying from heart disease by 58 per cent, making this problem more deadly than smoking.

Have low-fat milk or dairy foods two or three times a day A low-fat yoghurt, fruit smoothie, or hot chocolate made with low-fat milk and dark chocolate are not only delicious treats, they're also an essential part of a strategy to keep your blood pressure normal. Dairy foods are a top source of calcium, which some research suggests may help to prevent artery walls from stiffening. Choose low-fat or skimmed products to keep the saturated fat in your diet low. If you cannot tolerate dairy products, take 600–900mg of calcium a day in supplement form.

Put on your walking shoes Half an hour of brisk walking three to five days a week can keep your blood pressure five to six points lower than if you took no exercise. And when UK researchers checked the blood pressure levels of 106 government workers on a walking programme, they found that those who took their exercise in short bursts enjoyed the same blood pressure-lowering benefits as colleagues who had one longer exercise session a day.

Other research suggests that exercising in short bursts is actually better. In one study, the blood pressure levels of people who used this strategy stayed lower for longer during the day compared to people who took all their activity in one go.

Kick the habit Puffing on just one cigarette a day makes arteries less elastic, allowing blood pressure to rise even if you're young, slim and fit. Smoking 15 cigarettes a day raises your risk of high blood pressure by 11 per cent; smoking 25 cigarettes raises it by 21 per cent.

Snorers, ask your bedmate a question 'Do I seem to stop breathing, then catch my breath, during the night?' If the answer is yes, or if you wake up tired despite a full night of rest, you may have obstructive sleep apnoea, which makes your risk of high blood pressure up to seven times higher than normal. In one large study, having mild sleep apnoea increased the risk by 2.5, and even snoring, without apnoea, doubled it. What's more, disturbed sleep raises levels of artery-constricting stress hormones in your body.

Prevention boosters

Drink coffee instead of diet cola Drinking just one diet cola drink a day raised the risk of high blood pressure by 5 per cent, and four a day increased the odds by 19 per cent in a landmark US study. Risks were even higher for women who drank cola on a regular basis. Experts can't explain the association, but suggest that coffee might be a better alternative; women who drank coffee every day had no added risk of hypertension. Coffee triggers a temporary rise in blood pressure, but it doesn't persist in those who drink coffee regularly.

Try to relax Practising meditation, yoga or another relaxation technique on a regular basis can help keep your blood pressure low. When US scientists analysed 107 studies of the effect of meditation on blood pressure, they concluded that it produces significant drops (one of the studies found a 10-point drop in systolic pressure and a 6-point drop in diastolic pressure). When other researchers tested the blood pressure of 33 people taking a yoga class that met three times a week, they found improvements after just six weeks. Average blood pressure fell from 130/79 to 125/74mmHg. Tai chi has also been shown to be effective.

Sip beetroot juice UK researchers report that drinking 480ml of beetroot juice a day can lower your blood pressure by 8 to 10 points, fast. Volunteers who sipped two 240ml glasses a day saw their pressure drop significantly after 3 hours, and stay lower for up to a day. Emerging research suggests that nitrates in beetroots (and in green leafy vegetables) keep the lining of your arteries (endothelium) supple.

Have a piece of dark chocolate When people with slightly elevated blood pressure ate about 5g (30kcal) of dark chocolate each night after dinner for 18 weeks, their blood pressure fell by two to three points. Artery-friendly compounds called flavonols may be responsible for the improvement. And dark chocolate is also a source of magnesium.

Is your diet too salty?

Most people eat double or even triple the amount of salt recommended by blood-pressure experts. You could be one of them if you answer yes to one or more of these questions.

1. Do you often eat processed foods, such as frozen dinners; packet or canned goods (including soups and vegetables); processed meats such as ham, sausages and salami; cheeses; or bottled salad dressings or sauces?
2. Do you often eat salty snack foods, such as potato crisps, salted nuts or bar snacks?
3. Do you often eat in fast-food or other restaurants?
4. Do you often add salt to your food during cooking and/or at the table?

See also:

Cause 1: *Hypertension, page 22*
Step 1: *Exercise, page 62*
Step 3: *Quit smoking, page 66*

High cholesterol

Cholesterol is necessary to make cell membranes as well as hormones, and your body produces this cholesterol. What you eat also contributes to blood cholesterol levels. Some cholesterol is 'bad' (LDL attacks arteries and contributes to plaque build-up), while some is 'good' (HDL escorts the bad cholesterol out of the body). Only about half of people who have heart attacks have high cholesterol, but it's still important to keep your levels healthy.

17%
The amount you can lower 'bad' cholesterol if you have 2 servings of soluble fibre every day.

What causes it

For most people, a high-fat diet and a sedentary lifestyle combine to raise levels of LDL and reduce those of HDL. Cholesterol levels also rise with age. Your genes play a role, too: a few people inherit a genetic mutation that raises total blood cholesterol to dangerously high levels.

Key prevention strategies

Eat less saturated fat This is the fat found in fatty meat, butter, cheese and dairy ice cream. To reduce your risk of heart attack, switch to skinless chicken breasts, olive or rapeseed oil, oily fish and low-fat dairy foods. Experts estimate that every 5 per cent increase in consumption of saturated fat raises your risk of heart disease by 17 per cent. And one US study found that eating just one meal high in saturated fat had an adverse effect on the elasticity of arteries. Keep your daily intake of saturated fat to less than 10 per cent of your daily calorie intake – that's an intake of 20g for women and 30g for men – and you could lower your LDL by 9 to 11 per cent.

Avoid foods with 'hydrogenated' on the label Read the back of a packet of crisps or biscuits, crackers, cakes or pastries, and you may well see 'partially hydrogenated oil' on the list. These oils, also known as trans fats, extend the shelf life of a product, but they can spell disaster by raising LDL and triglycerides, reducing HDL, and increasing your risk of having a heart attack. In one study of 50 men with healthy cholesterol levels, eating trans fats for five weeks raised LDL 5 per cent and lowered HDL a heart-damaging 11 per cent.

Food served in restaurants and at fast-food chains – especially fried food – can also be high in trans fats; ask how food is cooked before you order it,

Cholesterol targets

Total cholesterol Under 4.0mmol/1.

LDL ('bad' cholesterol) Under 2.5mmol/l for people at higher risk, and under 3.0 mmol/l for those at lower risk.

HDL ('good' cholesterol) Over 1.0mmol/l.

Triglycerides Like cholesterol, these blood fats are dangerous to the heart. Ideal levels are below 2.0mmol/l.

Note: Any reduction in total or LDL cholesterol, or increase in HDL cholesterol, is likely to be of benefit, even if the desired targets aren't reached.

The heart-friendly fruit

If you haven't yet discovered the rich, creamy flavour of avocados, it's time you did. Slice one up and enjoy a few pieces as a snack, add it to a salad or use it in sandwiches or to make a delicious guacamole dip. In a study from Mexico's Instituto Mexicano del Seguro Social, women and men who ate one avocado a day for a week reduced their total cholesterol levels by 17 per cent. 'Bad' LDL cholesterol fell, and 'good' HDL rose. The reason? Avocados are rich in heart-healthy monounsaturated fat and contain significant amounts of beta-sitosterol, an ingredient of some cholesterol-lowering margarines.

and find out what oils are used and how often they're replenished. Even if they have made the switch to healthier oils, fried food is still generally too high in fat and calories to eat safely except on the odd occasion.

Stop smoking Smoking depresses levels of HDL cholesterol by 7 to 20 per cent and at the same time can raise your LDL cholesterol 70 per cent, according to one analysis of several studies. It also unleashes toxic chemicals that make LDL more dangerous to your arteries. By giving up smoking, you'll see benefits surprisingly quickly: blood levels of heart-protecting HDL bounce back within a month or two of making this one change.

Eat oats or pulses every day These 'superfoods' are packed with a type of soluble fibre called beta-glucan. It acts like a sponge, trapping cholesterol-rich bile acids in your intestines so they can be eliminated before they have the chance to raise your cholesterol. Whole grains such as wholemeal bread and brown rice, which are rich in insoluble fibre, just can't perform that trick. In one study of 36 overweight men, those who ate two large servings of foods rich in soluble fibre every day lowered their LDL by 17 per cent. Here are three delicious ways to include more soluble fibre in your diet:

○ **Have porridge for breakfast** Oats contain more soluble fibre than any other grain. Having just two servings of porridge a day can lower your cholesterol by 2 to 3 per cent. You can increase the benefit by adding grated apple – also rich in soluble fibre.

○ **Serve pearl barley instead of rice** In a US study from the Beltsville Human Nutrition Research Center, 25 people with slightly high cholesterol who ate pearl barley daily for several weeks saw their LDL drop significantly.

Symptoms to watch for

Usually none. If you have an inherited tendency to high cholesterol known as familial hypercholesterolaemia, you may develop small, bumpy cholesterol deposits on your elbows, knees and buttocks. If you have them, get your cholesterol checked; diet and exercise can help, but it's likely you'll need medication to bring levels back down to normal.

Latest thinking

Don't worry (too much) about cholesterol (as opposed to fat) in food. Studies show that for most people, foods such as eggs and prawns won't raise LDL cholesterol. US researchers have found, for example, that eating up to seven eggs a week doesn't raise LDL levels. And despite the fact that 12 large prawns contain 200mg of cholesterol, a US study found that while people who ate prawns did experience a slight rise in LDL levels, their cholesterol ratios improved because HDL rose even higher and levels of triglycerides fell.

○ **Combine the benefits** Try to eat a combination of soya protein, almonds, oats, barley and plant sterols at the same meal. Studies show that this can reduce LDL by 28 per cent in people with high cholesterol who also have a diet low in saturated fats.

Snack on nuts It may seem odd, since nuts are fatty, but they really are excellent for your cholesterol levels, thanks in part to the cholesterol-lowering monounsaturated fats they contain. Choosing a handful of almonds instead of a cake, crisps or biscuits for your afternoon snack every day could cut LDL cholesterol by nearly 10 per cent. A bonus is that vitamin E in the almond's 'meat' plus flavonoids in its papery skin protect LDL from oxidation, a process that is the first step in the development of artery-clogging plaque.

If you want to raise your HDL at the same time, choose walnuts. 'Bad' cholesterol fell 10 per cent and 'good' cholesterol rose 18 per cent when 58 women and men in one study snacked on about 14 walnut halves a day for six months.

Nuts are high in calories, so control the portions. A 15g/90kcal serving is about 12 almonds, 8 whole cashews, 8 pecans, 26 pistachios or 7 walnut halves. Limiting yourself to a small handful of any type of nut is a good rule of thumb when it comes to portion control.

Feast on fruit, double your vegetables Eating nine servings of fruit and vegetables a day can reduce your LDL by as much as 7 per cent. Researchers aren't sure why, but it could be because of soluble fibre, which blocks the reabsorption of cholesterol found in the bile acids (digestive juices) that make their way into your intestines. This effectively lowers your LDL levels. Apples, pears and prunes are all good fruit sources of soluble fibre. Or it could be that people who tend to eat lots of fresh fruit and vegetables also eat less fatty meat, snacks and desserts.

Get moving to boost good cholesterol Recently, doctors have discovered that having high levels of 'good' cholesterol is every bit as important as having low levels of the 'bad' kind. Aerobic exercise, whether it's walking, swimming, cycling or even working hard in your garden, can raise HDL by 5 to 10 per cent. If you're also following a healthy diet, adding exercise can nudge LDL down 0.075 to 0.4 points, other studies suggest. A recent Japanese study of 1,400 people found that those who took a 40 minute brisk walk four times a week raised their HDL by about 0.05 points – enough to reduce the risk of heart disease by about 6 per cent. For raising HDL, longer workouts are better than several short ones.

Mind over cholesterol?

Stress can raise levels of 'bad' LDL cholesterol – and relaxation exercises such as yoga and tai chi can lower them, studies suggest. In one study of 113 people with heart disease, researchers from India report that those who added regular yoga sessions to a healthy diet lowered their LDL by 26 per cent after one year. If yoga isn't your thing, try to find another soothing activity.

Prevention boosters

Have up to two glasses of alcohol a day, with food Studies suggest that people who drink alcohol in moderation (no more than two units a day, for both men and women, with food) get a double cholesterol benefit. In one study, one drink a day lowered LDL nearly 0.2 points. Drinking moderately also increases HDL; in one Dutch study, HDL was shown to rise by a respectable 7 per cent for moderate drinkers.

Get trim Losing about 6 per cent of your body weight – about 9lbs (4kg) if you now weigh 14 stone (70kg) – could lower your LDL by 12 per cent and raise your HDL by 18 per cent, researchers say. The best weight-loss strategy for making your cholesterol levels healthier is a relatively low-fat diet with lots of fresh fruit, vegetables and unsaturated fat from fish, nuts and olive and rapeseed oils. Don't go for an extremely low-fat diet: while research shows that this approach can make plaque in arteries shrink, a very strict low-fat regime is often difficult to follow. And plenty of studies show that a moderate-fat diet not only protects your heart well, but is also much more pleasurable and therefore easier to stick to.

Lower your LDL with plant sterols and stanols These natural compounds, found in cholesterol-lowering margarine spreads, block the absorption of some cholesterol in your intestines. In one study, people with normal cholesterol levels who used margarine spreads fortified with sterols, such as Flora pro-activ or Benecol, saw their LDL cholesterol decrease 7 to 11 per cent after three months. Experts recommend an intake of up to 2g of sterols and stanols a day, about the amount in 2 tablespoons of fortified margarine. Eat an extra serving of red, yellow or orange fruit or vegetables a day if you use these cholesterol-lowering spreads, as they can reduce absorption of heart-friendly compounds called carotenoids from foods you eat.

See also:

Cause 1: Bad cholesterol balance, page 30
Step 7: Cut back on saturated fat, page 72

Hip fractures

The most common reason for hip fractures is falling, particularly if you're 65 or older. In fact, about 1 per cent of all falls in older people result in hip fractures. This kind of injury means more than time lost to healing or surgery; it also increases the risk of dying during the following year by 20 to 36 per cent. There are two main ways to prevent hip fractures: prevent falls and maintain your bone density so that if you *do* fall, you wind up with a bruised – not broken – hip.

19%
The amount you can cut your risk of fractures by taking daily calcium and vitamin D supplements.

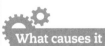

What causes it

Ninety-five per cent of hip fractures are due to falls. Fractures are most common in older people because they are more likely to have lower bone density, making their bones more likely to break.

Symptoms to watch for

Dizziness and problems with your vision are warnings that you are at risk from falls. While osteoporosis has few symptoms, any fracture after the age of 50 is a warning sign that you may have a bone-density problem. If you do fracture your hip, you'll have pain and be unable to walk.

Key prevention strategies

Take a daily calcium and vitamin D supplement Aim for a total intake of 1,200mg of calcium (taken in two doses) and a minimum of 1,000IU of vitamin D. (Anyone with darker skin and/or living in northern climates needs 2,000IU of vitamin D a day). This combination of nutrients provides a two-pronged attack on the bone-thinning disease osteoporosis, which weakens bones (see page 288). One analysis of eight studies found that these supplements reduced the risk of hip fractures by 19 per cent. Vitamin D may even help to prevent falls. One large study found that women with low blood levels of this vitamin were 77 per cent more likely to fall than women with normal levels.

Get walking Weak legs can increase your risk of falling fourfold. Boost your leg strength with that most basic yet effective exercise: walking. Aim to walk for at least 30 minutes a day on most days. To further protect yourself, add a few lunges and squats to your programme. Another good form of exercise for improving balance and leg strength is tai chi. Studies find it effective for improving balance, strengthening legs and reducing the risk of falls.

Get your vision checked You're two and a half times more likely to fall if you have problems with your eyesight than if you don't. This means getting the right prescription for your glasses or having your cataracts removed could prevent a broken hip.

Ask your doctor to review your medication Certain drugs, including tranquillisers, some antidepressants, anti-arrhythmic drugs, digoxin (used to treat congestive heart failure) and diuretics significantly increase the risk of a fall. What's more, regardless of what they are, if you take three or more medicines, you're also more likely to fall than someone who takes fewer. But never stop taking a prescription drug without talking to your GP first.

Get rid of clutter Rugs, plants and coffee tables filled with pictures and knick-knacks can all trip you up. If you find it hard to tackle this problem on your own, ask friends or family for help in decluttering your house. There are professional decluttering services that can help, too. For ideas and advice, visit www.cluttergone.co.uk.

Prevention boosters

Install bright bulbs No matter how good your eyesight is, if it's too dark to clearly see obstacles in your way, you're heading for a fall. Make sure all reading lamps have at least 60-watt (11-watt low-energy equivalent) bulbs, but preferably install 75-watt (15-watt low-energy) bulbs; put 100-watt (18-watt low-energy) bulbs in all overhead fixtures and turn on the main light when you enter a room.

Check your mood Are you depressed? If you are, see your GP. Depression doubles your risk of falling. Researchers don't know why, but it could be related to paying less attention, drinking more alcohol, eating less food, or even side effects of medication.

Sip water all day Although the old target of drinking eight glasses of water a day is no longer considered essential, staying hydrated is still important, particularly as you age. One reason is that it becomes harder to recognise thirst as you get older; also, many older people don't want to drink too much because they're afraid they might not make it to the toilet in time. (If that's your worry, see page 224.) Dehydration contributes to low blood pressure and dizziness, which, of course, contributes to falls. A good strategy is to keep a water bottle with you and make it a point to empty it by the time you go to the bathroom.

Strap on some hip pads Sold at some pharmacies and online, these are worn over the hips but under clothing. An analysis of 11 studies found they could reduce the risk of hip fractures in nursing-home patients by 23 per cent.

Latest thinking

Research has suggested that intravenous infusion of zoledronic acid (Zometa), a drug used to treat bone loss in cancer patients, could be helpful for reducing bone loss –and therefore hip fractures – following a stroke. However, further research is needed to confirm these results.

See also:

Cause 3: *Depression*, page 26
Exercises: *Better balance*, page 330
Joint strength, page 334

Hot flushes

A hot flush usually begins as warmth in the chest region, then slowly rises up into your neck and face. And just a few minutes later, you're chilled and shivering. Mimicking a fever, hot flushes are a symptom that some 80 per cent of women experience as they go through menopause. Most women aren't overly bothered by them, but for some, hot flushes and their nocturnal counterparts – night sweats – can make life miserable and difficult. Here are some ideas how you can try to keep hot flushes to a minimum.

up to **90**%
The amount by which hormone replacement therapy could reduce hot flushes.

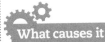

What causes it

Fluctuating levels of oestrogen. These fluctuations affect the temperature-control system in the brain so that it overreacts to minimal changes in temperature by dilating blood vessels in a mistaken attempt to cool down.

Key prevention strategies

Take hormone replacement therapy (HRT) Nothing works as well as oestrogen supplements to prevent hot flushes, with studies finding it reduces episodes by up to 90 per cent. The key is to take the lowest possible dose for the shortest possible time. Although a major study found higher rates of breast cancer, heart disease and stroke in women who took an oestrogen-plus-progesterone medication (progesterone is included with oestrogen therapy to reduce the risk of uterine cancer) and higher rates of stroke in women who took an oestrogen-only medication, major medical organisations say it's safe to use HRT in the short term (up to five years) to get you through the worst of the menopausal transition. The risks of any associated health problems are low if you're under sixty.

Take a supplement Many supplements have been investigated for possible hot flush-fighting activity, but few proved effective, despite promising initial results. Options include herbs such as black cohosh, dong quai and chasteberry, and supplements containing phyto-oestrogens, such as those based on soya products, which contain isoflavones or aglycones, or those containing red clover extracts. Phyto-oestrogens are similar in some ways to natural oestrogens and, like them, may increase breast cancer risk. Of all the supplements investigated to date, black cohosh has the best evidence to support its use, but even here the evidence is weak and there is a small risk of serious liver damage.

Antidepressant benefits Researchers trying to find non-oestrogen options to relieve hot flushes in women with breast cancer stumbled onto the benefits of certain antidepressants prescribed in lower-than-normal doses. These include fluoxetine (Prozac) and paroxetine (Seroxat).

Studies find they can reduce the number of hot flushes by up to 63 per cent compared to a placebo. So if you are also depressed, discuss medication with your GP. You may be able to gain a double benefit.

Prevention boosters

Lose fat, gain muscle Researchers used to think that having a bit of extra padding would actually reduce hot flushes because hormones in body fat called androgens are converted to oestrogen, which helps to prevent hot flushes. It turns out they were wrong. A study of women aged 47 to 59 found that those with the highest percentages of body fat were about 27 per cent more likely to have hot flushes than those with lower percentages. Ideally, aim for body fat levels below 33 per cent (but above 5 per cent). There are devices you can buy to measure your body fat percentage; your gym may have one. Your doctor can also perform a more accurate test.

While losing weight will certainly reduce your overall body fat, strength training is your best option for building muscle and therefore changing your body fat percentage. Consider investing in a couple of sessions with a personal trainer to get you started.

Take up yoga Australian research suggests yoga may be an effective and inexpensive way to control hot flushes. But don't forget to tell your instructor about any pre-existing injuries you may have.

Consider vitamin E Studies into its benefits for preventing hot flushes have mixed results, but one recent study in which 51 women received either 400IU of vitamin E or a placebo found that those taking vitamin E had about two fewer hot flushes a day compared to when they took a placebo, and the flushes they did have were less severe. High doses may increase stroke risk, so talk with your doctor before taking a vitamin E supplement, and don't take more than 400IU daily.

Symptoms to watch for

A feeling of warmth, flushing, heavy perspiration. When hot flushes occur at night, they can disrupt sleep.

Latest thinking

Ultra-low doses of oestrogen – as little as 25 per cent of the dose previously used – can still significantly improve a woman's hot flushes.

223

Incontinence

This emabarrassing problem is remarkably common – even in relatively young people. The reality is that it affects up to 25 per cent of women and 5 per cent of men under 65, and much higher numbers of those who are older. Yet there is plenty you can do to prevent or minimise this troublesome condition. Follow these recommendations to avoid embarrassment and incovenience and stay dry.

81%
The amount by which you could reduce your risk of incontinence by doing pelvic-floor exercises several times a day.

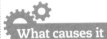
What causes it

There are numerous causes, ranging from urinary tract infections and pregnancy to being overweight. Over time, particularly after the menopause, bladder muscles can thin and weaken. In men, prostate surgery can lead to incontinence. And in both men and women, weak pelvic-floor muscles often play a role.

Key prevention strategies

Do pelvic-floor exercises every day These exercises strengthen the pelvic-floor muscles, which help control the release of urine. The stronger the muscles are, the less likely you are to have an accident. In fact, these exercises are even better than medication at reducing existing incontinence. They are particularly effective for pregnant women and for men who have undergone surgery for prostate cancer.

You can do them anytime, anywhere because no one knows you're doing them. First, work out which muscles to target by stopping in midstream when you're urinating. The muscles you use to do this are your pelvic-floor muscles. Squeeze those muscles and hold for a count of ten. Relax, then repeat. Perform at least three sets of ten contractions a day. If you're unsure whether you're doing them properly, check with your doctor or a physiotherapist – doing them incorrectly can worsen any existing problems.

Eat smaller portions Studies find that losing weight is one of the most effective ways, next to pelvic-floor exercises, to prevent incontinence. Always serve appropriate-sized portions onto your dinner plate and leave the serving dish on the worktop or elsewhere in the kitchen – not on the dinner table, where you may be tempted to have seconds. Another trick is to use the smallest dinner plates you own. The plate will look full, so it doesn't seem as if you're eating a reduced amount.

Put your bladder on a schedule Doctors think one reason for incontinence is that some people tend to urinate too often. This can reduce the amount your bladder is able to hold and teaches your bladder muscles to send 'must go' signals even when the bladder is barely half full. If you find yourself going every hour or two, try bladder training.

*" **Weight loss** is one of the most **effective** ways to prevent incontinence. "*

Numerous studies find that this approach, which strengthens bladder muscles, improves incontinence, so there's good reason to think it could help prevent it in the first place.

One way to train your bladder is to start out by going to the toilet every hour whether you have to or not. The next day, go every hour and a half. Continue to increase the time between toilet visits by 30 minutes a day until you're going every few hours, or whatever time frame works best for you to prevent incontinence.

Prevention boosters

Avoid caffeine If you're a tea drinker, you're more likely to develop incontinence, according to a large Norwegian study. It may or may not be due to the caffeine; researchers suspect that tea contains other chemicals that contribute to incontinence, although they don't yet know what they are. However, there is a link between caffeine and incontinence if you drink more than 4 cups of caffeine-containing drinks a day.

Avoid a hysterectomy Studies suggest that women who have a hysterectomy (removal of the womb), one of the most common types of gynaecological surgery, are twice as likely to later require surgery for urinary incontinence than women who don't have this operation. Some hysterectomies may be unnecessary, so if your doctor recommends one, ask about other options and get a second opinion.

Symptoms to watch for

Releasing small amounts of urine when you laugh, sneeze, cough or otherwise exert yourself and/or a sudden urge to urinate that you may or may not be able to control until you get to the toilet.

Latest thinking

An injection of botulinum A (Botox) into the bladder muscle can improve incontinence even in people who haven't responded to medication or other treatments.

Infertility

Within a year of trying, nine out of ten healthy young couples will conceive. The others, however, face the possibility of needing medical help for one or both partners, and infertility may be due to a combination of factors unique to a couple. The advice below for reducing the risk of infertility includes options for both men and women.

30%
The reduction in the time it could take to get pregnant if you floss regularly.

What causes it

In women, common causes include problems with ovulation, such as polycystic ovary syndrome (PCOS), blocked fallopian tubes and endometriosis, in which uterine tissue grows outside the uterus. In men, the most common causes are slow sperm, low sperm count and malformed sperm.

Key prevention strategies

Start trying to conceive early The odds of getting pregnant plummet with age. In men, the decline in fertility usually begins in the early forties, when their sperm start to move more slowly. Women are most fertile between 19 and 26, when they have a one-in-two chance of getting pregnant if they have sex when they're most fertile (typically, two days after ovulating). A woman aged 35 to 39 has only about a one in three chance of getting pregnant during that time, and less if her partner is at least five years older.

Maintain a healthy weight In women, obesity plays havoc with reproductive hormones, more than doubling the risk of infertility and making it ten times more likely to take longer than usual to get pregnant. In men, a 22lb (10kg) weight gain increases the risk of infertility by about 10 per cent. Consider a high-protein, low-carbohydrate approach to weight loss, which several studies suggest works best for returning reproductive hormones to their normal levels.

Quit smoking Smoking is definitely out for women trying to conceive, but it also reduces a man's fertility. This is because smoking creates free radicals (molecules that damage healthy cells) and therefore has a negative impact on the number of sperm that are made and how fast they swim.

Brush and floss your teeth daily Women who are trying to get pregnant should make sure they look after their dental hygiene. A Swedish study

Boxers or briefs?

As it turns out, it probably doesn't matter. For a long time, experts advised men to switch to boxer shorts since briefs, which are tighter, trap more heat in the groin area. This heat was thought to cause a drop in sperm count, but recent studies discount this theory. Researchers measured scrotal temperatures among 97 men who wore either boxers or briefs and found that those who wore boxers were just as warm as those who wore briefs.

suggests that gum disease can lengthen the time it takes for a woman to become pregnant. Those who flossed regularly reduced the time it took to get pregnant by 30 per cent. This may be because of the low-grade inflammation created by infected gums.

Prevention boosters

Chill out It's not clear whether stress contributes to infertility or vice versa, but studies find that infertile women who seek help from assisted reproductive techniques such as in-vitro fertilisation (IVF) have much higher levels of stress hormones than women who aren't infertile. Studies also find higher levels of stress hormones in women with disturbances in their menstrual cycles that could affect fertility.

Switch from wine to water Women trying to become pregnant shouldn't wait until they conceive to stop drinking alcohol. One study of healthy women, who were not alcoholics, found that those who had more than three drinks a day had disrupted menstrual cycles and temporary infertility.

Consider some supplements A German study of 7,900 women found that taking a daily multivitamin for a month before trying to become pregnant increased women's fertility rate by 5 per cent compared to taking a placebo. Studies have also found improved fertility in men and women who take vitamin C supplements. In men, taking daily supplements of 200-1,000mg of vitamin C increases sperm production. Buy a vitamin C supplement that contains flavonoids; the two together may work better than either alone to reduce oxidative damage to sperm. In women, the amount required was 750mg a day. But don't take more than 500mg in a single dose, as your body can't absorb more than that.

Men should also consider taking selenium and vitamin E. A study of 54 infertile men found that those who took supplements of 400IU of vitamin E and 225mcg of selenium for three months had healthier, faster sperm. Talk to your GP before taking any supplements.

Get regular screenings Women who have multiple sexual partners should be screened at least annually for sexually transmitted infections (STIs) that can result in pelvic inflammatory disease. This can create scarring of the fallopian tubes, which can prevent conception. Men should be checked regularly for inflammation of the prostate gland as this can also lead to damaged sperm.

Symptoms to watch for

If you are under 35 and have been trying to get pregnant for a year or more with no success, or if you're 35 or older and have been trying for at least six months, you should see a doctor. Also see a doctor if you or your partner has any known fertility risk factors (such as previous cancer treatment, endometriosis, blocked fallopian tubes, etc.) or other reproductive-system disorders (uterine fibroids or ovarian cysts, or testicular problems in men).

Latest thinking

Chlamydia reproduces inside the early bundle of cells that forms after conception and replicates. This hinders the cells' production of oestrogen and progesterone, hormones needed to maintain the pregnancy. This can lead to early miscarriage.

See also:

Step 3: *Quit smoking*, page 66
Step 8: *Reduce chronic stress*, page 74

Inflammatory bowel disease

Inflammatory bowel disease (IBD) encompasses two painful and sometimes life-threatening conditions: ulcerative colitis and Crohn's disease. Both trigger chronic inflammation of the intestinal system, leading to pain, sometimes-debilitating diarrhoea and infections. For many, surgery to remove parts of the intestines brings relief. While most cases of IBD begin in young adulthood, experts have noticed an increasing prevalence among people in their fifties and sixties. If you don't have IBD, the following strategies may reduce your risk of getting it, which is particularly important if close family members have it. And if you have IBD, our advice may help you avoid relapses and complications.

76%
The potential risk reduction if you eat plenty of whole grains, fish and nuts – and avoid meat and sweets.

What causes it

Inflammation of the intestines. Experts don't know what triggers it, but suspect that genetics and an immune system response – perhaps to 'unhealthy' bacteria in the intestinal tract, or perhaps to nothing at all – are responsible.

Key prevention strategies

Stop smoking Smoking cigarettes tripled the risk of Crohn's disease in one Scandinavian study of 317 sets of twins. If you already have Crohn's, continuing to smoke raises your risk of relapses and of the need for bowel surgery or aggressive medical treatment. Experts suspect that the reason for this is that smoking reduces blood flow to your intestines or somehow puts your immune system on high alert, making the intestinal walls extra sensitive. Strange as it may seem, smoking seems to slightly reduce the number of flare-ups for people with ulcerative colitis – but that's no reason to light up. Smoking is devastating for your health in every other way.

Eat more vegetables, fruit, olive oil, fish, grains and nuts
Eat less red meat and fatty foods (such as burgers and fry-ups). Canadian researchers who studied 400 children found that those who had diets high in fruit and vegetables, whole grains and 'good' fats from fish, nuts and olive oil cut their IBD risk by three quarters compared to those whose diets included more meat, saturated fats and sweets. Eating an unhealthy diet raised risk nearly five times higher than normal, according to researchers from the University of Montreal.

When the scientists looked more closely, they found that the most protective dietary components were fibre (fruit, vegetables and whole grains) and omega-3 fatty acids. You'll find those in fish, walnuts, freshly ground flaxseeds (linseeds), rapeseed oil and, if you can't eat a source of 'good' fats every day, in fish-oil capsules.

" *Be sure to drink* **plenty of clear fluids** *every day.* "

Kick the sugar habit Many people are addicted to sugar and don't even realise how much they're consuming. Instead of a biscuit or chocolate bar in the afternoon or cake for dessert, have fresh fruit instead. Eating more fruit cut the risk of IBD in several studies, while eating more desserts and refined sugar tripled the odds of developing Crohn's disease and ulcerative colitis. In one study, people who developed Crohn's reported eating twice as much refined sugar in the months and years before their diagnosis as people who did not suffer from this painful condition.

Use pain relievers sparingly Aspirin and other nonsteroidal anti-inflammatory pain relievers such as ibuprofen (Nurofen) can raise the risk of a relapse of IBD, probably because they can damage the lining of the upper intestinal tract. In one study 28 per cent of people with IBD who took these medications had a relapse within nine days. If you have arthritis or another painful chronic condition as well as IBD or if you just need occasional relief for a headache, talk to your doctor about your options. There's some evidence that paracetamol and the prescription pain reliever celecoxib (Celebrex) don't trigger relapses.

Cut back on red meat and processed meats When researchers at the University of Newcastle in the UK followed 191 people with ulcerative colitis for one year, they found that those who ate red meat (roasts, hamburgers and steaks) and processed meats (sausages, bacon and salami) most frequently were five times more likely to have painful relapses than those who ate very little of these foods.

Limit your alcohol intake In the same UK study, people who drank the most alcohol were four times more likely to have relapses of ulcerative colitis compared to those who drank little, if any, alcohol.

Avoid cola drinks and chocolate When researchers from the Netherlands checked on the eating habits and relapse rates of 688 people with IBD and 616 people without it, they discovered that both cola and

Got the gene?

Having a parent or sibling with Crohn's disease raises your own risk six times higher than that of the population as a whole; having a close family member with ulcerative colitis raises your risk two and a half times. Scientists have begun to identify the genes behind IBD, and they hope their discoveries will yield new treatments. In a study of nearly 2,000 people, US researchers have uncovered a genetic variation that appears to play an important role in raising risk. Those with an 'unhealthy' version of a gene called IL23R were two to four times more likely to develop IBD than those with a 'healthy' variant. This gene helps to regulate inflammation, the core problem in IBD.

chocoate were linked to health problems. Drinking cola and nibbling on chocolate doubled the risk of developing both ulcerative colitis and Crohn's disease.

Prevention boosters

Snack on yoghurt Your intestines are home to millions of bacteria. Some of them are there to help digest the food you eat and keep your bowels healthy. But 'unhealthy' bacteria may contribute to or even cause IBD problems. Having enough beneficial bacteria in your body keeps the unhealthy types in check. You can make sure you have sufficient by eating yoghurt that contains active cultures or by taking a probiotic ('healthy' bacteria) supplement.

When researchers at the University of Alberta in Canada gave a probiotic supplement to 34 people with mild to moderate ulcerative colitis, 53 per cent felt completely better after eight weeks, and 24 per cent felt somewhat better. The supplement, called VSL, contained eight species of lactobacillus bacteria, a type also found in yoghurt with live active cultures. In another study, researchers found that when people with ulcerative colitis and Crohn's disease ate yoghurt every day for a month, blood tests showed that inflammation levels in their intestinal tracts were reduced. Some studies suggest that probiotics are more helpful for preventing relapses of ulcerative colitis but are less helpful for Crohn's.

Take a break Stress doesn't cause IBD, but it may make it worse. Some studies suggest that stress increases levels of inflammation in the intestines and that the inflammation persists even when your stress levels are reduced. It makes sense to find time to unwind on a regular basis, in whatever way works for you – spending time in the garden, practising yoga, taking a hot bath or breathing deeply as you let tension flow out of your body.

Protect your bones

As many as 60 per cent of people with IBD may have low bone density, raising the risk of bone fractures. The reason is that long-term use of steroid medications (such as prednisone and cortisone) to reduce intestinal inflammation can also interfere with your body's ability to maintain healthy bones. And if you have severe IBD or have had surgery to remove part of your intestines, your body may not absorb enough calcium and vitamin D, nutrients needed for strong bones.

It's a good idea for everyone to aim for an intake of 1,000mg of calcium a day (1,200mg a day after the age of 50). You'll get this with three servings of low-fat dairy foods a day or a mix of dairy plus calcium supplements (don't have more than 600mg in a single meal, since your body can't absorb more than that at once). And aim for 800IU of vitamin D daily if your skin isn't regularly exposed to sunlight, to help your body absorb and use all that calcium. Weight-bearing exercise such as walking also helps. Talk to your GP about whether you need a bone density test or bone-strengthening medications.

Drink lots of water If you already have IBD, you're at risk of dehydration due to frequent and severe diarrhoea, which flushes fluid from your body. Be sure to drink plenty of fluids every day; some experts recommend 30ml a day for each kilo of body weight. If you weigh around 11 stone (70kg), that's about 2 litres of water or other clear fluids a day. And watch for signs of dehydration such as a dry mouth, extreme thirst or weakness.

Avoid dietary irritants If you have Crohn's disease that isn't improving, cutting back on sources of insoluble fibre – whole-grain bread, fruit and vegetable skins, nuts and seeds – could give your intestinal tract the break it needs. Instead, eat more soluble fibre (see below). However, consult your doctor before eliminating foods from your diet. It's important to make sure that the diet you're getting is nutritionally balanced.

For ulcerative colitis, consider soluble fibre Soluble fibre forms a protective gel in your intestinal tract and releases compounds that soothe inflammation and promote healing of the intestinal wall. Ask your doctor if you should eat foods such as potato salad (with the skin off), barley, porridge and cooked pulses, or if you would be better off trying a soluble-fibre supplement such as psyllium (Metamucil).

Watch your reaction to dairy foods An estimated 35 per cent of people with Crohn's disease and 12 to 20 per cent of those with ulcerative colitis are lactose-intolerant (lactose is a sugar found in milk and milk products). If milk, ice cream or cheese cause discomfort, try low-lactose milk (available from some supermarkets and health food shops). Yoghurt and hard cheeses are usually low in lactose.

Symptoms to watch for

Diarrhoea, which can range from slightly loose stools to dozens of liquid bowel movements per day, abdominal pain and cramping, blood or mucus in the stool, lack of appetite and weight loss. You may also have fatigue, night sweats and/or fever.

Latest thinking

If you have Crohn's disease or ulcerative colitis, your risk of developing colon cancer is up to five times higher than normal. Experts recommend early checks for this cancer, with a colonoscopy eight to ten years after you first have IBD symptoms.

See also:

Cause 6: Inflammation, page 32
Step 2: Fruit and vegetables, page 64

Insomnia

Having trouble falling asleep may seem minor, but insomnia raises the risk of depression, makes you more sensitive to pain, compromises concentration and memory, and significantly increases the risk of driving accidents. There's even evidence that it wreaks havoc with hormones that control appetite and metabolism, and may be partly responsible for obesity. The following advice should help to prevent or combat sleep problems.

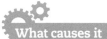

What causes it

Anyone can have trouble falling asleep at times of stress. Other causes include chronic pain, depression and anxiety disorders. You might also be inadvertently causing insomnia by worrying so much about whether you'll fall asleep that it becomes self-fulfilling.

Key prevention strategies

Stick to a regular sleep schedule That means going to bed at the same time every night and waking up at the same time in the morning, even on weekends. Think of it as training your body to fall asleep when it should.

Create the perfect sleeping environment If you have bills stacked on your bedside table or piles of laundry collecting around the bed, your bedroom is hardly an oasis for sleep. Clear the clutter, then remove the TV and computer from the bedroom, because to encourage good sleep, bedrooms should be used only for sleeping and intimate time with your partner. Don't eat or work in there, either. Don't even talk on the phone in your bedroom. This way, when you enter the room at night, you are conditioned to expect to go to sleep.

If your windows let in too much light, it may also help to invest in light-excluding curtains or blinds. And keep the room cool, but not too cold, which also helps to induce sleep.

Limit your time in bed The harder you try to fall asleep, the less likely you are to succeed. If you haven't fallen asleep within 15 minutes, get out of bed and move to another room. Do something quiet, such as reading or knitting, until you feel sleepy enough to nod off, then go back to bed. Continue this pattern until you finally fall asleep.

Go to the gym or take a jog One of the best ways to get a good night's sleep is to exercise. A study by the American Sleep Disorders Association found that depressed older people who exercised with weights three times a week experienced a 51 per cent improvement in their sleep

51%
The possible improvement in sleep quality if you exercise three times a week.

quality. Other studies have found that athletes who miss out exercise for just one day experience worse sleep and an increase in the time they take to fall asleep.

Most researchers think that exercise reduces insomnia, in part, by raising body temperature. If you exercise vigorously enough to raise your temperature in the late afternoon, it will fall around bedtime – and a drop in body temperature naturally triggers sleep. Exercise also helps by reducing stress hormones. Most people with insomnia have high levels of these hormones, or they release them with very little provocation. Exercise initially increases levels of these hormones, but a few hours later, seeking to return to balance, your body sends out signals to reduce them. That's why you shouldn't exercise in the evening; try to end your workout at least 6 hours before bedtime.

Spend time outside Exercise can improve sleep, and outside activities in bright sunlight can have an even greater effect by ensuring that your body clock is properly set. In one study, people who received 30 minutes a day of bright light therapy with full-spectrum lamps that mimic sunlight (available online and from lighting shops) increased their total sleep time by 44 minutes.

Prevention boosters

Talk to a therapist A form of treatment called cognitive behavioural therapy (CBT) can help with insomnia by teaching you techniques to overcome it – and your anxiety about it. For instance, after a few sleepless nights, many people begin to worry about their ability to ever fall asleep, starting what becomes a self-perpetuating cycle. They may also underestimate how much sleep they actually get and overestimate how much time they spend lying awake feeling anxious about how to fall asleep. CBT helps put things into perspective by teaching you more about insomnia and how to address it.

Limit alcohol intake While alcohol may help you fall asleep, you're likely to wake up again as the effects wear off and find yourself unable to fall back to sleep. If you want a drink, have it in the late afternoon or early evening.

Stay away from cigarettes Nicotine is a central nervous system stimulant, which means it keeps you awake. Even just being around cigarette smoke within a couple of hours of bedtime could interfere with your ability to fall asleep or stay asleep.

Symptoms to watch for

An inability to fall asleep or stay asleep, or waking up too early in the morning. Trouble falling asleep may be related to anxiety, whereas waking up too early could be related to depression. Watch out for daytime sleepiness and snoring; the two together are often a sign of sleep apnoea, which contributes to many medical conditions.

233

Latest thinking

Treating the insomnia that exists alongside another medical or mental health conditions not only relieves the sleeplessness but can actually improve the coexisting condition. However, most doctors still treat only the coexisting condition, believing that once it improves, so will the insomnia.

Check your medications Numerous medications, particularly some prescribed for high blood pressure, asthma, underactive thyroid, depression, attention deficit disorder (ADD) and neurological problems such as Parkinson's disease, can keep you awake at night. If you're having trouble drifting off or staying asleep throughout the night, ask your doctor whether one of your medications may be to blame and what you can do about it.

Consider a sleeping pill To prevent occasional insomnia, sleeping pills can help and, if you use them only for the short term, probably won't hurt. Ask your doctor if one of the newer prescription sleeping drugs such as zaleplon (Sonata) or zolpidem (Stilnoct) might be suitable in your

Ten ways to fall asleep

1. Sip chamomile tea before bedtime

2. Cover your eyes You can find eye masks in most pharmacies. They can work wonders and banish even the tiniest glow of a night-light.

3. Don't overheat your bedroom Keep your bedroom cooler than your sitting room. If it's hot, open the windows. A reduction in your body temperature prompts your brain to release the sleep hormone melatonin.

4. Read a book of poetry The cadences of the lines can be much more calming than a novel. Better still, listen to poetry on CD or an MP3 player – it's almost like hearing a bedtime story.

5. Make a list Before you get into bed, make a list of everything that's on your mind. Then you don't have to lie awake worrying about it.

6. Listen to white noise Tune in to radio static or buy a white-noise machine.

7. Spray lavender scent on your bed linen Lavender is known for its calming effects.

8. Try progressive muscle relaxation Starting with your feet and working up to your eyes, tense and relax one group of muscles at a time. This forces every muscle in your body to relax.

9. Wear the right nightclothes Keep warm nighties and pyjamas for the coldest nights only. Choose light fabrics for the warmer summer nights.

10. Wear earplugs They block out any noise from the street or from your partner's snoring.

> **" Soothing music** *really could succeed in sending you off to* **sleep. "**

case. Be aware, though, that all sleeping pills carry the risk of 'hangover' drowsiness the following day, which could affect your ability to drive or perform other activities that demand close concentration.

Get treated for allergies Sneezing because of pollen and other seasonal allergens may keep you up at night. French researchers found that about 42 per cent of people with seasonal allergies said they had trouble falling asleep compared with around 18 per cent of those who didn't have allergies. The study also showed that the worse the allergies, the longer it took people to fall asleep.

Turn on some music A study by Taiwanese researchers compared the effects of soft music on sleep in 63 people who had trouble sleeping. Half listened to 45 minutes of music when they went to bed; half listened to nothing. The result is that those who listened to music slept better and longer, took less time to fall asleep and functioned better the next day. Overall, sleep quality improved 45 per cent in the music group compared to the control group. What's more, the group's quality of sleep improved more with each week of music.

Take an afternoon nap Long naps will only keep you up at night, but short naps could make a positive difference. A very small Japanese study found that a 30 minute nap after lunch, followed by some stretching and flexibility exercises in the early evening, significantly improved sleep quality and reduced the amount of time it took to fall asleep.

Join a tai chi class When researchers assigned 118 older adults to either a tai chi or another low-impact exercise class for three 1 hour sessions a week over 24 weeks, they found that people taking tai chi improved significantly more than the control group in quality of sleep, the time it took to fall asleep and the total time spent asleep. In fact, the tai chi participants fell asleep an average of 18 minutes faster than those in the other group and slept nearly an hour longer per night. This may be the result of improved relaxation and diaphragmatic breathing.

See also:

Cause 3: Depression, page 26
Step 5: Sleep, page 70

Irritable bowel syndrome

Irritable bowel syndrome (IBS) is a frustrating mystery. Experts say the pain, cramps, diarrhoea and constipation that characterise this problem seem to be the result of bowels that move too quickly or too slowly and nerves that become excessively sensitive to the slightest pressure after you eat a meal. The following solutions have all been found to work, but be patient – you may have to try a few to find a plan that works for you.

58%
The improvement in pain when people with IBS took enteric-coated peppermint oil.

What causes it

The root cause of IBS remains a mystery. Experts suspect that an overgrowth of bacteria, gastrointestinal infection or other factors make muscles in the intestinal wall move too quickly or too slowly; in addition, nerves in the intestines seem to become oversensitive.

Key prevention strategies

Pinpoint trouble foods Many people with IBS know from experience which foods trigger problems. Common foods include alcohol, chocolate, caffeinated drinks, dairy products and sugar-free sweeteners such as sorbitol and mannitol. People who have problems with wind and bloating may be bothered by beans, broccoli, cabbage and cauliflower, too. For others, high-fat foods can cause intestinal pain.

When researchers at St George's Hospital Medical School in London tested the blood of 132 people with IBS and 42 healthy people who had been exposed to 16 common foods, people in the IBS group had higher levels of an antibody called IgG4 (associated with food intolerances) in response to beef, lamb, pork, soya beans and wheat, which suggests that if you have IBS, you should pay careful attention to how you feel in the hours after eating these foods. Here's how to pinpoint your trouble foods:

- **Step 1: Track your symptoms** Write down the date, the type of symptoms you're having, how long they last, what you ate (and how much) during the preceding day or two, any medications you took and what you were doing just before your discomfort began. After 14 days, look for patterns.
- **Step 2: Eliminate one suspected trigger food at a time** In another UK study, people who eliminated problem foods saw symptoms improve by 26 per cent. Cutting out one food at a time will give you a clearer picture of what helps and what doesn't.

Try a little fibre Until recently, digestive disease experts strongly recommended an increase in fibre intake for people with IBS. Conventional wisdom said that soluble fibre – the type found in beans, pears, barley and some fibre supplements – could firm up the stools of people with diarrhoea, while soluble and insoluble fibre (the type found in wholemeal bread and many vegetables) would counter constipation. Sometimes it works; in one US study of 81 people with IBS, 26 per cent reported less abdominal pain and bloating when they switched to a diet with more than 25g of fibre per day. But other studies show that fibre makes pain worse for some people and has little effect for others.

If you'd like to give it a try, go slowly. Swap one low-fibre food for a high-fibre one (replace white bread with wholemeal, for example) every day for a week and monitor how you feel. If you're feeling well, make another swap. And make sure you drink plenty of water to ensure that the fibre doesn't cause constipation.

Relax all over Progressive muscle relaxation eases stress, which in turn seems to reduce the pain of IBS. In one small US study, people with IBS who practised this technique daily for a month were five times more likely to experience improvement in pain and cramping than those who didn't use the technique.

Sit or lie down in a comfortable place and shut your eyes, breathe deeply and imagine stress flowing out of your muscles. Beginning with your feet, tense each muscle group tightly, then let the tension go so the muscles feel more relaxed than when you started. Move on to your calves, upper legs and up to your neck, face and head.

Prevention boosters

Get moving Exercise eased gastrointestinal symptoms in one large US study. The researchers weren't looking specifically at IBS, but there's plenty of other proof that being active can help by relaxing your bowels. Intestinal activity often slows during exercise, allowing your body to shunt more blood to your legs and arms. It also relieves stress and boosts mood, making pain easier to bear.

Take peppermint-oil capsules for spasms Peppermint oil relaxes muscles in your gastrointestinal tract. In one well-designed study of 57 people with IBS, 75 per cent of those who took peppermint-oil capsules saw symptoms improve by 50 per cent or more after four weeks, compared to 38 per cent who took a placebo. Study volunteers took two capsules twice a day. Use enteric-coated capsules to ensure that the oil is released in your intestines, not your stomach.

Try hypnotherapy In one UK study, people with IBS who tried five sessions of hypnotherapy had less pain and diarrhoea after three months than study volunteers who didn't have therapy. Benefits faded over time;

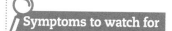
Symptoms to watch for

Abdominal pain and cramping, bloating, flatulence, diarrhoea or constipation (or alternating bouts of both), and mucus in the stools.

237

Latest thinking

Slow down and rest when you have a bout of diarrhoea. There's new evidence that trying to 'tough out' a gastrointestinal infection raises your risk of developing IBS afterwards. When researchers at the University of Southampton in the UK contacted 620 people with past gastrointestinal infections, they found that those who had pushed themselves hard (for example, they kept working until they collapsed in bed) during their illnesses were more likely to develop IBS than those who took it easy.

after a year, the hypnosis group needed less medication to control IBS, but their symptoms were about the same as the non-hypnosis group. In another study, people who had 12 sessions over three months were still feeling better five years later. Ask your doctor to refer you to trained hypnotherapist who is familiar with 'gut-directed' hypnotherapy, a technique that teaches you how to ease your own symptoms.

Soothe with yoga In one study from India, men with IBS had equal reductions in diarrhoea after two months of daily yoga or two months of daily doses of the over-the-counter medication loperamide (Imodium). Yoga seemed to soothe overactive nerves that stimulate bowel activity,

Drugs that prevent disease

A wide variety of medications can help prevent and control the most difficult IBS symptoms, from constipation and diarrhoea to pain and cramps.

Antidepressants Even if you aren't depressed, antidepressants can block pain signals travelling between the intestines and brain, and can even help your bowel movements become more normal. In one study, people with IBS who took citalopram (Cipramil) reported that abdominal pain and bloating improved significantly in just a few days. Which one's best for you? Expect pain and cramp relief with any of them. Constipation seems to improve more with selective serotonin-reuptake inhibitors (SSRIs) such as citalopram, escitalopram (Cipralex), fluoxetine (Prozac), paroxetine (Seroxat) and sertraline (Lustral). Diarrhoea seems to ease more with tricyclic antidepressants such as amitriptyline, imipramine and nortriptyline (Allegron).

Antispasmodic drugs These medications – for example, hyoscine (Buscapan) – are useful in treating pain and cramping. They work by relaxing the walls of the intestines. You may have to try several to find the one that's best for you.

Diarrhoea medications The over-the-counter diarrhoea medication loperamide (Imodium) works for many people. It shouldn't be used for acute infectious diarrhoea.

Mild laxatives Plain old milk of magnesia is often effective for the treatment of constipation. If it doesn't help, see your doctor. If your constipation is severe, he or she may suggest a different medication or approach.

Peppermint oil This old-fashioned remedy, available over-the-counter, was effective in several clinical trials. Choose an enteric-coated preparation such as Colpermin.

according to researchers from the All India Institute of Medical Sciences in New Delhi. Meanwhile, a Canadian study of teenagers with IBS found that doing yoga routines from a video daily for a month eased anxiety.

Talk with a cognitive behavioural therapist This practical type of counselling is aimed at helping you perceive and respond to everyday problems in new ways and to find solutions that really work. You may also work on relaxation skills. Some studies have found a benefit for IBS, while others haven't. Further research has found that CBT works for a little while, but then the effects wear off. It may be worth a try if you find it hard to cope with your IBS or if it prevents you from doing all the things you want or need to do in your life. It seems to work best as an add-on therapy along with medications.

Try biofeedback If you're bothered by constipation, learning how to use your abdominal muscles properly during a bowel movement could improve results -- and make you feel better. In one Australian study, 25 women with IBS used biofeedback to help them as a doctor and nurse gave them 'advanced training' in the proper way to push out stools without straining, using small water balloons. This type of biofeedback uses a probe inserted into the rectum to measure pressure exerted on stools. The result: 75 per cent reported that things had improved. Other types of biofeedback can help people with IBS learn to control stress, too.

Send in the 'healthy' bacteria Digestive disease researchers are beginning to suspect that an overgrowth of bacteria in the upper intestines – a place where few bacteria should be living – may explain many of IBS's confusing and hard-to-treat symptoms. In one study, US researchers found evidence that 84 per cent of study volunteers with IBS had an overgrowth of bacteria in the small intestine. In the future antibiotics may have a place in the treatment of this condition, but meanwhile, probiotics – as supplements or in yoghurt with active cultures – could help IBS symptoms by raising levels of healthy bacteria in your intestinal tract. In one study, 44 people with IBS took a supplement containing *Lactobacillus acidophilus* and Bifidobacterium (also found in yoghurt containing live active cultures) for a week. Typical IBS symptoms such as pain, spasms, constipation and diarrhoea improved by 50 per cent.

See also:

Step 8: *Reduce chronic stress, page 74*

Jet lag

If you've ever taken an overnight flight to America or Asia and have spent the following day in a stupor, you know the effects of jet lag. Even flying through just two time zones – especially if you're travelling east – is enough to confuse your body clock so that you can't fall asleep or wake up at the 'right' time, leaving you bleary eyed and exhausted. Chronic jet lag experienced by airline personnel and frequent business travellers even plays havoc with women's menstrual cycles and can increase the risk of cancer, heart disease and peptic ulcers. The next time you travel by plane, take these steps to keep jet lag from ruining your trip.

What causes it

Travelling to a destination several time zones ahead or behind the one you're used to. This disrupts your internal body clock.

Symptoms to watch for

Poor sleep during the 'new' night-time. If you fly east, you'll probably have trouble falling asleep; if you fly west, you're likely to wake up too early, regardless of when you went to bed. Other symptoms include poor performance on physical and mental tasks, fatigue, headaches, irritability and problems concentrating. You may also experience indigestion, changes in bowel habits and reduced appetite.

Key prevention strategies

Sleep on the plane This works only if you sleep when it's night-time at your destination – for instance, if you're travelling from London on an overnight flight to Delhi. Use earplugs and eye shades to block out light and sound. You can also try taking 3mg of melatonin, which some studies suggest may help you fall asleep. If you think this may help you, ask your GP, as this is a prescription-only preparation in the UK.

Turn on the lights If you're exhausted when you arrive, it's tempting to nap, even if it's morning. Do your best to resist the urge. Instead, go for a walk outside and try to get at least 3 hours of sunlight to help your body adjust more quickly to the new time zone.

Reset your body clock before your trip The idea is to start shifting your bedtime and wake-up time towards the schedule you'll be on at your destination before you leave. If you're travelling east through several time zones, go to sleep one hour earlier each night for three days before your trip – and get up an hour earlier, too. When you wake up, try to expose yourself to bright light for several hours, which helps to reset your body clock. While sunlight is best, a full-spectrum light or light box can also work. You can buy them online. One study recommends combining this strategy with taking 5mg of melatonin at bedtime and at 6pm on the day of your flight to increase the hormonal signals that tell your body it's time for bed, so you can fall asleep at the right time. Melatonin (Circadin) is not licensed in the UK for the prevention of jet lag, but if you feel it might help you, discuss treatment with your doctor.

> " **Sunlight** helps your body adjust more quickly to the **new time zone**. "

If you're flying west across several times zones, delay your sleep by an hour a night. If you're traveling through eight or more time zones, go to bed 2 hours earlier each night.

Prevention boosters

Take a sleeping pill when you arrive One study of travellers whose journey took them eastwards across five to nine time zones found that those who took 10mg of zolpidem (Stilnoct) for three or four nights once they arrived slept better and longer than those who didn't take the medication. However, if you're taking melatonin as part of a body clock re-adjustment programme, don't take a conventional sleeping pill as well.

Drink a little coffee in the morning It sounds simple, but caffeine is one of the best ways to improve your energy and concentration after flying across time zones. Don't drink too much, however, or it may affect your sleep that night.

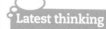

Latest thinking

Cells have their own built-in 'clock' that reacts to light, affecting their functioning throughout the day and night. Repeated disruptions to this clock – as a result of jet lag, sleep disorders, or even blindness – can increase the risk of numerous illnesses, even cancer.

Kidney disease

Chronic kidney disease is on the rise in large part due to the prevalence of diabetes and high blood pressure, both of which are leading causes. One out of six adults has kidney disease, yet many people with weak or failing kidneys have no idea that anything's wrong. Chronic kidney disease (CKD) occurs when the kidneys gradually lose their ability to filter waste and toxins from the blood. It can eventually cause fatigue and shortness of breath, and it's the main reason why people end up needing dialysis. Once you have CKD, you can't cure it, but you can halt or slow its progression.

20% The amount by which you could reduce your risk of kidney disease by maintaining normal blood pressure.

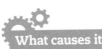

What causes it

Damage to blood vessels in the kidneys. The damage is most often caused by high blood pressure or diabetes but may also be the result of lupus, infections, inherited diseases, long-term use of NSAIDs such as aspirin or ibuprofen, kidney stones, an enlarged prostate that obstructs urine flow from the kidneys, or cancer.

Key prevention strategies

Prevent diabetes and hypertension These conditions damage the tiny blood vessels in the kidneys and your risk of chronic kidney disease doubles if you have both of them. If you already have both of these conditions, talk to your doctor about treatment with an ACE inhibitor. Studies find this group of antihypertensive drugs works best for preventing kidney disease or at the very least preventing it from advancing to the point where dialysis or a transplant is required. ACE inhibitors are particularly recommended for the treatment of high blood pressure in those with diabetes. (For more information on how to prevent these two serious conditions and the health risks associated with them, see *Diabetes*, starting on page 156, and *High blood pressure*, starting on page 212.)

Get a simple kidney check-up If you're at risk of kidney disease – you have diabetes or high blood pressure, or a family history of kidney problems – your doctor should test your kidney function regularly. In the past, doctors used a blood test that measured a protein called creatinine. But because creatinine levels vary among individuals, the test can be somewhat unreliable. Now doctors screen kidney function with the estimated glomerular filtration rate (eGFR) test, a blood test that measures how well the kidneys filter waste from the blood.

Keep a regular check on your blood pressure Many pharmacies and doctors' surgeries have blood pressure monitors available for customers and patients to test themselves. Pay special attention to your systolic blood pressure, the top number in your reading; it's a good indication of your vulnerability to kidney disease. A major study of

8,093 men who were followed for 14 years found that a systolic pressure between 130 and 139mmHg increased the risk of kidney disease by 26 per cent, and one of 140mmHg or higher increased it by 69 per cent.

Prevention boosters

Prevent kidney stones Blockages caused by kidney stones can increase the risk of chronic kidney disease. (See *Kidney stones* on the following page for some prevention tips.)

Spend the night in a sleep lab If you snore loudly, your partner says you make loud choking or gasping noises while you sleep, and/or you're exhausted during the day, you could have a condition called obstructive sleep apnoea, which may mean you're more likely to develop chronic kidney disease, though experts aren't sure why. Being overweight and having high blood pressure increase the risk of both conditions, but researchers also note that people with sleep-related breathing disorders often have anaemia or low levels of oxygen-carrying blood cells, both of which are associated with chronic kidney disease. It can't hurt – and will certainly help your overall health – to deal with your apnoea. The only way to diagnose obstructive sleep apnoea for certain is with polysomnography, a test that evaluates your breathing as you sleep. (For more information and advice, see *Snoring*, starting on page 296.)

Skip dessert Or find other ways to lose weight. Not only does being overweight make existing kidney disease worse, but it can also increase the risk of developing the condition in the first place. A study in 11,000 healthy men that found those whose body mass index (BMI), increased 10 per cent or more over 14 years were 27 per cent more likely to develop chronic kidney disease than those whose BMI either dropped or increased by a maximum of 5 per cent. The risk remained even if the men had normal blood pressure and blood glucose levels, and exercised on a regular basis.

Symptoms to watch for

The early stages have no symptoms. In later stages, you may experience fatigue, frequent hiccups, feeling 'fluey', itching, headache, foot and ankle swelling, nausea and vomiting, or weight loss. In the late stages, symptoms include blood in vomit or stools, decreased alertness, reduced sensation in your hands or feet, easy bruising, an increase or decrease in urine production, muscle twitching or cramps, seizures, or white crystals in and on your skin.

Latest thinking

A recent study found that people with gum disease were 60 per cent more likely to have chronic kidney disease. Researchers suspect that the chronic inflammation caused by the bacterial infection responsible for gum disease may play a role.

See also:

Cause 1: Hypertension, page 22

Kidney stones

One out of every 10 adults will experience at some point in their lives the excruciating pain of a kidney stone lodged in the urinary tract. Kidney stones result from microscopic deposits in urine that eventually solidify, much like the salt left at the bottom of a glass of salt water after the liquid evaporates. There are several types of kidney stones. If you have passed a stone, your doctor can test its composition and measure chemicals in your blood and urine to decide on the best way to prevent stones from developing in the future.

up to 39%
The reduction in the risk of developing kidney stones by drinking 1.3–2.5 litres of fluids a day.

What causes it

Genetic disposition, urinary tract infections, kidney disease, chronic dehydration and certain metabolic conditions that affect the make-up of urine. Certain medications, including diuretics and calcium-based antacids, can also contribute.

Key prevention strategies

Drink lots of fluids Drinking plenty of fluids is the best way to prevent all types of kidney stones. One study found that men who produced a prodigious 2.5 litres or more of urine a day (the average is 1.4 litres) were 29 per cent less likely to develop symptomatic stones than those who produced 1.2 litres or less. In women, urinating 2.6 litres or more reduced their risk by 49 per cent compared with urinating less than 1.4 litres a day. To lower the risk of kidney stones, aim to drink 2 litres of non-alcoholic fluids a day (more in hot weather) to ensure that you produce plenty of pale-coloured urine.

Eat yoghurt Doctors used to warn all patients at risk of kidney stones to limit their calcium intake. But it turns out that people who have the least calcium in their diets can have the highest risk of kidney stones. (A few patients, those with absorptive hypercalciuria, are still asked to reduce their calcium intake.) It is important to note that this research relates to dietary calcium; there's no evidence that calcium supplements reduce your risk. In fact, in women, supplements could increase the risk of stones by about 20 per cent.

Researchers think that calcium protects against stones by binding to oxalic acid, which is present in certain foods and contributes to some types of kidney stones. The best dietary sources of calcium are low-fat milk, yoghurt and cheese. Edamame (green soya beans) are also high in calcium. An unexpectedly good source is whole-grain cereal, which can contain up to 1,000mg in a single serving. Most people need an intake of 1,200mg of calcium a day to protect their bones; there is no specific level recommended to reduce the risk of kidney stones.

Limit high-oxalate foods This advice is for people who have already had calcium oxalate stones. Researchers have found that certain high-oxalate foods – spinach, rhubarb, beetroot, strawberries, figs, chocolate, wheat bran, peanuts and almonds – increase the risk of stones. If you can't bear to give up any of these foods, increase the amount of calcium you take in when you eat them. For instance, slice strawberries into a bowl of cereal with milk, sprinkle almonds over yoghurt and top a spinach salad with low-fat grated cheese.

Prevention boosters

Drink a glass of orange juice every day Experts have long prescribed lightly sweetened lemonade as a way to keep stones at bay. But recent studies suggest that orange juice may be an even better choice. Both are great sources of potassium citrate, which is often prescribed to prevent kidney stones. Just stay away from grapefruit juice: it seems that having as little as 250ml a day can increase the risk of kidney stones, though researchers have no idea why this should be the case. Apple juice may also increase your risk.

Lose weight if you need to When researchers analysed study results, they found that men who were over 15½ stone (100kg) were 44 per cent more likely to develop kidney stones than those who weighed less than 10½ stone (168 kg). For women, the danger of being overweight was greater: those who weighed more than 15½ stone (100kg) were between 89 and 92 per cent more likely to develop kidney stones than those under 10½ stone (68kg).

Avoid high-fructose corn syrup Numerous packaged foods and drinks contain corn syrup, but avoiding sweetened fruit drinks and eating fewer packaged snacks is a good first step towards reducing your intake. Cutting back may significantly reduce your risk of stones. Researchers suspect the connection has to do with fructose's tendency to increase the amount of calcium in urine.

Symptoms to watch for

Initially, none. In fact, the majority of stones pass without any symptoms. Larger stones, however, can cause sudden, intense pain in your back, side and lower abdomen, as well as nausea and vomiting. You may also notice blood in your urine, feel that you have to urinate more often than usual and/or feel burning when you urinate.

Latest thinking

People with metabolic syndrome – a constellation of symptoms that include high blood pressure and triglycerides, abdominal fat, insulin resistance and low levels of 'good' HDL cholesterol – have a much higher risk of developing kidney stones.

See also:

Cause 1: Hypertension, page 22
Cause 2: Intra-abdominal fat, page 24
Cause 4: Insulin resistance, page 28

245

Knee pain

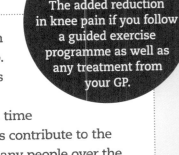

14%
The added reduction in knee pain if you follow a guided exercise programme as well as any treatment from your GP.

The human knee is built to withstand forces four times greater than your body weight – and to support you as you bend, twist and jump. However, its complex arrangement of bones, ligaments and tendons works best when the muscles around it are also strong and flexible. If they go soft, then even carrying heavy bags can lead to pain. And time isn't always kind to knees, either. Since ageing, genetics and injuries contribute to the wide variety of problems that can cause pain, it's no wonder that many people over the age of 55 complain of chronic knee pain. Here's how to avoid it.

What causes it

Osteoarthritis, rheumatoid arthritis, overweight, falls and accidents, overuse, weak muscles, or not warming up before starting a challenging exercise routine.

Key prevention strategies

Lose unwanted weight Each pound (500g) of excess weight you lose reduces the pressure on your knees by nearly 4½lbs (2kg). And exercising while you diet not only makes permanent weight loss much easier to achieve but also translates into bigger benefits for your knees. In a study that followed 316 women and men with painful knees, those who took a knee-friendly low-impact aerobics and strength-training class for an hour three times a week, and also lost weight, reported a 30 per cent drop in knee pain and a 24 per cent improvement in their ability to do everyday things such as climbing stairs.

Don't smoke Chemicals in tobacco smoke interfere with the process that heals torn ligaments, including those in the knees. (A symptom of a torn knee ligament is pain, tenderness or stiffness on the outside of the knee that you feel mostly when you're moving around.)

US researchers found that smoking tobacco reduced the number of infection-fighting cells called macrophages that arrive at the site of ligament injuries and release chemical signals that summon other cells needed for making repairs. Any shortening of the time it takes for healing to take place is of course of benefit to the affected person and thousands of people endure knee pain each year due to damaged ligaments.

Avoid high-impact exercise If running, step aerobics or even star jumps (jumping jacks) hurt, it's time to switch to a lower-impact fitness routine. Walking, swimming, cycling and water aerobics are great work-outs that burn calories, boost cardiovascular fitness, and have even been shown to reduce knee pain in studies. Stop doing an activity if it hurts your knees and choose something different.

Strengthen all the muscles that support your knees Strong quadriceps (the big muscles that run down the front of your thighs) and hamstrings (at the back of your thighs) act as shock absorbers that take some of the pressure put on your knees when you walk, jump and bend. They also keep the bones in your knees properly aligned, which reduces the risk of pain and excess wear and tear. In one study women with stronger thigh muscles were 55 per cent less likely to develop knee pain. Strengthening your 'core' abdominal and back muscles, as well as those in your hips and buttocks, is also important for reducing knee pain.

Prevention boosters

Wear joint-friendly footwear The best shoes for your knees are flat and flexible, according to researchers from Rush Medical College in the USA. The scientists analysed pressure on the knees of 16 volunteers as they walked in clogs, flip-flops, walking shoes and the shoes often worn by older people with balance problems. The surprise winners were flip flops and walking shoes, which allowed the feet to bend and flex naturally with each step, taking pressure off the knees. We recommend the walking shoes. While flip flops are comfortable on the beach, they don't protect your feet or stay in place very well as you walk.

If you have flat feet, over-the-counter shoe inserts or custom-made orthotics can help keep the bones in your knees better aligned, helping to prevent pain.

Measure your legs Or better still, ask your doctor to do it. It's surprisingly common to have legs of unequal length and this can contribute to osteoarthritis as well as knee and hip pain, say US researchers from the University of North Carolina at Chapel Hill School of Medicine. Apparently, having one leg as little as 8mm shorter than the other can increase the risk of knee pain by 50 per cent. The answer is to ask your doctor about shoe inserts.

Symptoms to watch for

Knee pain due to osteoarthritis is usually deep and achy, is felt around the knee joint and is often worse at night. Sudden, severe pain can be the result of injured ligaments (which attach the bones in your upper and lower legs), irritation or inflammation of tendons (which attach muscle to bone), or a dislocated kneecap.

Your knee may also lock in place, often due to a torn meniscus, the curved piece of cartilage inside your knee joint. If your knee swells (often called water on the knee), it may be a sign that fluid-filled sacs called bursae that act as joint cushions have become inflamed. You may also have pain just below the knee. See your doctor if your knee is hot, swollen or extremely painful, has locked in place or if you can't stand or walk.

Latest thinking

Low vitamin D levels can make knee pain worse. If you have osteoarthritis of the knee, be sure you're getting 1,000 to 2,000IU of vitamin D a day.

See also:

Exercises: *Back strength and flexibility*, page 324
Joint strength, page 334

Lung cancer

up to **50**%
The amount by which your risk of lung cancer drops 10 years after quitting smoking.

Unless you've been on a desert island for the past 40 years, you know that smoking is the leading cause of lung cancer (although 2 to 10 per cent of lung cancers occur in people who have never smoked, particularly women). To help prevent lung cancer, don't smoke, and stay away from smokers – an hour spent inhaling someone else's cigarette smoke damages your lungs as much as smoking four cigarettes yourself.

What causes it

Smoking causes 90 per cent of lung cancers. Other possible causes are radon and exposure to asbestos, other chemicals, and breathing in secondhand tobacco smoke.

Key prevention strategies

Quit smoking Your risk of developing lung cancer if you smoke a pack of cigarettes a day for 40 years is about 20 times that of someone who never smoked. It's not easy to kick the habit; typically it takes most smokers several attempts before they succeed. To help your efforts, do consult your GP. Working with your doctor increases your chances of success by 75 per cent compared with trying on your own. The doctor will probably prescribe a nicotine-replacement product. Whether you choose gum, a patch, lozenges, an inhaler or a nasal spray, studies find that the products can double the odds of quitting successfully (defined as being smoke free for a year). Your doctor may also prescribe bupropion (Zyban) or varenicline (Champix), both of which help people give up. Only bupropion can be used in conjunction with nicotine-replacement products.

Should you try to quit slowly or all at once? Research shows that quitting 'cold turkey' works better, but starting nicotine-replacement therapy a couple of weeks before you stop may help.

Test your house for radon Radon, a colourless, odourless gas that is emitted by decaying radioactive elements in the earth, is found in most homes but in very low levels. Much depends on where you live. Radon is the second leading cause of lung cancer (albeit way behind smoking). The best

Drugs that prevent disease

Researchers evaluating the use of statins (medications widely prescribed to reduce cholesterol in the blood) in nearly half a million patients found that taking them for at least six months reduced the risk of lung cancer by 55 per cent. Researchers suspect that statins protect against lung cancer by countering inflammation in the body, which contributes to the development of cancer. The next step is clinical trials to confirm these preliminary findings.

Another drug that may help prevent lung cancer is the pain reliever celecoxib (Celebrex). In one study, researchers found that heavy smokers who took a high dose were less likely than those who didn't receive the medication to develop the kind of pre-cancerous cellular changes seen in smokers. Like statins, celecoxib reduces inflammation. Both have potential side effects, so talk to your doctor.

> **Broccoli** is high in compounds called isothiocyanates, which **prevent lung cancer** in animals.

way to find out if you have radon in your house is to arrange for a professional to test for it. You can find out more about radon in the home by visiting www.hse.gov.uk/radiation/ionising/radon.htm.

Prevention boosters

Eat lots of vegetables Start with broccoli, cabbage and Brussels sprouts. These cruciferous vegetables are high in compounds called isothiocyanates, which have been shown to prevent lung cancer in animals. In humans, research suggests that eating these vegetables at least once a week could cut the risk of lung cancer by 33 per cent.

Brush and floss regularly Losing your teeth, which is usually due to bacterial infection in the mouth, increases your risk of lung cancer by 54 per cent even if you don't smoke. The reason? It could be related to the inflammation that leads to gum disease and tooth loss, or to the fact that people who lose their teeth are more likely to have an unhealthy diet than those who retain their teeth.

Symptoms to watch for

Chronic cough, hoarseness, coughing up blood, weight loss, loss of appetite, shortness of breath, unexplained fever, wheezing, bouts of bronchitis or pneumonia, or chest pain.

Latest thinking

Vitamin E supplements don't protect against lung cancer and may even increase your risk of the disease. A large study involving more than 77,000 people found that taking a 400mg daily dose increased risk by 28 per cent over 10 years. Don't worry about dietary vitamin E, though; there's no evidence that it – or levels of any other vitamin or mineral in food – increases the risk of lung cancer.

See also:

Step 2: Fruit and vegetables, page 64
Step 3: Quit smoking, page 66

Lyme disease

It's hard to believe that something the size of a poppy seed could trigger such a big health problem. A single bite from a deer tick infected with the bacterium *Borrelia burgdorferi* is enough to cause Lyme disease and the various miseries that come with it. Most cases are easily cured with antibiotics, but if untreated, the disease can eventually lead to serious heart, joint and nervous system complications. The Health Protection Agency has estimated that there are between 1,000 and 2,000 cases of Lyme disease in the UK each year. Follow these precautions to reduce your exposure.

40%
The amount by which you can reduce your risk if you dress protectively.

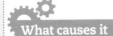

What causes it

A bite from a tick infected with *Borrelia burgdorferi* bacteria.

Key prevention strategies

Understand the risk The ticks that carry the Lyme disease bacterium are particularly prevalent on heathland and in woods, especially where there are deer and other tick-carrying animals. So it is important to take care when out walking in these areas. For further information, visit www.nhs.uk/Conditions/Lyme-disease/Pages/Introduction.aspx.

Cover up Wherever you are walking in the countryside, regardless of the temperature, protect yourself with long-sleeved shirts and long trousers tucked into socks. Choosing light-coloured clothing will help you to see any ticks. Dressing this way can reduce your risk of Lyme disease by 40 per cent.

Be repellent Using an insect repellent reduces your risk of infection by 20 per cent. The most effective repellents contain 10 to 35 per cent DEET. Ten per cent DEET products work for about 2 hours; be sure to reapply after that. Don't use repellents with more than 30 per cent DEET on children. If you expect to be heavily exposed to ticks, in addition to spraying yourself with DEET, consider spraying your clothing (especially socks and trousers) with the pesticide permethrin, which remains effective through several washes. Never use permethrin on your skin.

What to do if you find a tick

The best way to remove a tick is with a special tick-removal device (available from vets) or fine tweezers. Grasp the tick as close to your skin as possible, near the tick's head or mouth, then pull the tick straight out – don't twist. Don't squeeze it, rub petroleum jelly on it, touch it with a hot match or cigarette, or pour paraffin or nail polish on it. Place the tick in a small jar or resealable plastic bag and take it with you to the doctor.

Check yourself After a walk in a potentially tick-infested area, examine your whole body for any small, round, black or brown bumps. Don't forget to check between your toes, on the bottoms of your feet, and in your groin. Stand in front of a long mirror to look at your back, and ask someone to check your scalp. If you see a tick, don't panic. You have up to 24 hours to remove it before the infection is transmitted, and 96 per cent of people who find and remove a tick within this time avoid getting infected.

Know the signs of a tick bite At first, a tick bite causes a hard bump. About 70 to 80 per cent of people with Lyme disease develop a circular rash at the site of the bite within 3 to 30 days of being bitten. As the rash expands, the centre may become paler. But you can have Lyme disease without developing the rash. Other early symptoms include fever, chills, body aches and headache.

Seek help early If you've been bitten or suspect you have Lyme disease, go to your GP, who is likely to prescribe antibiotics. A single 200mg dose of doxycycline within three days of removing the tick can reduce the risk of serious disease by 87 per cent. This treatment can help prevent the infection, but some experts recommend a longer course of treatment even if a potential infection is caught early, just in case the infection has already taken hold.

Prevention boosters

Stay in the middle of the path When you're walking, avoid the footpath edges. Ticks inhabit shrubby vegetation anywhere from ankle to waist high. If you avoid brushing against the greenery at the edge of the path, you're less likely to come home with a tick.

Do some landscaping If you live in the country, get rid of any brush and leaf litter (where ticks love to hang out) and create a one-metre buffer zone of wood chips or gravel between any woodland and your garden. Keep your lawn cut short.

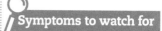

Symptoms to watch for

Early symptoms include fever, headache, fatigue and a characteristic skin rash. Left untreated, the infection can spread to the heart, joints and nervous system. Complications include arthritis, heart rhythm abnormalities, encephalitis and facial paralysis.

Latest thinking

The antibiotic doxycycline, used to treat the disease in its earliest stage, could one day be used to protect against it, perhaps as a slow-release patch that you put on before going into tick-infested areas.

Macular degeneration

There's no cure for age-related macular degeneration (AMD), so called because it usually strikes after the age of 60. It destroys the macula – the centre of the retina, an ultra-thin layer of light-sensitive tissue deep in the eye. People who have it find that vision erodes so gradually that it's easy not to notice anything at first, and, in fact, most people with AMD have this slow-moving 'dry' form. However, 1 in 10 develop 'wet' AMD, in which blood vessels in the macula leak, and vision deteriorates rapidly. The best advice is to have regular eye tests and try the following tips to reduce your risk.

33%
The reduction in your risk of progressive vision loss if you keep your plate piled high with colourful fruit and vegetables.

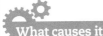

What causes it

Experts don't know what triggers the damage, but smoking and being over the age of 60, Caucasian or female raises the risk.

Symptoms to watch for

Distorted vision in one or both eyes; or straight lines that look wavy. Over time, central vision grows worse, and it becomes difficult to see objects far away, to read or do close work, or even to distinguish faces and colours.

Key prevention strategies

Don't smoke The more you smoke, the higher your risk. In fact, when US scientists at the University of Wisconsin tracked the health of nearly 5,000 women and men for 15 years, they found that smoking raised the risk of developing this condition by 47 per cent. Smoking robs your eyes of antioxidants that protect against cell damage, reduces blood flow to the eyes and may even affect the pigments in your irises that not only determine your eye colour but also act as a natural sunscreen.

Eat the right vegetables Spinach, pak choy and Swiss chard are rich in the eye-protecting nutrients lutein and zeaxanthin. These compounds concentrate in the macula of the eyes, filtering out the sun's destructive blue light before it can harm delicate light-sensitive cells deeper in the retina. They also neutralise damaging free radicals produced when light hits the eye. Other good food sources include brightly coloured fruit and vegetables such as sweetcorn, red peppers and mandarins.

At this point, experts say there's no evidence that antioxidant supplements help prevent AMD, though recent research suggests they may slow its progression if you already have it.

Eat smarter carbs 'White' foods such as white bread, white rice and pasta, potatoes, cakes or sweetened fruit drinks may be harming your eyes because of the rapid rise in blood glucose levels they produce. When US researchers looked into the diets of 526 people with AMD, they found that those who ate the most foods that produced rapid rises in blood glucose were 2.7 times more likely to develop AMD than those who ate the fewest.

The answer is to eat plenty of fresh fruit, vegetables and dried beans; choose whole-grain bread and cereal; drink water or unsweetened tea; and avoid crisps, crackers and biscuits. Experts think that lower blood glucose helps to maintain a healthy flow of blood and oxygen to the eyes, keeping them healthy.

Eat oily fish, not fatty meat In one Harvard Medical School study, eating two or more fish meals a week cut the risk of AMD by an impressive 60 per cent. The researchers think that the omega-3 fatty acids in oily fish promote good blood flow to the eyes and cool inflammation, an emerging risk factor for AMD. The catch is that fish helped only those people who also limited their intake of omega-6 fatty acids. These are found in corn, safflower and sunflower oils as well as fried foods and margarines made with these oils.

Other foods to avoid include cheese, ice cream, hamburgers and anything else rich in saturated fat, and also alcohol. People who ate these foods had twice the risk that early macular degeneration would progress compared to people who ate a healthier diet.

Prevention boosters

Snack on nuts The same Harvard study found that people with AMD who ate more than one serving of nuts each week cut their risk of the progression of AMD by 40 per cent. (A serving is a small handful of any type of nut.) Scientists speculate that the reason for this helpful effect is that nuts contain resveratrol, an antioxidant that can protect against cell damage, soothe inflammation and promote healthy blood flow.

Watch your weight The eyesight of overweight people with AMD worsens up to twice as fast as that of people of normal weight. Research shows that exercising as part of your weight-control strategy pays dividends for your eyes. In one study, people with early AMD who took at least half an hour of vigorous exercise three times a week cut their risk of developing advanced AMD by 25 per cent.

Supplements for vision loss

If you already have macular degeneration, taking an antioxidant supplement could cut your risk of deteriorating vision by 33 per cent, according to a recent UK review of eight well-designed studies. (They didn't help prevent AMD in people whose eyes were healthy.) You may want to consider taking a supplement if you have been diagnosed with intermediate or advanced AMD. The formula recommended by experts contains 500mg of vitamin C, 400IU of vitamin E, 15mg of beta carotene, 80mg of zinc (as zinc oxide) and 2mg of copper (as cupric oxide). The latter is added to prevent copper deficiency, which can occur if zinc intake is high.

Latest thinking

Avoid second-hand smoke. Nonsmokers who lived with smokers raised their risk of AMD by 87 per cent in one recent UK study. Don't wait for someone to give up in order to clear the air and guard your eyesight: ask them to smoke outside to protect your health.

See also:

Cause 6: Inflammation, page 32
Step 3: Quit smoking, page 66

Menstrual problems

Compared to our ancestral grandmothers, who spent most of their reproductive years pregnant or breastfeeding, women today have about three times as many menstrual periods. The reality is that we don't *need* to menstruate. In fact, the manufacturers of birth control pills originally included one week of placebo pills mainly because they thought that women would find it 'reassuring' to have a regular period. Today women can choose a range of treatments for painful or heavy periods. And there are always new approaches and treatment options being tested to help women with heavy menstrual bleeding. One such technique currently being researched is using sound waves from high-intensity ultrasound to destroy fibroids, which are a common cause of heavy menstrual bleeding.

91%
The amount by which you could reduce cramps by taking vitamin E supplements before and during your period.

What causes it

Hormonal changes during your menstrual cycle trigger the production of hormone-like chemicals called prostaglandins that make the uterus contract, causing cramps. Endometriosis, a condition in which the tissue that lines the uterus grows outside the organ, also causes painful periods. Heavy periods are caused by an imbalance between oestrogen and progesterone, most often during puberty and the years just before menopause; fibroids; and, rarely, endometrial cancer.

Key prevention strategies

Use the contraceptive hormones to treat problem periods
If you're not trying to get pregnant, starting on oral contraceptives (the Pill) is the most effective way to prevent severe menstrual cramps and excessive bleeding. Standard birth control pills contain a synthetic progestogen hormone that thins the lining of the uterus over time. A thinner lining produces less arachidonic acid, which contributes to the production of prostaglandins, hormone-like chemicals that cause cramps. And shedding a thin uterine lining causes less blood loss. Studies find that the oral contraceptive pill can reduce menstrual bleeding by up to 60 per cent. If you take oral contraceptives, be sure to tell your doctor if you start to experience severe headaches; there is a slightly increased risk of stroke.

A hormone-impregnated or IUCD (intrauterine contraceptive device) is another option. The IUCD Mirena releases a progestogen hormone called levonorgestrel, which is highly effective for reducing heavy periods. Other contraceptive options that can be used include the vaginal ring (NuvaRing), the contraceptive implant (Implanon) and the injectable contraceptive (Depo-Provera).

Take painkillers early Start taking an over-the-counter nonsteroidal anti-inflammatory (NSAID), such as ibuprofen (Nurofen) and naproxen (Naprosyn), following the directions on the label, one to two days before your period is due. A review of 51 studies involving 1,649 women found that 72 per cent experienced significant pain relief with this approach

> " *Menstrual **bleeding can be reduced** by up to 50% by taking prescription medication.* "

compared to women taking a placebo. Continue for the first two or three days of your period. The pain relievers act by reducing levels of prostaglandins, which cause cramping. As these hormone-like chemicals also interfere with blood clotting, taking NSAIDs for pain relief can help prevent heavy menstrual bleeding.

Ask your doctor about prescription medication Mefenamic acid (Ponstan), another NSAID, can be helpful and is often prescribed for painful, heavy periods because it seems to be less likely to irritate the stomach and can reduce bleeding by 22 to 46 per cent. Avoid aspirin, which may increase bleeding. Tranexamic acid (Cyklokapron) is the most effective medical treatment available for preventing heavy bleeding. It is an antifibrinolytic, which means it prevents blood clots from disintegrating. It also stimulates clot formation. And more clotting means less bleeding. Studies have found that this medication can reduce heavy menstrual bleeding by as much as 50 per cent.

Prevention boosters

Feast on fish or take fish oil Fish rich in omega-3 fatty acids, such as salmon, trout, sardines and mackerel, may help ease menstrual cramps and have the added benefit of improving your levels of blood fats, including cholesterol. A study of 181 Dutch women found that those with the lowest levels of omega-3 fatty acids in their diets had the greatest amount of menstrual pain.

Even if you don't like fish, you can still be sure to get enough omega-3s by taking fish-oil capsules. A study of 70 women, half of whom received fish oil, found that pain levels in those taking the oil dropped by 33 per cent compared to a 20 per cent improvement in the women who took placebos. The women took 2g of fish oil every day for a month. The next month, they took 2g a day for eight days before their period and two days after their period. Check with your doctor before taking fish oil supplements.

> " Women who **exercise** regularly, are **less likely** to have pain during their period. "

Symptoms to watch for

Lower-abdominal pain during your period. With heavy bleeding, if you are changing your tampon and/or pad every hour during the first couple of days of your period, you have an abnormally heavy flow. Also watch out for any unusual fatigue or dizziness – a heavy menstrual flow could lead to anaemia from iron loss. But don't take iron supplements on your own; always talk to your doctor first.

Try a low-fat vegetarian diet Researchers asked 33 women with bad menstrual cramps to follow such a diet (no animal products, fried foods, avocados, olives or nuts, but plenty of grains, vegetables, pulses and fruit) for two menstrual cycles, then eat their regular diet for two cycles and take a placebo pill. During the vegetarian diet phase, the duration and intensity of the women's menstrual pain dropped by about a third. And there was a bonus: they lost weight. The diet probably triggers beneficial changes in the metabolism of oestrogen and/or cuts down on the production of prostaglandins.

Take vitamin E with caution Regular long-term use of vitamin E supplements, which may slightly increase the risk of early death, are not recommended. But some research suggests that taking vitamin E just before and after your period begins can bring significant relief from painful periods.

One study involving 278 adolescent girls found that taking 400IU of vitamin E a day, beginning two days before their period began and for the first three days of their period, relieved cramps better than a placebo. After four months, girls who took the vitamin E had average pain scores nearly six times lower than those who took placebos, and their pain lasted an average of 1.6 hours compared to 17 hours in the placebo group. Vitamin E may work to relieve cramping by affecting the action of prostaglandins.

Run (or walk) off cramps There is a strong likelihood that if you are a woman who is physically active, you don't get debilitating menstrual cramps. Studies find that women who exercise regularly – regardless of what kind of activity they do – are less likely to have pain during their period, so make an effort to be active throughout the month, and try to keep it up during your period.

Try chasteberry to stem heavy bleeding *Vitex agnus castus*, better known as chasteberry, is often used by herbalists to treat problems affecting the reproductive organs in women. Scientific studies suggest

When to get medical advice

While most menstrual problems are not serious, there are times when you should seek a doctor's advice in order to get the most effective treatment and to rule out the possibility of a more serious underlying condition. The NHS Choices website (www.nhs.uk/Livewell/menstrualcycle/Pages/DoIneedtoseeadoctor.aspx) recommends that you see your GP in the following cases:

- **You experience bleeding between periods or after sex**
- **You have bleeding after the menopause (after you have had no periods for 12 months)**
- **Your periods suddenly become heavier or longer**

And of course if your periods are very painful, you should also see your doctor.

Latest thinking

Menstrual blood is a rich source of stem cells, which in the future could be used to create a variety of tissue such as insulin-producing cells to benefit people with Type 1 diabetes.

that as little as 15 drops of a tincture can significantly reduce the number of days of heavy bleeding, though it may take several months before you experience a benefit.

Get tested for a bleeding disorder Blood clotting disorders such as von Willebrand's disease often underlie heavy menstrual bleeding, yet many doctors don't always think to check for this possibility. This diagnosis is particularly likely if you have had heavy periods since you were in your teens. If you have a clotting disorder, regular injections or infusions of missing clotting factors could make your heavy periods a thing of the past.

See also:

Step 1: Exercise, page 62

Migraines

Migraines are a problem for 1 in 6 women and 1 in 16 men. But as many as half of all sufferers don't understand what triggers their pain. As a result, they may be missing out on strategies that could stop the downward spiral before it starts. If your symptoms match some or all of those listed on the opposite page, try the following prevention measures.

40%
The drop in the number of migraines among people who switched to a low-fat diet for eight weeks.

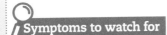

What causes it

No one's sure. Experts suspect that the trigeminal nerve system, which sends and receives pain signals involving the face and head, is involved, as is the brain chemical serotonin. Levels of serotonin fall during a migraine and may prompt the trigeminal nerve to send out chemicals that dilate blood vessels, causing pain.

Symptoms to watch for

Moderate to severe pain on one or both sides of the head. It may throb or pulse, feel worse with physical activity and come with nausea, vomiting and sensitivity to light and sound. Some people experience auras just before the pain begins. These can include flashing lights, blind spots, tingling in arms or legs, or feeling extremely weak. (Those who have migraines with auras are also at increased risk of cardiovascular problems, studies show, so follow the book's advice for preventing heart disease and stroke.)

Key prevention strategies

Discover your personal migraine triggers Certain foods, some medications, stress, changes in sleeping patterns, cigarette smoke and a variety of other things can result in a migraine. Triggers vary, so keeping a headache diary may help you to determine yours, but be aware that some triggers are unidentifiable. Record when you get a migraine and what you were taking, eating, drinking, feeling and doing for the 24 hours before the pain began.

Common medication culprits include some antidepressants, bronchodilators, contraceptives containing oestrogen, and diet pills. Food triggers include caffeine, most alcoholic drinks, aged cheese, processed meats, MSG (monosodium glutamate), nuts, dairy foods, tropical fruits and most dried fruit, onions, bread products containing fresh yeast, and the artificial sweetener aspartame.

Step off the painkiller merry-go-round Taking any painkillers more than twice a week can cause problems. These medications constrict swollen blood vessels, which makes your head feel better. But when they wear off, blood vessels swell again, and you could end up with a migraine as a result. End the cycle by stopping your pain medications. It will probably hurt at first, but experts say you'll start feeling better after a week to 10 days. Then you can focus on prevention strategies such as the ones outlined here. However, when you do need to take a painkiller, take it promptly, because the longer you leave it, the less effective it will be.

Cut back on dietary fat Drastically reducing the amount of fat you eat could cut the number of migraines you have by 40 per cent. That was the finding from a US study involving 54 migraine sufferers who followed extremely low fat diets (they obtained just 10 to 15 per cent of their energy intake from fat each day) for eight weeks. When the participants in the study did get headaches, they were 66 per cent less intense and their duration was reduced by 70 per cent. The subjects also used 72 per cent less headache medication.

The researchers suspect that eating less fat improves the flexibility of blood vessels so they expand and contract more easily. They also discovered that study volunteers replaced fat with carbohydrate-rich foods such as bread and pasta, which raise levels of the brain chemical serotonin, linked to lower migraine risk.

If you think this kind of diet may be too strict for you, work on cutting back on saturated fat – the kind found in fatty meat, full-fat milk and cheese, and tropical oils (such as palm and coconut oil) – and getting most of your fat from oily fish, rapeseed or olive oil, walnuts and flaxseeds (linseeds). In some studies, these good fats reduced the frequency of migraines.

Prevention boosters

Give ginger a try Research shows that this warming spice contains potent compounds that are similar to those in NSAIDs. It may work against migraines by blocking inflammatory substances called prostaglandins. Although ginger hasn't been rigorously tested for its ability to subdue a migraine, it may well relieve the nausea that often comes with this kind of severe headache. Try taking ginger as a tea made by steeping fresh ginger root in boiling water, or use it in cooking.

Ask your doctor about taking riboflavin supplements In one Belgian study, 60 per cent of people who took 400mg of riboflavin (vitamin B_2) every day for three months had half as many migraines as they had before the study started.

Relax your mind and body You can do this with yoga, meditation, deep breathing or any other therapy that helps to relieve tension. In one interesting study from India, 72 migraine sufferers who practised yoga for an hour five days a week reduced the frequency and intensity of their migraine attacks.

Drugs that prevent disease

If you get two or more migraines a month, ask your doctor if you might benefit from taking migraine medication such as pizotifen (Sanomigran), the beta-blocker propranolol or possibly low-dose tricyclic antidepressants such as amitriptyline and nortriptyline. The right treatment could cut your risk of future migraines dramatically, but it can take four weeks before you begin to see improvements and up to six months to know whether a medication is really working for you.

Latest thinking

Think twice before taking feverfew. It probably won't do any harm, but this popular anti-migraine herb did little to prevent migraines or lessen pain in a UK review of five well-designed studies.

See also:

Step 7: Cut back on saturated fat, page 72
Step 8: Reduce chronic stress, page 74

Mouth ulcers

Mouth ulcers are tiny white sores inside your mouth or on the gums, and they can be painful, as well as making it difficult to eat or even to talk. Mouth ulcers can be triggered by anything from food to toothpaste ingredients and sharp-edged potato crisps to stress. Researchers aren't sure what causes them, but the following tips may help you avoid them.

64%
The potential reduction in your odds of recurrent mouth ulcers if you switch to a sodium lauryl sulfate-free toothpaste.

What causes it

No one knows. Experts suspect that mouth ulcers are caused by several factors, including tiny immune system attacks on healthy mouth tissue, allergic reactions, low levels of B vitamins and iron, injury and irritation of the lining of the mouth, additives in foods and toothpaste, hormonal changes related to the menstrual cycle in women, and stress.

Key prevention strategies

Avoid toothpaste containing sodium lauryl sulfate (SLS) This ingredient can irritate the delicate lining of the mouth and trigger mouth ulcers in some people. In a Norwegian study of 10 people who suffered from recurrent mouth ulcers, switching to an SLS-free toothpaste cut their rate of new sores by nearly two-thirds. But don't skimp on dental hygiene. Brushing and flossing twice a day can keep your mouth free of tiny food bits and bacteria that can irritate the lining of your mouth and kick-start a new mouth ulcer. Brush gently to avoid activating a new sore.

Swish with an antibacterial mouthwash Rinses containing triclosan, chlorhexidine and other antibacterial ingredients can significantly reduce the number of mouth ulcers in people who get them repeatedly, according to several studies. They may work by washing away debris from hard-to-reach spots as well preventing the bacteria that are always present in your mouth from multiplying, thereby preventing the flare-up of tiny infections that could trigger a mouth ulcer and helping to prevent infection if you do get a sore.

The gluten connection

An estimated 1 in 20 people who suffer from recurrent mouth ulcers have coeliac disease, an intolerance to the gluten protein found in wheat and some other grains. But don't give up wheat yet. If you think you may have coeliac disease, talk to your doctor about the possibility of testing and treatment, if necessary. Other symptoms of gluten intolerance include diarrhoea, abdominal pain, weight loss, fatigue and wind.

Avoid these food culprits Some mouth ulcers are caused by a food or food additives. Citrus fruits, tomatoes, aubergines, tea and cola drinks all triggered mouth ulcers in one study from Turkey, presumably because these foods irritated the lining of the mouth. Benzoic acid (a food preservative), cinnamon, milk, coffee, chocolate, potatoes, cheese, walnuts and figs are said to be other culprits.

Avoid spicy foods, which can also irritate the sensitive tissue of the lining of the mouth. And avoid sharp-edged foods such as corn chips, potato crisps and crackers.

Before eliminating these foods from your diet, look for connections between foods you've eaten recently and the onset of a new sore. Experts recommend removing a food for a few weeks, taking note of whether you get fewer sores, then introducing the food again to see if it triggers a the formation of a new sore.

Prevention boosters

Be calm Stress seems to be a classic instigator of mouth ulcers. In one study of people with mouth ulcers, 16 per cent said that extreme stress triggered outbreaks. Experts think stress may be a factor in up to 60 per cent of first-time mouth ulcer episodes. Irish researchers have found higher levels of the stress hormone cortisol in the saliva of people who get the sores, too. Try a relaxation technique such as yoga.

Take a supplement When Israeli researchers gave 15 people with recurring mouth ulcers either an injection of vitamin B_{12} or a daily vitamin B_{12} tablet, mouth ulcers dropped from an average of 10 per month to about one every three months. Several studies have found low levels of vitamin B_{12} in people who get mouth ulcers regularly. People in the study took 1,000mcg of vitamin B_{12} daily, but talk to your doctor before taking that much. (Some experts recommend a more conservative 100mcg per day.) Top food sources include fortified cereals, lamb or veal kidneys, mussels, chicken livers and salmon.

Clear up other nutritional deficiencies About one in five people with recurring mouth ulcers has a nutritional deficiency. Some need more B vitamins or have iron-deficiency anaemia. Studies show that correcting low iron stores could cut your risk of developing more mouth ulcers by 71 per cent. It's not advisable to take extra iron without medical advice; for some people, it can be harmful. Ask your doctor whether you need a blood test to check for deficiencies.

Symptoms to watch for

Small round sores under your tongue, inside your cheeks or lips, or at the base of your gums. Most are less than 1cm in diameter, but some mouth ulcers can be large and can take up to a month to heal.

Latest thinking

Some children get recurring mouth ulcers along with a fever and sore throat on a regular basis between the ages of three and ten. This newly recognised condition, called periodic fever, aphthous-stomatitis, pharyngitis and adenitis (PFAPA) syndrome, returns like clockwork every few weeks or months. No one's sure what causes it, and there's no recognised treatment, though new research from Children's Hospital Boston, USA, suggests that removing the tonsils of a child with PFAPA can stop future attacks.

Neck pain

The average human head weighs about as much as a 10-pin bowling ball, yet it is supported by seven of the smallest, lightest vertebrae in your spine. Nature designed the neck to curve slightly backwards to keep your head from flopping over, but years of bad posture, driving, computer work and sleeping on sagging mattresses or big pillows can flatten that curve, leading to pain. Injuries, such as whiplash, and stress also contribute. Here's how to reduce your risk of neck pain.

40%
The amount by which an intensive programme of stretching and relaxation exercises could reduce your risk of neck and shoulder pain.

What causes it

Trauma, such as whiplash from a car accident; excessive strain on the neck or shoulder muscles; emotional stress that causes you to tighten your shoulder or neck muscles; and degenerative changes in the vertebrae and discs in your neck, which are common with age.

Key prevention strategies

Pull up on your string Think of yourself as a puppet with a string coming out of the top of your head. Now imagine that someone's pulling on that string, causing you to sit (or stand) straight and hold your head high, with your chin tucked in slightly. That's the position you want to be in most of the time. Instead, many of us sit, drive and even walk with the head thrust forwards, which puts added strain on the neck. To help you sit up straight at the computer, use armrests and adjust your monitor so that your eyes are looking near the top of the screen. While driving, adjust your seat and headrest so you don't have to crane your neck forwards to see the road.

Keep your head held high by balancing an object Most music CDs come in hard plastic cases that are quite light, so place one on top of your head and see how long you can keep it balanced there. Eventually, sitting straighter should become second nature.

Downsize your pillows Sleeping on a big pile of pillows or just one big pillow means your neck will be out of alignment with the rest of your spine while you sleep. It's better to use a relatively flat pillow and sleep on your back or side, not on your stomach. For many, a neck pillow is the best solution, but you'll need to sleep on your back.

Move every 20 to 30 minutes If you're sitting at a computer, knitting or working at a drawing board, it's easy to get lost in the flow and sit in an

Help for a stiff neck

Wet a towel, wring it out and warm it in the microwave for 30 seconds on *High*. Then wrap it around your neck and keep it in place until it loses its heat. Do this before performing neck exercises to loosen up the muscles. (Never put a dry towel in a microwave oven.)

> **Backpacks** *evenly distribute the weight of what you're carrying, helping you to* **avoid neck pain.**

unnatural position for too long, straining your back, shoulder and neck muscles. Set an alarm or kitchen timer to ring every 20 to 30 minutes. Each time it goes off, stand up, walk around for a few minutes and practise the neck exercises starting on page 338. An Italian study found that when office workers were trained to practise relaxation and stretching exercises several times a day to stop 'clenching' their neck and shoulder muscles, they had 54 per cent less neck and shoulder pain compared with a control group, whose pain dropped by only 4 per cent.

Prevention boosters

Lighten the load Carrying a heavy bag slung over one shoulder is a leading cause of neck pain for many women because it pulls the body out of alignment. One doctor, tired of hearing his patients complain about neck pain, started weighing their bags and found that many tipped the scales at 3kg to 4.5kg. If you need to carry a lot of things, use a backpack to distribute the weight evenly on both shoulders.

Watch your phone posture If you often spend a long time making phone calls on a conventional telephone handset, avoid scrunching the phone between your ear and shoulder. And use an earpiece with your mobile phone.

Symptoms to watch for

Pain and difficulty turning your head to the right or left or moving it up or down; frequent headaches.

Latest thinking

In the case of severe neck pain, a surgeon may perform an anterior cervical discectomy (ACD) to remove a damaged disc and replace it with a metal or synthetic implant or small piece of bone. The procedure can relieve pain while retaining mobility. Surgery is a last resort when nothing else helps.

See also:

Exercises: *Neck strength and flexibility, page 338*

Obesity

Obesity can have a devastating effect on your health. It's linked not only to an increased risk of the problems you'd expect – heart disease and diabetes, as well as joint pain – but also to numerous others you might not think of, such as cancer, hearing loss, Alzheimer's disease and gastrointestinal problems. For some people, keeping their weight under control seems almost impossible – but it's not. Just don't make the mistake of relying on short-term dieting, which is surprisingly ineffective. The trick is to combine balanced nutrition and sensible portion control with exercise – something you simply can't leave out of the equation.

22%
The reduction in your risk of becoming overweight if you eat whole-grain cereal every morning over a period of eight years.

What causes it

While genetics plays a role in weight gain, the greatest contributor is eating more calories than your body burns for energy. The excess is stored in the body as fat.

Key prevention strategies

Exercise for 30 minutes a day Exercise, even more than cutting calories, is key to losing weight and keeping it off. Any amount helps, but a good, easily reached goal is 30 minutes on most days. Surprisingly, a 30 minute workout is almost as effective as a 60 minute workout, according to a study published in the *Journal of the American Medical Association*. When 184 women walked either outside or on a treadmill at various intensities for 30 or 60 minutes a day, five days a week for a year, researchers found that it didn't matter how hard or how long the workout was – the women still lost nearly the same amount of weight. Those who exercised for an hour a day lost about 10 per cent more than those who did it for half an hour a day. Given that the average weight loss was 19lb (8.5kg), that's a difference of only about 2lb. But why? The researchers speculate that the more you exercise, the more you think you can eat – and by eating more, you offset some of the weight loss you would have achieved. The moral of the story is to go ahead and get as much exercise as you can (some people will need more than 30 minutes a day to get rid of stubborn fat or keep weight off); just don't raid the fridge as a reward.

Don't skip breakfast We've known for a long time that people who eat breakfast every day (a whole-grain cereal with at least 4g of fibre per serving) are more likely to maintain a healthy weight or, if they're trying to lose weight, lose more than those who don't eat breakfast. The reason has to do with how your body reacts to any shortage of food, even a brief one. If you skip breakfast in the morning, not only do you feel as if you're starving by lunchtime, your body actually thinks it's starving and reacts by slowing down the rate at which it burns food for energy to conserve its resources. Most experts agree that eating breakfast every day is simply one of the best things you can do for your weight.

Some researchers now even think that your breakfast should be a large one – your biggest meal of the day, in fact. They point to studies that suggest a big breakfast does a better job of regulating appetite and reducing cravings for sweets and starches later in the day, helping you keep your weight under control.

Practise portion control In the developed world, we're eating as much as 25 per cent more food per person than we did 40 years ago. One reason is 'portion distortion' – we've become used to the vastly oversized servings at some fast-food and sit-down restaurants, making it difficult for us to recognise a 'normal' portion at home. Here's a new way of thinking you could try: when you eat, consider quality rather than quantity, and stop eating when you're only 80 per cent full. The point is to give your body the nutrition it needs, not to overstuff yourself as if food may never again be available. Try these tips:

- **Use smaller plates** Studies find that if you use large plates, you not only put more food on the plate but eat more of what's in front of you.
- **Don't eat in the kitchen** Serve in the kitchen, then go to another room to eat. You'll be less likely to go for seconds if you have to get up and go back the kitchen to refill your plate.
- **Slow down** Most of us eat too fast. This doesn't give the brain time to receive the hormonal signals from the stomach that it's full. For this reason, wait at least 20 minutes after eating before helping yourself to a second helping or dessert. The chances are that you'll find you don't want to have either.

Fill half of your plate with non-starchy vegetables Most vegetables, excluding potatoes and sweetcorn, fill you up on very few calories – far fewer than whatever other food your plate contains. Fill another quarter of your plate with unrefined carbohydrate such as wholemeal pasta or brown rice and the rest with lean meat, chicken, fish or another protein food. It's the simplest way to avoid excess calories.

Join a weight-loss support group If you've managed to lose weight and want to keep it off, it helps to have support, preferably in person, from a group such as Weight Watchers. When researchers compared people who attended support groups with those who received online help or just a newsletter about maintaining weight loss, they found that the live-meeting group regained an average of 5½lb (2.5kg); the other

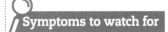

Symptoms to watch for

A body mass index (BMI) of 30 or more, which indicates obesity. Find out what your BMI is at www.bmi-calculator. net/metric-bmi-calculator.php.

two groups regained an average of just under 11lb (5kg). The online support did provide some extra benefit, however: just 54.6 per cent of those participants regained weight compared with 72.4 per cent in the newsletter group.

Prevention boosters

Support healthy-weight habits One major study that followed a group of people for more than 30 years found that a person's risk of obesity increased by 57 per cent if a close friend became obese and by 37 per cent if their spouse became obese. So if you or your spouse or close friend is gaining weight, join a workout/weight-loss group together (there are plenty to choose from); studies find that 'buddying up' like this can lead to both of you shedding more pounds than either of you would if you tried alone.

Weigh yourself often It's much easier to lose 1lb than 10, and unless your clothes are tight-fitting you may not notice that you've put on a few pounds. A study of more than 3,000 people found that the more often people weighed themselves, the more weight they lost or the less weight they gained.

'Fast food' in the freezer

Eating out – particularly fast food – is a major cause of weight gain. One study found that people who ate fast food more than twice a week gained 10lb (4.5kg) more over a 15 year period than those who ate fast food less than once a week. To reduce the incentive to eat out, keep the freezer stocked with these 'convenience' foods:

- Frozen prawns
- Frozen fish (no sauce)
- Frozen vegetables (no sauce)
- Boneless skinless chicken breasts
- Homemade soup
- Frozen lean mince
- Pork loin (thinly sliced for quick cooking)

Combine them with larder items such as whole-grain pasta, brown rice, olive oil, homemade pesto, tinned tomatoes, beans and lentils, along with washed salad leaves from the fridge, and you have the makings of countless emergency meals.

Watch it when you're pregnant It's important to be careful about exactly how much weight you gain during pregnancy. It turns out that pregnancy itself may leave a 'legacy' of extra pounds. For instance, in one study, a year after women delivered, they still weighed between 4½ and 6½lb (2-3kg) more than women of the same age who had not been pregnant. To maintain a healthy weight during pregnancy, keep physically active, weigh yourself regularly and don't fool yourself that you need to eat more 'for the baby' – although, of course, you do need to make sure that what you do eat is high in healthy nutrients.

Eat less and exercise more when you quit smoking Nicotine suppresses weight gain, so if you're giving up smoking, plan to get more exercise and stock up on low-calorie foods that you can use to help you through the times when you really want to light up. Also, weigh yourself regularly to make sure that you are aware of any extra pounds. The prescription medication bupropion (Zyban) may help you to quit without gaining weight. (See page 67 for more information.)

Seek professional advice If you've got more than a few pounds to lose, it's a good idea to talk to your GP about the right approach for you. Your doctor can give you advice about diet and nutrition and, if appropriate, refer you to a dietitian for further guidance. What's more, a GP can provide a 'fitness prescription' for you to participate in exercise sessions at your local gym.

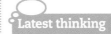

Latest thinking

A virus known as human adenovirus-36 may be partly responsible for obesity in some people. A study involving 502 unrelated thin and obese people found that 30 per cent of those who were obese had at one point been infected with adenovirus-36 compared with 11 per cent of those who were not obese. The researchers also looked at 28 pairs of twins and found that people with antibodies to the virus (meaning that they had been infected at some point) tended to weigh more than their identical siblings who didn't have the antibodies.

See also:

Cause 2: Intra-abdominal fat, page 24
Step 1: Exercise, page 63
Step 2: Fruit and vegetables, page 64

Osteoporosis

40%
The amount by which you can reduce your risk of hip fracture by walking for at least 4 hours a week.

After about the age of 30, the body breaks down old bone faster than it can build new bone. And since the hormone oestrogen works to keep bones strong, women have even more rapid bone loss after the age of 50 or when they have passed the menopause. Men develop osteoporosis, too. Medications are available to slow the process in people at high risk of fractures, but generally speaking, once bone is lost, it's gone for good. (And some bone-building medications come with serious side effects, including an *increased* risk of certain fractures.) That's why prevention is so important. While about 60 per cent of your bone density is determined by genetics, that still leaves 40 per cent you can affect.

Key prevention strategies

Get enough calcium and vitamin D If you're not getting enough calcium in your diet, your body takes what it needs from your bones, putting you at risk of osteoporosis. To protect your bones, add more low-fat dairy foods, such as low-fat or skimmed milk and low-fat yoghurt, to your diet. Aim for about 1,200mg a day (200g of low-fat yoghurt or a 250ml glass of skimmed milk has 300mg). Spread out your intake through the day in amounts of 500mg or less for the best use of calcium (See also *Getting your calcium from food,* page 270.)

It's also critical to get enough vitamin D, which helps your body to use calcium. Sunlight is the best source, but if you don't get sufficient sun exposure, there is a risk that your vitamin D levels may suffer. Experts sometimes recommend getting 10 to 15 minutes of sunlight – without sunblock – a day. Unfortunately, as you age, your body's ability to synthesise vitamin D from sunlight decreases, so you may want to think about taking a daily supplement of 400IU of vitamin D, especially if you don't want to expose yourself to sunlight because of fears about its effects on your skin. As insurance you might also consider calcium

Drugs that prevent disease

If you're a postmenopausal woman with a high risk of osteoporosis – because it runs in your family, you're underweight, you smoke or used to smoke, and/or you don't get much weight-bearing exercise, you have had long-term treatment with oral corticosteroids for a disease such as asthma or arthritis – talk to your doctor about getting a bone-density scan. You may benefit from treatment with raloxifene (Evista), which works by mimicking oestrogen in your body, slowing the action of bone-destroying cells. Or you may be prescribed one of the bisphosphonate medications – alendronate (Fosamax), risedronate (Actonel) or etidronate (Didronel). These work by suppressing the bone-destroying cells directly. These medications have side effects, so your doctor will assess their risks and benefits in your case.

" The **best** kinds of exercises are those that **work muscle.** "

supplements, although calcium from food is the most effective. In the huge US Women's Health Initiative study, women who took 1,000mg of calcium and 400IU of vitamin D every day for seven years had a hip bone density 1.06 per cent higher than that of those who took a placebo, plus a 29 per cent lower risk of hip fracture.

You can take up to 1,200mg of calcium a day in two doses (up to 600mg each, which is all the body can absorb at one time). Calcium citrate, though it costs more than other forms of calcium, is absorbed better by your body, especially if you're taking a proton-pump inhibitor such as omeprazole (Losec) or esomeprazole (Nexium) or an H2 blocker such as famotidine (Pepcid) or ranitidine (Zantac), which reduce the production of stomach acid, which breaks down nutrients.

Strengthen your bones through exercise When astronauts go into space, they lose up to 1.5 per cent of their total bone mass for each month in orbit. Why? Because at zero gravity, there's no weight pressing on their bones, and bone-building cells do their work only when they feel some 'strain'. That, in a nutshell, sums up the reason why exercise is so important to bone strength.

An analysis of 25 major studies on the effect of exercise on bone found it could prevent or reverse almost 1 per cent of bone loss a year in the lower spine and hip for pre and postmenopausal women. That may not sound like a lot, but it's enough to make a huge difference in your risk of fracture, given that with age, between 0.5 and 1 per cent of bone density is lost per year.

The best kinds of exercises are those that work muscle (and therefore bone), such as heavy gardening, lifting weights or jogging. You can even just hop up and down. When researchers asked pre-menopausal women to hop on one leg for a few minutes (50 hops) daily for six months, they found increased hip-bone density on the side of that leg compared to no change in the other hip. And simply walking also helps. A study of more than 61,000 postmenopausal women found those who walked for 4 hours or more a week had a 40 per cent lower risk of hip fracture than those who walked for an hour or less a week.

What causes it

Bone is constantly being built up by cells called osteoblasts and broken down by cells called osteoclasts. Until about your thirties, the osteoblasts are in the lead, but sometime during that decade you reach 'peak bone mass', and for the next decade or so, the two run neck and neck. From about the age of 50 onwards, as levels of oestrogen (in women) and testosterone (in men) drop, the osteoclasts pull ahead and bone density declines.

Get treated for depression If you have even mild depression – feeling less interested in things you usually enjoy, changes in your sleep and eating patterns, fatigue and so on – your bones may suffer. It turns out that premenopausal women with even mild depression have less bone mass than women of the same age who aren't depressed. It doesn't seem to be related to antidepressants but to changes in the immune system that increase underlying inflammation. In fact, some experts suggest that depression should be viewed as an early symptom of osteoporosis, which typically has no symptoms. It appears to be just as serious a risk factor as low calcium intake, smoking and lack of exercise.

Foods full of calcium

Getting calcium from food sources is generally better for your bones than getting it from supplements. Here are some easy ways to get more calcium every day, and to reach your daily target of 1,000mg.

- **Start with cereal** Choose one that is low in sugar and salt, and add just 200ml of semi-skimmed milk to get 240mg of calcium.

- **Snack on low-fat dairy foods** A 150ml pot of low-fat yoghurt also provides about 240g calcium. If you can't tolerate dairy foods, try calcium-enriched soya yoghurts and milk.

- **Eat your greens** 200g of raw spinach contains 340mg of calcium, although only 5 per cent of this can be absorbed because spinach also contains calcium oxalate – a salt that makes calcium less available to your body. Pair it with a vitamin C source, such as red peppers, to absorb more of the calcium. 100g of uncooked soya beans contains about 240mg calcium and 175g of raw broccoli has about 98mg.

- **Lunch on canned fish** About 100g of sardines, with bones, provides 500mg of calcium, and 100g tinned salmon, with bones and liquid, has about 300mg.

- **Look for fortified foods** About 100ml of fortified orange juice has up to 80mg calcium. Bread is also a good source as white flour is fortified with calcium.

- **Opt for low-fat cheese** About 30g of low-fat cheese (less than 10 per cent fat) on whole-grain crackers or toast makes a calcium-rich healthy snack or breakfast, and contains about 250mg of calcium, whereas 30g of full-fat cheddar cheese has less than that – only 220mg.

- **Snack on nuts** Eating almonds is an easy way to get more calcium in your diet; a 30g serving (about 23 nuts) provides about 72mg. Brazil nuts and tahini (sesame paste) are other good sources.

- **Whip up a smoothie** Blend a banana, 250ml low-fat milk or calcium-fortified soya milk, 80g strawberries and 1 tablespoon honey on High for 30 seconds for a delicious drink that is full of bone-strengthening calcium.

Prevention boosters

Stop smoking Studies find that smoking increases the risk of a spinal fracture by 13 per cent in women and 32 per cent in men and increases the risk of a hip fracture by 31 per cent in women and 40 per cent in men. Once you quit, that risk begins to drop quickly.

Stock up on spinach Spinach is packed with vitamin K, an often-forgotten vitamin that is important for preventing fractures. One study found that taking 45mg of vitamin K a day reduced the rate of spinal fractures by 65 per cent in women with osteoporosis compared to women who didn't take a supplement. Aim for 90 to 120mcg of vitamin K daily, about the amount in 2 tablespoons of chopped parsley and in 45g of cooked spinach.

Reduce your risk of falls Taking a few simple precautions can dramatically reduce your risk of falls and therefore your risk of fractures to high-risk areas such as the wrist and hip. For advice on how to prevent hip fractures and the falls that cause them, see page 220.

Symptoms to watch for

None. Osteoporosis is typically identified with a bone density scan or when you fracture a bone. If you have a fracture, particularly if it occurred as a result of something relatively minor, such as tripping over a step, ask your doctor for a scan to measure your bone density. Consider asking for a bone scan at the age of 65, or earlier if your GP recommends it or if you have other reasons to be concerned.

Latest thinking

Men should also be screened for osteoporosis. If risk factors exist, men should consider having a scan to measure bone density. Medication may be appropriate if it's low. About 6 out of 100 men will have osteoporosis by the age of 65.

See also:

Step 1: Exercise, page 62
Exercises: Back strength and flexibility, page 324
Better balance, page 330
Joint strength, page 334

Ovarian cancer

Don't shrug off persistent back or abdominal pain, especially if you've also been feeling bloated and tired. It could be a sign of ovarian cancer. While breast cancer is far more common in women, ovarian cancer is far more deadly. That's because most of the time, it isn't discovered until the late stages, when it's much more difficult to treat. However, this cancer isn't inevitable for women; researchers have found numerous steps you can take to reduce your risk.

20%
The amount your risk of this cancer drops for every five years of taking oral contraceptives.

What causes it

The precise cause is still under investigation, but there are two main theories. One is that ovulation leads to trauma and repair of ovarian cells; the more you ovulate, the more repair is required, providing more opportunities for genetic errors to occur when cells divide. The other theory suggests that long-term exposure to reproductive hormones like oestrogen, which contribute to cell division, triggers those cellular errors.

Symptoms to watch for

Bloating; persistent pain in the pelvis, abdomen or lower back; feeling full quickly; urinary symptoms, such as the urgent or frequent need to urinate; and persistent fatigue. If these symptoms occur suddenly and are present nearly every day for several weeks, consult your doctor.

Key prevention strategies

Take oral contraceptives The link between oral contraceptives and a reduced risk of ovarian cancer is so strong that a recent editorial in a leading medical journal suggested that all women for whom there is no medical reason for not taking it, should be prescribed the Pill – unless, of course, they want to get pregnant. An analysis of 45 studies from 21 countries found that women who had used oral contraceptives at any time had a 27 per cent lower risk of developing ovarian cancer than women who had never used them. Every five years of use reduced the risk by about 20 per cent; after 15 years of use, the risk was halved. And the protective effect of oral contraceptives lasts 30 years after a woman stops taking them. The downside is that they carry a higher risk of blood clots.

Breastfeed if you can Because breastfeeding suppresses ovulation, it can also reduce your risk of ovarian cancer. One study of nearly 150,000 nurses found that women who had breastfed a baby – no matter for how long – reduced their risk by 14 per cent. Those who breastfed for 18 months or longer cut their risk by a third. Overall, each month of breastfeeding reduced the risk of ovarian cancer by 2 per cent.

Prevention boosters

Avoid talcum powder Made from magnesium silicate, talcum powder has been controversially linked with an increased risk of ovarian cancer in some studies and has even been found embedded in some ovarian cancers. One study found that women who used talcum powder in the genital area or on sanitary pads had a 50 to 70 per cent increased risk of developing ovarian cancer. The link may be related to the inflammation

> " Because **breastfeeding** suppresses ovulation, it can also **reduce your risk** of ovarian cancer. "

that results if particles of talc travel through the reproductive tract to the ovaries or to the fact that, decades ago, the powder was contaminated with asbestos, a known carcinogen. While today's manufacturers are careful to keep any asbestos fibres out of the powder, it's still worth finding another alternative for staying dry.

Shed a few pounds If you have a body mass index (BMI) of 30 or more, you also have about a 30 per cent increased risk of developing ovarian cancer. And if you do get the cancer, your risk of dying from it is 50 per cent higher than that of women with a healthier BMI. The reason is probably related to the fact that fat cells release chemicals that are eventually converted to oestrogen, a hormone that fuels the growth of reproductive cancers such as ovarian cancer.

Get your tubes tied Many studies find that having a tubal ligation – an operation in which the fallopian tubes are cut and sealed shut – reduces the risk of ovarian cancer by at least a third overall and by up to 60 per cent in women who carry the BRCA1 genetic mutation. One reason may be that when the tubes are closed off, cancer-causing substances can't travel from the vagina and cervix through the tubes to the ovaries. This operation should normally only be considered by women who have completed their families or who are sure that they do not want to have children.

Got the gene?

If your mother, sister or mother's sister had ovarian cancer or breast cancer before the menopause, talk to your doctor about the possibility that you might carry a mutation of the BRCA1 or BRCA2 gene. Such mutations significantly increase your risk of developing ovarian cancer as well as breast cancer. If genetic screening shows that you carry the gene, you may want to consider having your ovaries removed, which studies find can reduce the risk of ovarian cancer by 96 per cent and of breast cancer by 50 per cent.

Latest thinking

A simple screening test for early ovarian cancer is every doctor's dream, but so far no test or combination of tests (e.g. regular pelvic ultrasound or blood tests for a cancer marker called CA125) has proven reliable.

Peripheral vascular disease

Think of peripheral vascular disease (PVD) as heart disease in your legs. The same factors that clog your coronary arteries with plaque, from eating saturated fat to being inactive, also lead to narrowing of your leg arteries. This can eventually shut off the blood supply to leg muscles and trigger intense pain when you walk. PVD is a problem for two reasons: it causes circulation problems that keep you off your feet and increases the risk of developing persistent sores on your feet and lower legs, and it's a warning sign that arteries throughout your body are being narrowed by plaque. People with PVD have a one-in-five chance of having a heart attack or stroke within a year. The following advice will help to keep the blood vessels in your legs clear.

33%
The reduction in your risk of peripheral vascular disease if you eat 10g of cereal fibre per day.

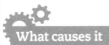

What causes it

Deposits of plaque in the walls of the arteries that supply blood to your legs and/or arms. These deposits narrow arteries and restrict the flow of blood to your muscles. They can also trigger the formation of artery-blocking clots.

Key prevention strategies

Stop smoking Nothing's worse than tobacco smoke for the arteries in your legs. The thousands of toxic chemicals in cigarettes narrow your arteries so much that smokers have a tenfold higher risk of PVD than nonsmokers do. Nicotine and other chemicals in tobacco also stiffen the normally flexible inner lining of artery walls, raising blood pressure and helping to trigger changes in cholesterol levels that prompt the build-up of plaque in artery walls. If you already have signs of PVD, such as leg pain, stopping smoking can double or triple the distance you could walk without pain.

Control your blood glucose Having diabetes raises your risk of PVD two and a half times higher than normal (see *Diabetes*, starting on page 164). If your blood glucose remains high (7mmol/l or higher on a fasting blood sugar test), it may be time for blood glucose-lowering medication. In a UK study of people with diabetes, those who kept their blood glucose under tight control reduced their risk of serious consequences of PVD, such as leg pain or the need for blood vessel surgery or even amputation, by 22 per cent.

Lower LDL, raise HDL Unhealthy cholesterol levels clog the walls of arteries in your legs (or arms) just as they do in your heart. Having high total cholesterol (over 5.5mmol/l) increases your risk of PVD by an incredible 90 per cent. The best solution is to use the same strategies that protect the arteries in your heart and brain: reducing your 'bad' LDL cholesterol and boosting your 'good' HDL cholesterol (see *High cholesterol* on page 216 for more information) and eating more healthily – choose heart-healthy salmon instead of steak, switch from refined grains to whole grains, eat plenty of fresh fruit and vegetables, drink lots of water, and take at least 30 minutes of exercise on most days of the week.

Follow advice if you've had a stroke or have heart disease A history of heart attack or stroke more than triples your risk of PVD. If you've survived one of these life-threatening events, it's time to look after your entire cardiovascular system so that you can live well. That means getting regular physical activity, eating healthily, trying not to get stressed and taking any medications your doctor prescribes.

Get rid of that spare tyre If you have a beer belly or any other form of extra fat around your middle, it's time to get rid of it. When Spanish researchers weighed and measured 708 men with and without PVD, they found that those carrying more fat around their waistlines had a 32 per cent higher risk than those with trim waistlines. Experts recommend waist measurements less than 102cm (40in) for men and 88cm (34½in) for women. (For people of Asian descent, risk rises with measurements over 95cm/37½in for men and 80cm/31½in for women.)

Prevention boosters

Eat more fibre Men who consumed 29g of fibre a day had a 33 per cent lower risk of developing PVD compared to men who had just 13g a day (closer to the amount the average person eats), according to US researchers from the Harvard School of Public Health who tracked the health of more than 44,000 men for 12 years. The men with a high fibre intake had a diet that included lots of whole grains, fruit and vegetables; those with a low fibre intake also tended to exercise more and eat less fat, all strategies that also help to keep blood vessels healthy.

Symptoms to watch for

Numbness or weakness in your legs; cold feet or legs; sores that won't heal on your toes, feet or legs; hair loss or changes in the colour of the skin on your legs and feet; pain or cramping that starts when you're active and disappears at rest. Half of the people with PVD have very mild symptoms or no symptoms at all.

Latest thinking

Exposure to lead and cadmium could raise PVD risk. In one US study, researchers found that those with the highest lead exposures – from sources such as lead paint, lead-glazed pottery and contaminated drinking water – had a 65 per cent higher risk than people with the lowest exposures. High exposure to cadmium, found in the emissions from coal-fired power plants and rubbish incinerators and in cigarette smoke, raised risk 86 per cent compared to people with the lowest exposures. Avoiding cigarette smoke and following safety advice for removing lead paint are some ways to limit exposure.

See also:

Cause 2: Intra-abdominal fat, page 24
Step 3: Quit smoking, page 66

Premature skin ageing

Wrinkles are to some extent an inevitable consequence of ageing. But there's plenty you can do short of surgery, to reduce the impact of the passing years on your skin. The key? Pampering your skin's inner structure, the collagen and elastin fibres that keep your face looking smooth and firm.

11%
The reduction in your risk of deep wrinkles if you eat several servings of vitamin C–rich fruit and vegetables every day.

What causes it

In addition to the passage of time, sun exposure, smoking, genetics, skimping on fruit, vegetables and 'good' fats, eating a diet high in saturated ('bad') fats and refined carbohydrates all conspire to erode collagen and elastin, the fibres that keep skin smooth, flexible and firm.

Key prevention strategies

Wear sunscreen every day Sunlight causes 90 per cent of age-related damage to your skin, making sun protection the most effective anti-ageing measure you can take. The culprits are UVA rays – the longer, more penetrating ultraviolet light that's constant throughout the year – and UVB, the rays that cause sunburn and are strongest in summer. Your best protection comes from clothing – including a broad-brimmed hat – and a broad-spectrum sunscreen with SPF 30 or higher. For the most effective protection use a sunblocking product that protects against both UVA and UVB rays. Look for products that contain zinc oxide or titanium dioxide.

Kick the tobacco habit When University of Utah researchers compared facial wrinkling in 109 smokers and 23 nonsmokers, they found that heavy smokers were five times more likely to have deep, craggy lines. Chemicals in cigarette smoke seem to dismantle the internal structure of the skin -- which includes connective tissue made of the proteins collagen and elastin – that keeps it firm and smooth.

Put more fruit and vegetables on your plate When British researchers checked the diets and wrinkles of 4,025 middle-aged women, they found that eating vitamin C–rich foods reduced the risk of significant wrinkles by 11 per cent. This antioxidant vitamin may protect skin

The anti-wrinkle diet

When dermatologists checked the skin and diets of 453 people from Australia, Greece and Sweden, they found that while a healthy diet can't erase damage done by years of unprotected sunbathing or smoking, it can help. Here's what to eat and what to avoid.

Have more:
Olive oil
Fish
Low-fat milk
Water and tea
Fruit and vegetables
Eggs
Nuts and nut butters
Beans

Have less:
Butter
Red meat
Full-fat milk
Soft drinks
Cakes and pastries
Margarine
Potatoes

by mopping up free radicals, the unstable oxygen molecules that damage collagen. Increasing your intake of vitamin C is as easy as having berries or a glass of orange juice at breakfast, red peppers and grapefruit at lunch, and broccoli at dinner. Other studies show that the more fruit and vegetables of all kinds you eat, the fewer wrinkles you'll develop.

Order salmon when you're dining out This boosts your intake of the good omega-3 fatty acids that researchers say could reduce the rate of skin ageing. Walnuts, rapeseed oil, fish-oil capsules and flaxseeds are also excellent.

Cut back on white bread and sugar Each 50g increase in your daily carbohydrate consumption (the amount in four slices of white bread) increases your risk of significant wrinkles by 36 per cent, according to the British study mentioned earlier. The damage may be caused by 'advanced glycation end products', molecules made from sugars and proteins that attack collagen as well as elastin, the stretchy protein that keeps skin looking firm.

Prevention boosters

Have a cup of sugar-free cocoa In one study, antioxidants called epicatechin and catechin in cocoa protected skin from sun damage and boosted circulation to skin cells.

Use a facial cleanser instead of soap and water Soap strips away barrier oils and moisture that protect skin from wrinkling.

Shop for a smart anti-wrinkle product Confused by the countless anti-ageing creams on the market? A recent test by *Consumer Reports* magazine reports that most do very little to prevent wrinkles. But products containing these active ingredients may help.
- **Retinoids** Available in over-the-counter products, these vitamin A derivatives minimise fine lines and help to build new collagen.
- **Alpha-hydroxy acids (AHAs)** These natural acids minimise the appearance of fine lines and wrinkles, especially around the eyes, by lifting off the top layer of dead skin on your face. At higher concentrations, they may even spur the production of new collagen.
- **Antioxidants** Creams and lotions containing vitamin C, idebenone and other antioxidants may help reduce fine lines and wrinkles by counteracting cell damage from free radicals.

Symptoms to watch for

Fine lines around the eyes; furrows in the forehead and around the mouth; deepening wrinkles under the eyes.

Latest thinking

Driving your car could give you wrinkles. Dermatologists at the St. Louis University School of Medicine in the USA report an increase in patients with mysterious, lopsided facial wrinkles. These signs of ageing were usually worse on the left side than the right. The cause? Sun streaming through the driver's side window of the car (left side, of course, in the USA) – even for just a few minutes each day. The sun's UVA rays, which penetrate deeply into the skin and are a leading cause of the damage that leads to wrinkles, travel easily through window glass – a good reason to wear sunscreen every day.

Premenstrual syndrome

About one in three women experiences bloating, breast tenderness, insomnia, headaches and other symptoms of premenstrual syndrome (PMS) in the five to seven days before a period. Another 3 to 8 per cent experience a more severe version, premenstrual dysphoric disorder, or PMDD. Given that women will have on average 451 menstrual cycles in their lifetimes, feeling rotten for four or five days before each cycle adds up to more than six years of misery. Find out how to beat the averages with the following tips.

30%
The amount by which you may reduce your risk of PMS by getting enough calcium from your daily diet.

Got the gene?

In late 2007 medical research identified the first genetic link to PMS and its more severe cousin, premenstrual dysphoric disorder (PMDD). The gene in question affects how women respond to changes in oestrogen levels; in women with PMS, mutations in the gene make them respond abnormally. The mutations also lead to reduced levels of dopamine, a brain chemical involved in mood. The findings may provide some peace of mind to women who now know that the mood swings and other symptoms of PMS are not in their heads but at least partly in their genes.

Key prevention strategies

Follow a bone-strengthening diet That means one rich in calcium and vitamin D, which promotes the absorption of calcium by the body. No one is certain exactly why this combination works – it's possible that PMS actually stems from a lack of calcium – but it does help some women. A large study of about 3,000 women found that those whose diet supplied about 1,200mg of calcium and 400IU of vitamin D were about a third less likely to have PMS than those whose diet was considerably lower in those nutrients. Low-fat dairy foods such as skimmed milk and low-fat yoghurt are excellent sources of calcium and vitamin D, as is fortified orange juice.

While getting calcium from food provides the greatest benefit (both for preventing PMS and helping to keep bones healthy), there is also evidence that taking supplements can help. One study of 248 women found that taking 1,200mg of calcium carbonate in supplement form for three months cut the severity of PMS symptoms nearly in half compared to taking a placebo.

Turn to chasteberry Several studies find that an extract from the fruit of chasteberry trees (also known as vitex agnus castus) works fairly well at preventing PMS symptoms. In one study of 170 German women, 86 received the dried herbal extract and 84 were given a placebo.

Researchers tracked six PMS symptoms – irritability, mood swings, anger, headache, breast fullness and bloating – and found that these symptoms were improved by more than 50 per cent in the majority of the women taking the extract compared to no improvement in those taking the placebo.

Drugs that prevent disease

The antidepressant venlafaxine has been found to be of benefit for some PMS sufferers. It is not, however, suitable for those with a risk of abnormal heart rhythms. Your doctor will advise you.

Another possible form of treatment is the Pill. If you also wish to prevent pregnancy, oral contraceptives, taken for 24 days with four days off rather than the typical 21 days on and 7 days off, can reduce PMS symptoms. Discuss this option with your doctor.

Prevention boosters

Eat less fat and more vegetables A study of 33 healthy women found that reducing the amount of fat in their diets to 20 per cent by following a vegetarian diet, reduced duration and intensity of pain, improved concentration and reduced mood swings and bloating prior to menstruation. Overall, bloating incidence dropped from nearly three days to just over a day, mood swings from nearly two days to one day, and concentration problems from nearly two days to less than a day.

Why does this type of diet help? It could be that it flattens the hormone rollercoaster by lowering levels of oestrogen in the blood.

Consider these supplements Various studies suggest that taking either 100mg of vitamin B_6 a day or 200mg to 360mg a day of magnesium (in divided doses taken three times a day beginning 15 days after your period starts) can also relieve PMS. Check with your doctor before taking any of these supplements long term.

What causes it

There is probably a link between hormonal changes during the menstrual cycle and chemicals in the brain called neurotransmitters that affect mood, particularly serotonin and endorphins. There's some evidence that the autonomic nervous system, which manages involuntary processes such as breathing and heart rate, also plays a role (see *Latest thinking*, below).

Symptoms to watch for

Bloating, fatigue, breast tenderness, headaches, mood swings, irritability, depression, increased appetite, trouble concentrating, forgetfulness.

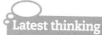

Latest thinking

Severe PMS may be a sign of a permanently depressed nervous system. Japanese researchers proposed this theory in late 2007 after measuring heart rates and hormone levels in 62 women and evaluating their physical, emotional and behavioural symptoms before and during their period. Women with PMS showed significant drops in heart-rate variability, a sign of how well the autonomic nervous system functions.

Prostate cancer

If you're a man and you live long enough, you'll develop prostate cancer. That's just one of the downsides of the hormone testosterone, which fuels the growth of prostate cells. The key to prevention is to keep this typically slow-growing cancer at bay long enough so that if you do get it, it remains so minuscule that it doesn't need treatment.

What causes it

Ageing. Over time, the cellular mechanisms that prevent abnormalities in dividing cells and destroy abnormal cells weaken. This increases the risk of cells whose 'off buttons' don't work. When that happens, the cells divide relentlessly, fuelled in part by male hormones such as testosterone. Two out of every three prostate cancers are found in men over the age of 65.

Key prevention strategies

Follow a prostate-protective diet Eating the right kinds of food can be protective. Here's what a typical day's diet might contain:

Breakfast

- **Half a grapefruit** It turns out that the pectin in citrus fruits – the substance that makes jam 'set' – destroys prostate cancer cells. It's also an important form of soluble fibre, which seems to bind to hormones such as testosterone to reduce the amount circulating in your body, and therefore the amount your prostate cells are exposed to. Studies have found that men whose diets are rich in soluble fibre (also found in pulses and oats) have lower levels of prostate-specific antigen (PSA), a protein released by prostate cells and often used to detect prostate cancer. Researchers suspect that a high-fibre diet is one reason why vegetarians are so much less likely to develop prostate cancer than meat-eaters.

- **A cup of green tea** Green tea contains substantial amounts of a powerful antioxidant called EGCG, which protects prostate cells from the type of biological damage that can lead to cancer. One study found that men who drank three cups of green tea a day were 73 per cent less likely to develop prostate cancer than those who didn't drink this tea at all; men who drank this amount of green tea for more than 40 years were 88 per cent less likely to develop the cancer. Overall, the more green tea the men drank and the longer the period for which they drank it, the lower their risk of prostate cancer. This area is so

Drugs that prevent disease

You may have heard of finasteride (Proscar), the medication used to treat prostate enlargement. It may help prevent prostate cancer, too. A major prostate cancer prevention trial involving nearly 20,000 men who didn't have prostate enlargement found that men who took finasteride for seven years had about a 25 per cent reduced risk of prostate cancer compared to men who took a placebo.

" *The **more tea** the men drank and the longer they drank it, the **lower their risk** of prostate cancer.* "

promising that the US National Institutes of Health is studying a green tea extract as the basis for a possible new medication for the prevention of prostate cancer.

Lunch

- **Soup or salad with edamame** People in Asian countries tend to eat a lot of soya beans, and men there don't develop prostate cancer as often as Western men do. Soya products such as edamame (immature soya beans still in their pods), tofu and soya milk contain plant-based hormones called isoflavones that help reduce levels of sex hormones like testosterone. The lower the testosterone levels in your body, of course, the less fuel is available to drive prostate cancer cell growth. Buy edamame frozen, thaw, then add to soups and salads, or steam lightly and enjoy them as a tasty snack.

Snack

- **A handful of nuts** Hazelnuts and almonds are excellent food sources of vitamin E, providing 6mg and 4mg, respectively, in just a small handful – and vitamin E may reduce your risk of prostate cancer. A major study of 29,000 Finnish males found that men who took 50IU of vitamin E (about 33mg) in supplement form were 32 per cent less likely than men not taking the supplement to develop prostate cancer and 41 per cent less likely to die from it during a five- to eight-year period. Vitamin E supplements have, however, been linked to premature death, so stick to natural food sources.

Dinner

- **Broccoli sautéed in olive oil** Broccoli, as well as cauliflower, cabbage and Brussels sprouts, contains the anti-cancer compound sulforaphane. One study found that men who ate three or more servings a week of these cruciferous vegetables were 41 per cent less likely to develop prostate cancer than those who ate less than one serving a week. The reason why you should use olive oil for sautéing is because it's made primarily of healthy monounsaturated fat, instead

Symptoms to watch for

Frequent urination, particularly at night; problems urinating (starting or stopping the flow); painful urination; or blood in the urine or semen.

Got the gene?

Many researchers are studying genes that may be linked to prostate cancer. A company in Iceland recently discovered a genetic mutation that may provide an early warning of risk – and help explain why men of Afro-Caribbean origin are more likely than Caucasians to develop the disease. The mutation is carried by about 13 per cent of men of European ancestry and 26 per cent of men of African ancestry. It increases the risk of prostate cancer by 60 per cent in either group, accounting for about 8 out of every 100 cases of prostate cancer overall. The mutation also appears to be associated with more aggressive forms of the disease. A test for the suspect gene is being developed, which may ultimately affect the treatment options of those carrying that gene.

of the polyunsaturated fat in corn, safflower and sunflower oil. Several studies have found that men whose diets are high in polyunsaturated fats are more likely to develop prostate cancer than those who consume less of this type of fat.

- **Baked salmon** Salmon is an excellent source of heart-healthy omega-3 fatty acids, which are also strongly linked to a lower risk of prostate cancer. A 30 year study of 6,000 Swedish men found that those who ate little or no oily fish had two to three times the risk of developing prostate cancer compared to those who ate moderate or large amounts of oily fish. Trout, sardines and mackerel are other good sources of omega-3s.

Get enough selenium The trace mineral selenium, found in brazil nuts, many types of white fish, salmon, oysters, wheat flour and pearl barley, is linked to lower rates of prostate cancer. But since levels of selenium in the soil vary widely throughout the world, selenium levels also vary widely in much of the food we eat. For example, a study conducted with people living in the southeastern USA, where soil levels of selenium are very low, found nearly half the rate of prostate cancer in people who took daily supplements of 200mcg of selenium compared to those who didn't take supplements. This and other studies found the benefits of selenium are even greater in ex-smokers.

Taking individual selenium supplements can be risky, though, since they can raise the risk of diabetes, according to new research (and side effects of excess selenium can include hair loss and brittle nails). It is best to take only the amount in a multivitamin product and add more fish to your diet, if you haven't already.

Get 10 minutes of sunshine (without sunscreen) a day You'll get valuable vitamin D, which the body manufactures when the sun's UVB rays strike the skin. Men in the UK – where vitamin D deficiency is fairly common – who took regular holidays in sunny climates, sunbathed regularly and had more overall exposure to ultraviolet rays were at far lower risk of prostate cancer than men who didn't do these things. Men with low levels of sun exposure also developed this form of cancer at a younger age (age 67.7) than those who got more exposure to sunlight (age 72.1). Of course, sun exposure raises your risk of skin cancer, so don't take this news as an excuse to sunbathe excessively; 10 minutes in the sun is all you need. If you spend most of your time indoors or covered up in the sun, you may want to consider supplementing with 1,000IU of vitamin D a day; it's also good for your bones.

" Salmon *is an excellent source of omega-3 fatty acids, which are strongly linked to a **lower risk** of prostate cancer.* **"**

Prevention boosters

Ask your doctor about a PSA test If your doctor suspects you have prostate cancer (or even if not), he or she may recommend a PSA test. This blood test measures levels of a protein called prostate-specific antigen, which is produced by prostate cells. The higher your levels, the more likely it is that you have prostate cancer. But the test isn't definitive; it sounds a lot of false alarms that can result in unnecessary needle biopsies. And since prostate cancer often grows so slowly that treating it isn't necessary, finding it early doesn't necessarily affect your risk of dying from it. That's why there's no consensus on whether doctors should use the test to screen men for the disease. Should you get screened? That's a decision you and your doctor should make based on your family history and your overall risk. Another test that's used to detect prostate cancer is the digital rectal examination, often used in conjunction with the PSA test.

Choose chicken Black skinned men who eat 650g or more of red meat a week – no matter what type – may be more than twice as likely to develop prostate cancer than those who eat less than 255g, according to a study that showed this difference in African-American men. Bacon, sausage and salami pose the greatest risk. So eat poultry and fish instead.

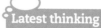

Latest thinking

Prostate cancer in many men does not require treatment. Older men with less aggressive forms of cancer can be simply monitored through check-ups and blood tests. In a major study of 9,000 men of an average age of 77, with early-stage prostate cancer who did not undergo treatment, researchers found that 72 per cent either died of other causes or didn't have enough cancer growth to warrant treatment. For the rest, about 10 years passed before the cancer grew enough to require treatment. Men with more aggressive forms of the cancer, however, do require treatment.

Psoriasis

In psoriasis, skin cells mature almost 10 times faster than normal. They pile up, creating silvery scales and patches of thick, red, scaly skin on the elbows, knees, legs, scalp and elsewhere. These steps can help you avoid the condition and, if you have it already, reduce the chances of a flare-up.

50%
The likelihood that using the drug etanercept will help prevent new psoriasis flare-ups.

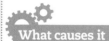
What causes it

Genetic factors raise your risk of psoriasis, but experts aren't certain what triggers the immune system malfunction that leads to the condition. It begins when infection-fighting T cells in the skin become too active, stimulating the overgrowth of skin cells.

Key prevention strategies

Quit smoking Tobacco use triples your risk of plaque psoriasis, the most common form of this condition, according to Swedish research. And if you already have psoriasis, smoking severely reduces the likelihood of you experiencing periods of clear, calm skin. When researchers asked 104 people if their psoriasis had ever gone into remission, 77 per cent of nonsmokers said yes, compared to just 9 per cent of smokers.

Think before you drink Alcohol appears to exacerbate and may even cause psoriasis in some cases. Finnish scientists have found that, for people who already had psoriasis, the extent of skin affected increased as their alcohol intake rose. If you're in the midst of a flare-up, abstaining makes sense. If your psoriasis is under control, and you find that an occasional drink doesn't aggravate your skin, enjoy it in moderation.

Maintain a healthy weight Gaining weight raised risk by 40 per cent in one Harvard Medical School study of more than 78,000 women. Doctors aren't certain how excess body fat contributes to psoriasis, but they do know that it can make existing skin problems worse and render psoriasis treatments less effective.

Try one of the newer treatments If you have psoriasis, your goal is to prevent flare-ups. Older medications were often too messy or risky for many people. For people with just a few spots of psoriasis, the latest sprays or foam products may be preferable. For

Dead Sea magic?

A month of sunbathing and swimming at one of the psoriasis spas along Israel's scenic Dead Sea is virtually guaranteed to improve or completely clear up your skin, studies show. A more affordable option is to fill a bath with warm water, sprinkle in Dead Sea salts (available from some health-food shops) and soak. In one German study, almost everyone who did this three or four times a week for a month saw their psoriasis improve significantly.

more severe forms of psoriasis or for psoriatic arthritis, newer injectable medications are available. One of them, etanercept (Enbrel), has been shown to improve psoriasis symptoms by 75 per cent in 57 per cent of the people who use it. Two others, adalimumab (Humira) and infliximab (Remicade), are even more effective.

Moisturise well Lubricating your skin every day can also help cut your odds of flare-ups prompted by dry skin.

Stress less Stress can trigger new outbreaks of psoriasis, so try to break the cycle by building relaxation into your day, even if it's just 10 minutes of quiet, calm breathing. Or try mindfulness-based stress reduction (MBSR). In one US study, people with psoriasis who listened to a MBSR tape while undergoing light therapy saw their skin clear up twice as fast as those who didn't hear the tape, researchers report.

Sunbathe, but safely Exposing your skin to sunlight for a few minutes each day can reduce inflammation and scaling. Eighty per cent of people with psoriasis who sunbathe every day see an improvement. Don't overdo it, though; for about 1 in 10 people, exposure to sunlight makes skin problems worse, and getting sunburnt raises the risk of skin cancer. Use a broad-spectrum sunscreen on skin that's not affected by psoriasis. Commercial tanning beds may help, but talk to your doctor first, as their use is controversial.

Steer clear of these medications Some medications can trigger a flare-up of this condition. If your doctor prescribes anti-malaria medication, beta-blockers, indometacin or lithium, ask whether a substitute is possible.

Prevention boosters

Avoid damage For about half of all people with psoriasis, it worsens 10 to 14 days after any sort of cut, bruise, insect bite or scrape. Even shaving or removing an adhesive bandage could trigger a flare-up, so take care with your skin.

Check your reaction to gluten In some studies, psoriasis symptoms decreased when people with coeliac disease avoided gluten – a protein found in wheat, barley and rye. You may have undiagnosed gluten intolerance if you frequently suffer diarrhoea, abdominal pain or wind.

Symptoms to watch for

Patches of thick red skin with silvery scales on the back of the elbows, front of the knees, other parts of the legs, scalp, lower back, face, palms and soles of the feet. Less often, they appear on the fingernails, toenails and genitals, and inside the mouth.

Latest thinking

In a recent survey, over half of people with moderate to severe psoriasis weren't getting the treatments that prevent future flare-ups. If your psoriasis isn't improving with lotions and topical medications, ask about light therapy and oral or injectable medications that help to regulate the overactive immune responses that trigger psoriasis.

See also:

Step 3: Quit smoking, page 66

Rosacea

Avoiding and treating flare-ups of this skin condition that only affects adults can help keep it from getting worse. Yet three out of four people don't recognise the early signs and symptoms. Flushing, blushing and persistently red skin on your cheeks and nose are major clues, but other hints are burning, stinging or itching facial skin as well as raised red patches and even swollen spots. In one survey, one in four sufferers had signs of rosacea on the neck, chest, scalp or ears, too. You may be more prone to rosacea if other family members have it.

45% The probable reduction in a recurrence of symptoms after using a skin-calming cream for six months following antibiotic therapy.

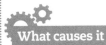

What causes it

Swelling of tiny blood vessels near the surface of the skin. Experts say that genetic factors and sun damage both play a role. There's also some evidence that microscopic mites that live in human hair follicles may clog oil glands and inflame skin.

Key prevention strategies

Avoid rosacea triggers The most important step in avoiding outbreaks is learning what triggers them. At the top of most people's lists are sun exposure, emotional stress and hot weather, but there are plenty more. In a survey of people with rosacea, about half said that wind, strenuous exercise, drinking alcohol, taking a hot bath, cold weather and spicy foods (including chillies and Indian food), as well as vinegar, white pepper and garlic set off a reaction.

To pinpoint your triggers, keep a rosacea diary. Every day make a note of common triggers you're exposed to and record days when symptoms flare up. After two to four weeks, you should see a pattern; triggers usually encourage redness within a few minutes to a day.

Avoid the sun The sun's ultraviolet rays aggravate rosacea simply by reddening the skin, but that's not all. US dermatologists from Boston University have found that sunlight also seems to trigger the production of compounds that encourage the growth of blood vessels close to the surface of the skin. So it is best to apply sunscreen to your face when you leave the house, stay in the shade during the brightest hours of the day in the summer and wear a broad-brimmed hat.

Don't let your sunscreen aggravate your skin, though. Choose a formula that contains dimethicone and cyclomethicone. In one study, these additives protected against the irritation caused by a common sun-blocking ingredient padimate-O. Or try a sunscreen formulated for babies, which may be milder. Also look for the ingredients zinc oxide and micronised titanium oxide, which deflect some of the sun's heat and therefore help prevent rosacea flare-ups.

Maintain healthy skin with a prescription cream or gel Many doctors begin treatment by prescribing antibiotics such as tetracycline for 12 weeks or so to help reduce bumps and redness. But that's not a cure. In one study, two thirds of the people who took a course of tetracycline for rosacea saw skin problems return within six months. That's why doctors also prescribe a skin-calming cream or gel containing metronidazole (Rozex) or azelaic acid (Finacea) for long-term use. In one study, people who used metronidazole for six months after antibiotic treatment were about half as likely to have redness or bumps return as those who didn't use it.

Consider laser therapy This may be the best way to treat broken blood vessels, persistent redness and a rosacea-induced swollen nose.

Prevention boosters

Be gentle to your skin Skin-care products such as cleansers, moisturisers, sunscreens and make-up can easily irritate and redden your skin if you have rosacea. To avoid irritation, choose mild, hypoallergenic cleansers and moisturisers, wash with lukewarm (not hot) water, and avoid contact with rough materials such as scratchy face washers, loofahs and abrasive skin-care products such as grainy skin scrubs and exfoliators. If your skin tends to sting when you apply sunscreen, make-up or medicated creams and gels, wait half an hour after washing so that your skin is completely dry before application.

Symptoms to watch for

Reddened skin, especially on your cheeks and nose. As rosacea progresses, you may notice small, spidery blood vessels appearing in these areas as well as bumps on your nose, cheeks, forehead and chin. You may also notice a gritty or burning feeling in your eyes. For a few people, rosacea triggers the buildup of tissue on and around the nose, too.

Latest thinking

Ask your doctor about a retinoid product. These vitamin A-based skin creams and gels speed cell turnover and are usually used to control acne and reduce wrinkles. Recent studies suggest they may reduce two visible signs of rosacea: redness and tiny blood vessels near the surface of the skin. Proceed with caution, though; retinoids can irritate the skin at first, so start with a low-dose product.

Sexually transmitted infections

Sexually transmitted infections (STIs) – including genital warts, herpes, chlamydia, gonorrhoea and syphilis – are common in young people, and also increasingly common among people over forty-five. As many STIs have no symptoms in the early or even late stages, you won't necessarily notice if a sexual partner is infected. But these tips might help you to avoid contracting an STI.

90%
The amount by which you could reduce your risk of HIV by always using a condom.

What causes it

Viruses, bacteria or protozoa (in the case of trichomoniasis) that are spread through sexual intercourse, oral sex or even skin-to-skin contact. Some, like HIV, are also spread through blood.

Symptoms to watch for

Many STIs don't cause any symptoms in the early or even late stages; infections like chlamydia can spread and permanently damage parts of your reproductive system without you being aware of it. See your doctor if you have genital itching or discharge; painful sex or urination; pelvic pain; a sore throat (if you have oral sex) or a sore anus (if you have anal sex); sores, blisters or scabs on your genital area, anus, tongue and/or throat; a scaly rash on the palms of your hands and soles of your feet; dark urine, light-coloured loose stools and yellow eyes and skin; swollen glands, fever and body aches; or unusual infections, unexplained fatigue, night sweats and weight loss.

Key prevention strategies

Be careful The fewer people you have sex with, the fewer of their sexual partners you're exposed to. And the less your exposure, the less likely you are to catch an STI. Abstaining from anal, oral or vaginal sex until you are in a long-term monogamous relationship is the safest policy. In some cases, you may want to ensure that a new partner has tested negative for any sexually transmitted infections.

Use condoms These simple sheaths have been around for more than 300 years, and they're still the best thing we have to protect against many STIs, including HIV/AIDS, gonorrhoea, chlamydia and trichomoniasis. They're not completely foolproof, but in the case of HIV/AIDS, for instance, properly used latex condoms could prevent 80 to 90 per cent of infections. However, it's important that a condom fits properly. If it doesn't, it's likely to slip off or break during intercourse. Try a regular size first, then adjust your choice accordingly.

Get vaccinated for HPV While progress on an HIV vaccine has been slow, there is a vaccine that prevents four of the most common types of human papillomavirus (HPV), including the ones that cause the majority of cervical cancers, not to mention genital warts. The three-dose vaccine is offered to girls at the age of 12 to 13 but can also be given to older girls or women. (See also *Cervical cancer*, starting on page 132.)

Prevention boosters

Get tested If you're sexually active and not in a monogamous relationship, you should be screened at least once a year for STIs, particularly gonorrhoea, chlamydia and trichomoniasis. A large

288

> *" **Condoms** are still the best thing we have to **protect** against many sexually transmitted infections. "*

The kindest cut?

A growing body of evidence suggests that circumcision may reduce the risk of STIs, particularly HIV, in men. For instance, a large Kenyan study showed that circumcision reduced men's risk of HIV infection from men or women by 53 per cent, while a Ugandan study showed a reduced risk of 51 per cent. Researchers think that circumcision protects against HIV because the foreskin of the penis contains a rich source of cells the virus likes to target; remove the foreskin, and you remove vulnerable cells. Other studies have found that circumcised men have a lower risk of infection with syphilis and chancroid (a bacterial infection). There is still no good evidence that circumcised men are less likely to infect women with HIV than uncircumcised men are.

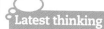

Latest thinking

One reason that men are at greater risk for AIDS than women are may be an enzyme produced by the prostate and found in semen; it appears to increase the risk of HIV infection. The finding, from German researchers, could open up a new avenue for prevention.

multinational study found that women infected with trichomoniasis are 50 per cent more likely to acquire HIV. Researchers don't know why, but they suspect that the infection may create minuscule areas in the vagina that provide entry points for the HIV virus.

Stop smoking We already know that smoking increases the risk of cervical cancer, but there's also intriguing evidence that smokers have a greater risk of HIV infection than nonsmokers, with the increase ranging from 60 per cent to more than threefold. Researchers suggest that the effects of tobacco smoke on the immune system may reduce the ability of immune cells to fight off the virus.

Shingles

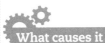

69%
The reduction in your risk of shingles if you eat a least five portions of fruit a day rather than one portion or less.

If you had chickenpox as a child or adult, the varicella-zoster virus responsible remains in your body, lying dormant in a bundle of nerves at the base of your spine. In one in five people, the virus reactivates perhaps decades later to raise a new red rash and blisters – often with excruciating skin pain – a condition called shingles. However, there's a host of immunity-bolstering strategies to deploy.

What causes it

The varicella-zoster virus, the same virus responsible for chickenpox. Once you've had chickenpox, the virus lies dormant in a bundle of nerve cells called the sensory ganglia, located near the spinal cord. It can re-emerge in the form of shingles decades later, often triggered by lowered immunity, physical or emotional stress, an injury or even dental work.

Key prevention strategies

Act fast if you notice shingles symptoms Shingles blisters heal in three to five weeks, but pain can linger for months or even years. Called post-herpetic neuralgia (PHN), this sharp, throbbing or stabbing pain affects up to 40 per cent of people who get shingles. PHN can make your skin so sensitive that wearing even the softest, lightest fabric is agony. Any skin contact – even a kiss or a cool breeze – can be excruciating. Living with this chronic pain can lead to depression, anxiety, sleeplessness and even weight loss.

Your best option for avoiding PHN is to recognise the early symptoms of a shingles outbreak and get to your doctor for treatment within 72 hours. Studies show that the antiviral drugs aciclovir (Zovirax), famciclovir (Famvir) or valaciclovir (Valtrex) can lessen PHN pain and shorten its duration if taken early. These medications seem to work by reducing the nerve damage caused by the virus. They also speed healing of the original shingles outbreak.

It sounds odd, but adding a tricyclic antidepressant such as amitriptyline or nortriptyline can help, too. In one study, people who took 25mg of amitriptyline daily were 50 per cent less likely to have lingering PHN pain after six months than those who were given a placebo. Study volunteers began taking the antidepressant, which calms nerve cells, two days after the rash came and continued for 90 days.

Other medications that have been shown to be effective are the anti-epileptic drugs gabapentin (Neurontin) and pregabalin (Lyrica). If you are suffering from PHN, discuss this option with your GP.

Look out for the new shingles vaccine A shingles vaccine which has recently been licensed in the UK could reduce your risk of developing this condition by 61 per cent. In studies of more than 38,000 women and men, the vaccine also reduced the severity of shingles outbreaks for people who developed it. The government's joint committee on vaccination and immunisation has recommended its use for people aged from 70 to 79 years, if it can be procured at a cost-effective price.

Consider the varicella vaccine if you are vulnerable Another vaccine is already available under the NHS for those with no antibodies to the varicella-zoster virus who work closely with people at high risk of developing shingles (for example, health workers looking after patients with lowered natural immunity).

Prevention boosters

Feed your immune system more fruit and vegetables In a study of 726 people, those who ate more than three servings of fruit a day cut their risk of shingles in half compared to people who ate fruit less than once a day, report researchers from the London School of Hygiene and Tropical Medicine. Study volunteers who ate five daily servings of vegetables reduced their odds by 70 per cent compared to people who had just one or two daily servings.

Learn the ancient art of tai chi In one US study of 112 healthy adults aged 59 to 82, this gentle, flowing exercise form boosted immunity against shingles dramatically. Compared to participants who took health-education classes, volunteers who practised tai chi three times a week for four months developed antibodies to the shingles virus on a par with those found in 30 to 40-year-olds who had received the shingles vaccine.

Symptoms to watch for

Burning, tingling or numb skin plus chills, fever, upset stomach and/or headache; after a few days, a red rash develops on one side of your body (commonly the torso), neck or face. The rash develops into fluid-filled blisters, which dry up in a few days. Shingles usually clears up completely in three to five weeks, but for 25 to 50 per cent of people who get it, severe nerve pain can linger for months or years after the rash has faded.

Latest thinking

Having just one close family member who has had shingles quadruples your risk of developing it, according to US dermatologists from the University of Texas Medical School in Houston. They asked 500 people with shingles about their relatives and discovered that, for 39 per cent, it ran in the family. The more relatives who've had it, the higher your risk.

See also:

Step 2: *Fruit and vegetables,* page 64

Sinusitis and sinus infections

Sinuses, the hollow cavities within the bones of the face, have a serious design flaw. When tiny sinus drainage holes swell shut, trapped mucus causes pressure and pain – and provides a home where viruses and bacteria can breed. Stop your next sinus infection before it starts by avoiding colds and flu, and treating or preventing respiratory allergy attacks. Follow these tips to ease congestion and promote drainage.

72%
The potential reduction in your risk of chronic sinus infections if you rinse your nose with salt water every day.

What causes it

When swollen nasal and sinus passages cause congestion, trapped mucus can become a breeding ground for viruses and bacteria.

Key prevention strategies

Rinse with saline For thousands of years, people have used saltwater rinses to prevent sinus problems. Now there's hard science to recommend this practice. When researchers from the UK's Royal National Throat, Nose and Ear Hospital reviewed eight well-designed studies, they concluded that a daily saline rinse cuts the risk of chronic sinus infections by up to 72 per cent. A rinse can also help prevent a cold from turning into a sinus infection. (Experts say you should use a decongestant first to reduce swelling so the fluid can drain out easily.)

You can buy a sinus-rinsing tool called a neti pot – it looks like a tiny watering can – at a health food shop, or use a bulb syringe to deliver the saline solution to your nose. Mix ¼ teaspoon of bicarbonate of soda and ¼ teaspoon of table salt in 250ml of lukewarm water. Lean over the sink. Tilt your head sideways and pour some of the solution into your upper nostril. Relax and keep breathing through your mouth as the liquid makes its way into the other nostril and back out. Spit out any solution that drains into your mouth. Repeat the process until you've used all the solution.

Blow gently

Blowing hard into a tissue is counterproductive because it triggers 'reflex nasal congestion', experts say. This natural reaction that happens when you sneeze involves an increase in blood flow, which makes nasal tissues swell. It serves a purpose by preventing anything going back up your nose or from travelling further up your nose. But it also happens if you blow too vigorously. The result is that your nose becomes even more stuffed up. Blowing gently is a better way to keep nasal passages open.

Thin nasal mucus Mucus trapped in your sinuses during a cold, flu or allergy attack is a breeding ground for viruses and bacteria. To keep it thin so it can drain easily, drink six glasses a day of water, hot tea or other clear liquids, unless your doctor has advised you to restrict your fluid intake. Also consider an over-the-counter remedy that contains the mucus-thinner guaifenesin, such as Robitussin. If you prefer a natural approach, inhale some steam for 10 minutes. Simply lean over a bowl of hot water with a towel over your head to trap the steam, stand in a steamy shower or sit in the steam room at the gym.

If the air in your home or office is very dry, increasing the humidity can help. Use a humidifier or vaporiser, and clean it regularly.

Warm your sinuses Placing a hot flannel on your face feels good if sinus pressure is building. It may also nudge microscopic hairs called cilia in your sinuses into action. They normally sweep back and forth at a brisk 700 beats per minute to whisk mucus along. When you have a cold or flu, the hairs move at a sluggish 300 beats per minute. Warmth seems to help them pick up the pace.

Use over-the-counter decongestants sparingly These tablets and sprays make blood vessels in your nose constrict, opening swollen nasal passages. Early in a cold or flu, using a decongestant could help promote drainage but it can backfire quickly, causing 'rebound congestion' as each dose wears off. Most experts believe that decongestants should not be used to help prevent sinus infections. The best advice is to never use an over-the-counter decongestant spray for more than three days, and use decongestants in tablet form sparingly; they can thicken mucus.

See your doctor for severe acute or chronic infections If you develop severe pain in your face or jaw and/or a fever higher than 38.5°C (101°F) when you have sinus congestion, consult your doctor. You may need an antibiotic.

Ask about preventive medication If you have multiple episodes of sinus congestion or sinusitis in a year, or your colds or allergy attacks regularly turn into sinus infections, you may benefit from long-term courses of appropriate antibiotics or from prescription steroid nasal sprays. The sprays soothe inflammation, which shrinks swollen nasal and sinus passages so they can drain, without risking the side effects of over-the-counter decongestant sprays.

Symptoms to watch for

Pressure and pain in your cheeks or behind your eyes (often on just one side) or in the upper teeth or jaw; green, yellow or brownish nasal discharge; fever higher than 38.5°C (101.5°F); extreme fatigue; reduced sense of taste and/or smell; cough from post-nasal drip; and new or unusual bad breath.

Latest thinking

Antibiotics inhaled as a mist via a device called a nebuliser could help if sinus surgery and other medical treatments don't cure chronic sinus trouble. In one US study of 42 people with repeated sinus infections, 76 per cent saw significant improvement with three weeks of nebulised antibiotics, and they remained free from infection for an average of 17 weeks. Before treatment, infections recurred every six weeks or so.

Skin cancer

Sunlight improves our mood and provides us with all-important vitamin D, but most of us are aware of the downside of over-exposure: skin cancer. The incidence of melanoma, the most serious form of skin cancer, is increasing faster than that of any other cancer. But it's impact varies from country to country. The UK has a rate of around 16 cases per 100,000 population, while Australia has a rate of about 28 cases per 100,000. UVB rays cause the majority of skin cancers, along with UVA rays, which make the damage worse (and may even cause cancer in their own right). Follow these strategies to reduce your risk.

40%
The amount you can reduce your risk of SCC, the second commonest skin cancer, by using sunscreen daily.

What causes it

UV rays from the sun or radiation. Your risk of basal cell skin carcinoma, the most common type, and squamous cell skin carcinoma (SSC), the second most common type, depends on cumulative sun exposure throughout your life. Your risk of melanoma, the deadliest form of skin cancer, seems to depend more on the intensity of the sun exposure. Even a single bad sunburn episode could lead to melanoma.

Key prevention strategies

Slap on the sunscreen If you're going to be out in the sun for more than 10 or 15 minutes, make sure you're wearing sunscreen. Apply it generously; most people don't use enough. It takes about 2 tablespoons just to cover your face and neck (don't forget the ears). And pay special attention to the danger areas; 55 per cent of skin cancers occur on the head or neck (balding men take note), followed by the hands, forearms and legs. Also use lip protection with an SPF rating of 15 or higher, and reapply sunscreen to all parts of your body every 2 hours (more often if you're in and out of the water).

Stay covered up Wearing protective clothing and a hat when you're in the sun is also important. These days, you can even find clothing with built-in sun protection; it's not cheap, but it's worth it if you spend a lot of time in places where the sun is strong. Regular cotton or linen clothing may not provide the physical protection from the sun that is necessary during prolonged periods of exposure, for instance, while playing or watching sport in full sun.

Be sure to protect your children's skin from an early age by covering up when the sun is strong. Don't forget sunglasses, too.

Use self-tanners, not tanning beds Tanning beds, which use UVA rays to darken your skin, can increase your risk of melanoma by up to 75 per cent, boost your risk of basal cell carcinoma by 50 per cent, and more than double your risk of squamous cell skin carcinoma (SSC). Stick to self-tanning creams, lotions and sprays, which safely provide a bronze glow.

" Wear **protective clothing** and a hat when you're **in the sun.** "

Shopping for sunscreen

Confused by the plethora of sunscreens on the supermarket shelf? Look for the following.

- **An SPF of at least 15** These products block 93 per cent of all incoming UVB rays, assuming you reapply often. SPF 30 blocks an extra 4 per cent, and SPF 50 an extra 6 per cent. SPF doesn't measure protection from UVA rays, only UVB.

- **UVA-filtering ingredients** Most sunscreens today offer 'broad-spectrum' protection, meaning they protect against both UVA and UVB rays. But some may not provide adequate UVA protection. For extra insurance, look for avobenzone or ecamsule, both of which absorb UVA light. (Unfortunately, they also add – sometimes significantly – to a product's price tag.) Also look for titanium dioxide or zinc oxide, which both scatter rather than absorb UVA light. If you have sensitive skin, look for a PABA-free sunscreen.

Prevention boosters

Quit smoking As with nearly every other cancer, your risk of skin cancer is higher if you smoke, with one study finding that the risk doubled in smokers.

Cook with turmeric This yellow spice, prominent in curry powder, contains the chemical curcumin, considered a strong cancer-fighting agent. Laboratory studies suggest that it may offer particular protection against melanoma.

Symptoms to watch for

Pearly or waxy bumps; a flat, flesh-coloured, or brown scar-like lesion on your chest or back; a red nodule on your face, lips, ears, neck, hands or arms; a flat lesion with a scaly, crusted surface on your face, ears, neck, hands or arms; an ulcer that won't heal; a large brownish spot with darker speckles; a mole that has one of the ABCDEs – asymmetrical shape, irregular border, a variety of colours, a diameter greater than 6mm or evolution (changes over time); dark lesions on your palms, the soles of your feet, fingertips and toes, or on mucous membranes lining your mouth, nose, vagina or anus.

Latest thinking

A skin cream under development could protect against certain types of skin cancer by making the outer layers of skin less vulnerable to damage from UV rays. The active ingredient, myristyl nicotinate, is derived from the vitamin niacin.

Snoring

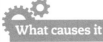

26% The potential reduction in snoring due to OSA if you're overweight and lose 10 per cent of your body weight.

If you've ever been banished to another room for snoring too loudly, it's time to take action. Loud night-time snorts and snuffling are a sign that tissue in the airway is vibrating with each breath at decibel levels that can keep your partner awake for hours. An estimated 50 to 60 per cent of loud snorers also have obstructive sleep apnoea (OSA), in which flabby tissue blocks the airway repeatedly throughout the night, leading to dozens or even hundreds of unrecognised partial awakenings and an increased risk of diabetes, high blood pressure, heart disease, depression, weight problems and dangerous daytime fatigue. OSA requires medical evaluation and treatment, but some of these measures may also help.

What causes it

The relaxation of your tongue as well as muscles in the roof of your mouth and throat during sleep, which causes throat tissues to vibrate as you inhale and exhale. The tissues may even collapse against your airway, restricting or blocking the flow of air. Being overweight or having enlarged tonsils, thick tissue on the roof of your mouth or an extra-long uvula all increase the chances that you'll snore.

Key prevention strategies

Prop yourself up Instead of lying flat on your back, sleep with your head, shoulders and upper back elevated on extra pillows or a foam wedge. Or raise the entire head of your bed by about 10cm by putting lengths of board (from a DIY shop or timber yard) under the legs at the top end of your bed. Elevating your head may keep flabby tissue in your throat from collapsing into your breathing passages and vibrating all night, alleviating regular snoring and even mild obstructive sleep apnoea.

Try the tennis ball cure Snoring tends to be worse when you sleep on your back because your tongue and soft palate crowd the back of your throat, blocking your airway. Sleeping on your side can help. To ensure you stay in that position, wear an old T-shirt with a front pocket (back to front) and put a tennis ball in the pocket (now at back), or put the ball in a bumbag and wear it to bed.

Lose weight When US researchers tracked 690 Wisconsin residents for four years, they found that people who gained at least 10 per cent in body weight were six times more likely to develop OSA. In people who already had it, whenever weight increased by 10 per cent, OSA worsened by 32 per cent. A 10 per cent weight loss reduced apnoea by 26 per cent.

Any weight loss relieved both OSA and ordinary snoring. Extremely overweight people who underwent surgical weight-loss procedures to lose 25 to 50 per cent of their body weight had a 70 to 98 per cent reduction in OSA in one study. And among people who lost just 7 to 9 per cent of their body weight, OSA fell by about 50 per cent.

> " **Elevating** your head may keep flabby tissue in your throat from collapsing into **your breathing** passages and vibrating all night. "

Avoid alcohol, sleeping pills and antihistamines at night All act as sedatives, which encourage snoring and apnoea by relaxing muscles in your mouth and throat. Sedatives such as these also make OSA worse, possibly by altering your ability to rouse yourself when your airway is blocked and making it more difficult to fall into the deep, restorative stages of sleep.

Relieve congestion before going to bed Inhale steam – in a hot shower, from a bowl of hot water or from the type of steam vaporiser that you can use as a facial sauna – to loosen mucus, then gently blow your nose. If you have seasonal allergies, keep the windows shut in your bedroom. Keep pets out, too, and remove throws and bedspreads – they can harbour allergens. Also, the next time you get new floor covering, choose something other than carpet.

Stop smoking Tobacco smoke irritates the mucous membranes in your throat. The result is that tissue swells, narrowing your airway and making snoring more likely. Smoking also increases your risk of heart disease, breathing problems and the irritation of seasonal allergies.

The risks of sleep apnoea

In a recent Hungarian study of 12,643 people, those with obstructive sleep apnoea had an increased risk of high blood pressure (40 per cent higher), of heart attack (34 per cent higher) and of stroke (67 per cent higher). The condition can also increase your odds of developing diabetes. A night of monitored sleep either with special devices brought to your home or in a sleep clinic, with monitoring of your breathing pattern, heart rate and blood oxygen levels, can help doctors determine whether you have apnoea. If you do, talk to your doctor about the advice outlined here, which may improve mild cases. If you're overweight, losing weight will help, but it may take months or years; treatment with medical solutions shouldn't be delayed while you slim down.

Symptoms to watch for

Light snoring may not disrupt your sleep or your partner's. But if you snore loudly and feel tired or have a headache when you wake up in the morning, or you gasp and choke or stop breathing for short periods of time during sleep, you may have obstructive sleep apnoea and should ask your doctor about testing and treatment.

Latest thinking

Obstructive sleep apnoea's immediate health risk is traffic accidents. People with OSA are twice as likely to be involved in crashes as those without the disorder, according to Canadian researchers who tracked the car insurance records of 1,600 people. And they're not just minor bumps: OSA was found to increase the risk of severe car crashes that caused physical injury and death to three to five times higher than normal.

Sleep with an oral appliance These devices, which look like a cross between a sports mouthguard and braces, reposition your jaw to prevent tissue in your mouth from flapping as you breathe. Custom-made versions, available from dentists, have a success rate of 70 to 80 per cent for ordinary snoring (and may also be effective for mild to moderate OSA). Off-the-shelf versions, sold online and in many pharmacies may be less effective.

Ask about surgery If you have a deviated septum, two surgical procedures – a submucous resection (SMR) and a septoplasty – can help to prevent the loud snoring this nasal defect may trigger. Both involve removing cartilage from the bony divider between your left and right nasal cavity. In one small study from Thailand, septum surgery significantly reduced snoring for 28 out of 30 study participants.

Try continuous positive airway pressure (CPAP) This is the 'gold standard' treatment for OSA. CPAP uses a small, quiet air compressor to gently push air through a mask over the sleeper's nose and keep the airway open during sleep. Studies show that CPAP can ease daytime sleepiness resulting from OSA by about 50 per cent, boost blood oxygen levels, reduce high blood pressure, improve heart function and reduce memory problems related to apnoea, and cut the number of sleep disruptions. It can also lower blood glucose levels in people who have both diabetes and apnoea.

Consider other surgical options If CPAP and oral appliances don't work, surgical removal of excess tissue from your nose or throat might. The most widely used technique, uvulopalatopharyngoplasty (UPPP) trims tissue from the rear of the mouth and top of the throat; tonsils and adenoids are usually whisked out at the same time. UPPP improves apnoea for just 40 to 60 per cent of those who have it, say Israeli researchers who reviewed many apnoea studies – but it's impossible to predict who it will work for.

Prevention boosters

Try a nasal strip These adhesive strips improve airflow through your nose by lifting the top of each nostril. Some research has found no benefit for snorers, but in one Swiss study, the strips reduced snoring after about two weeks of use. This inexpensive solution could work for you, especially if your snoring is caused by nasal congestion or mouth breathing. It may be worth a try.

" Playing a wind instrument can reduce snoring by about 22 per cent. ""

Sing loud, long and low When 20 chronic snorers practised singing techniques designed to tone the throat muscles, their snoring reduced, report researchers from the University of Exeter. The snorers agreed to keep voice-activated tape recorders by their beds for a week before and after their three months of daily 30 minute singing sessions.

Simply belting out your favourites from *The Sound of Music* won't do the trick. Exercises that work – such as energetically singing 'ung-gah' to familiar tunes – build strength in muscles that support your soft palate, the tissue at the back of your mouth that vibrates if you snore. You can order the programme at www.singingforsnorers.com.

Play a wind instrument When 25 snorers at a Swiss sleep clinic started playing the didgeridoo (an Australian wind instrument), daytime sleepiness improved by 12 per cent and snoring was reduced by about 22 per cent. If you don't have access to a didgeridoo, try playing a clarinet, flute or tuba instead.

Rest your head on an anti-snore pillow These pillows have many different designs; some elevate the head, while others have a hump in the middle and slanting sides so that you simply cannot sleep on your back. Do they work? Experts say there's no guarantee, but some types may work for some people.

Stomach bugs

All of us have at some time been hit by stomach bugs (gastroenteritis) that cause cramping, fever, vomiting and diarrhoea. The germ most commonly responsible for this misery is norovirus – a highly contagious virus that causes 90 per cent of gastric flu outbreaks, but other viruses and bacteria can cause such symptoms, too. It makes sense to take precautions to help prevent yourself falling victim to the next outbreak.

96%
The percentage of stomach-bug virus particles removed when you wash with soap and water for 20 seconds.

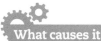

What causes it

Viruses and bacteria. Most stomach bugs are the result of infection with norovirus.

Symptoms to watch for

Nausea, vomiting, stomach cramps and diarrhoea that last for 12 hours to 3 days. Usually a bout of gastroenteritis is uncomfortable but not serious, but young children, older people and anyone with a weakened immune system should be watched for signs of dehydration or lingering infection. Drink plenty of clear fluids and call the doctor if you have any of the following signs: extreme thirst, dry mouth, dark or scanty urine, few tears, weakness, lethargy or dizziness.

Key prevention strategies

Wash your hands You can easily catch a stomach bug by touching a contaminated doorknob or shaking hands with someone who's carrying the infection. Soap, water and 20 seconds of vigorous scrubbing and rinsing can almost eliminate this risk. In one study, hand washing removed 96 per cent of viral particles compared to just 46 per cent removed with an alcohol-based hand sanitiser – the next best option.

If you're ill, stay out of the kitchen Many stomach-bug outbreaks have been traced to food prepared by people who were suffering from an active stomach infection or had just recovered from one. To reduce this risk, wipe down worktops and other kitchen surfaces with disinfectant wipes or a solution of 1 teaspoon of bleach in 1 litre of warm water. And be wary of any homemade food prepared by a friend or relative who's had a stomach bug.

Clean up fast after someone has been sick After a bout of vomiting and/or diarrhoea, a fast clean-up can help prevent the spread of germs. Wipe down exposed surfaces with a mixture of bleach and water. Wear rubber gloves and use paper towels (dispose of them outside the house). Wash the gloves before taking them off. The person who's been sick should also wash themselves and their clothes as soon as possible.

Stay safe at sea Cruise ships are far from the only places where you can contract stomach bugs such as norovirus; it spreads swiftly wherever there are many people in a confined area. But because health officials are obliged to report illnesses contracted on ships, outbreaks of stomach bugs on cruise ships tend to hit the headlines. Studies appear to show that the risk of contracting norovirus on board has increased over the past two decades. As elsewhere the best advice is to wash your hands

Infection know-how

Norovirus, a family of germs responsible for most cases of gastric flu, which isn't really the flu because it's not caused by the influenza virus, is highly contagious before anyone has warning signs. Here are some good reasons to protect yourself all the time:

- **Number of viral particles it takes to become infected** Less than 10
- **Percentage of infected people who are contagious but never have symptoms** 30
- **Length of time someone is contagious after vomiting ends** 2 to 3 weeks
- **Lifespan of the virus on floors, worktops and other hard surfaces** 3 days
- **Lifespan on 'soft' surfaces such as rugs** Up to 12 days.

often and use a hand sanitiser. If there is an outbreak of gastroenteritis onboard, it is wise to avoid uncooked food, use bottled water and never share glasses or eating implements.

Prevention boosters

Wash fruit and vegetables and handle food safely Viruses and bacteria that trigger vomiting and diarrhoea can live on virtually any food. Follow the advice of food storage and handling given under *Food poisoning*, starting on page 182.

Eat more 'good bacteria' Antibiotics taken for any reason can reduce the volume of beneficial bacteria in your intestinal tract, and getting more of these bacteria by eating yoghurt with live active cultures or taking a probiotic supplement can help keep your digestive system in good shape. When UK researchers studied 135 people taking antibiotics, those who also had a yoghurt drink daily cut their risk of diarrhoea by 21 per cent compared to those who had a placebo drink. The yoghurt drink contained the bacteria strains *Lactobacillus casei, L. bulgaricus* and *Streptococcus thermophilus*, commonly found in commercial yoghurts and in probiotic supplements available from health food shops and some pharmacies.

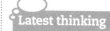

Latest thinking

While any food can carry viruses and bacteria that cause stomach troubles, bivalve shellfish (for example, oysters) can pose a special threat if they're uncooked. Substances in an oyster's gastrointestinal tract allow the norovirus to bind and accumulate, a recent US study showed, meaning you could get a large dose of the virus if you eat a contaminated one. So eat your oysters steamed, boiled, baked or fried, because thorough cooking destroys the virus.

See also:

Step 2: *Fight germs in key places,* page 80

Stomach cancer

Here's the good news about stomach cancer: ever since we discovered that most ulcers and the most common form of stomach cancer (non-cardia cancer) are caused by the bacterium *Helicobacter pylori* and began treating people who are infected with it with antibiotics, rates of stomach cancer have plummeted in most countries. The not so good news is that, at the same time, rates of the other form of stomach cancer (cardia cancer) are rising.

up to **33**%
The amount by which you could reduce your risk of this cancer by eating an orange three or more times a week.

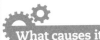

What causes it

The bacterium *Helicobacter pylori* causes the most common form of stomach cancer, non-cardia gastric cancer, or cancer anywhere in the stomach except the top 2.5 cm, where the stomach meets the oesophagus. Cancer in that area is called cardia gastric cancer. Ironically, the presence of *H. pylori* seems to reduce the risk of cardia cancer. Other risk factors include chronic gastritis, or inflammation of the stomach; age; being male; a diet high in salted, smoked or preserved foods and low in fresh fruit and vegetables; smoking; certain types of anaemia; and a family history of the disease.

Key prevention strategies

Avoid foods high in nitrites Most studies evaluating what people eat and their risk of stomach cancer find that diets high in salted, pickled or smoked foods (pickled vegetables, herring, smoked salmon, etc.) and preserved or salt-cured meat (such as ham and bacon) significantly increase the risk of stomach cancer. Foods of this type contain nitrites, which can form cancer-causing compounds, called nitrosamides, in the stomach.

Eat an orange a day Eating plenty of fresh fruit and vegetables, especially citrus fruits such as oranges, can reduce your risk of stomach cancer. Japanese research suggests that three or more servings of citrus fruit a week reduced the risk of stomach cancer by up to 33 per cent (though this may be a high estimate). Researchers suspect the antioxidant vitamin C and a carotenoid called beta-cryptoxanthin may protect stomach cells from cancer-causing damage.

Consume more whole-grain foods If your diet is packed with refined grains in the form of white bread, rolls and shop-bought cakes and pastries, and you avoid whole grains in the form of foods such as oats or wholemeal bread, you could be increasing your risk of stomach cancer by anywhere from 50 per cent to more than sevenfold. Conversely, the more fibre you eat, the lower your risk of stomach cancer – this is particularly true for women.

Cut out steaks and fatty takeaways A Mexican study of about 1,000 people found that those who ate an average of 25g of saturated fat a day were 3.3 times more likely to develop stomach cancer than those who kept their intake at 14g or less. Another study found that every 100g of meat eaten per day – no matter what type – increased the risk of stomach cancer nearly 2.5 times overall and more than five times in people infected with *H. pylori*.

Prevention boosters

Treat *H. pylori* infection early Infection with this bug is the leading cause of stomach ulcers; now it is known that it's also the leading cause of stomach cancer. Researchers think that inflammation related to *H. pylori* infection leads to changes in the stomach lining that make the stomach less acidic, encouraging the formation of the cancer-causing compounds, nitrosamides.

Getting rid of the infection can lower your risk A Chinese study randomly assigned 1,630 people infected with the bacteria to take either a placebo or therapy designed to eradicate the bacteria. After seven and a half years, six people in the placebo group had developed stomach cancer compared to none in the treatment group. The traditional treatment for *H. pylori* infection is 7 to 14 days of treatment with a proton-pump inhibitor such as omeprazole (Losec) or esomeprazole (Nexium) and the antibiotics clarithromycin and either amoxicillin or metronidazole. Ask your doctor if you should be tested for *H. pylori*.

Kick the habit The smoking habit, that is. As with so many other cancers, smoking increases your risk of stomach cancer; nearly one in five cases is related to smoking. Overall, European researchers found that people who had ever smoked had about a 40 per cent increased risk of stomach cancer; those still smoking had a risk 73 per cent (in men) to 87 per cent (in women) higher than that of people who never smoked.

Wash your hands thoroughly and often This is especially important before cooking and eating. Researchers suspect that one of the main ways *H. pylori* is transmitted is through person-to-person contact – such as inadvertently touching the vomit or stool of someone who has been infected by the bacteria.

Symptoms to watch for

Internal bleeding; it may not be noticed unless you have a faecal occult blood test or the bleeding becomes extreme, causing anaemia. Symptoms of more advanced cancer include an uncomfortable feeling in your abdomen that antacids don't improve and that worsens when you eat; black, tarry stools; vomiting blood (a medical emergency); vomiting after meals; weakness, fatigue and weight loss; and feeling full after meals even if you eat less than normal.

Latest thinking

In the near future, there will be a vaccine for *H. pylori*. It may need to be given early, however; studies have found children as young as seven who are infected with the bacteria.

Stomach ulcers

Eating bland food and taking stomach-coating antacids was once standard treatment for stomach ulcers, but now it is known that the bacterium *Helicobacter pylori* is responsible for two-thirds of all stomach ulcers and duodenal ulcers (those in the beginning of the small intestine). Use of nonsteroidal anti-inflammatory drugs (NSAIDs) such as aspirin and ibuprofen causes almost all the rest, with a smaller proportion caused by steroid medications such as prednisone.

What causes it

The bacterium *Helicobacter pylori*; regular use of non-steroidal anti-inflammatory drugs (NSAIDs), such as aspirin and ibuprofen; and regular use of oral steroids such as prednisone.

Key prevention strategies

Avoid aspirin and NSAIDs If you regularly take low-dose aspirin for your heart or an NSAID such as ibuprofen for pain relief – for example, for arthritis – you're raising your ulcer risk. These medications interfere with mechanisms that protect the stomach lining from corrosive acids. They thin the stomach's protective mucus coating, reduce production of an acid-neutralising chemical called bicarbonate and reduce blood flow, which helps stomach cells repair themselves. NSAIDs can also cause an ulcer to bleed more freely.

In one UK study of more than 3,000 people, those who had taken NSAIDs were 2 to 30 times more likely to have bleeding ulcers than those who didn't take these painkillers. So if you need to take painkillers, what should you do? Experts suggest the following three strategies:

○ **Switch to paracetamol for the relief of chronic pain** This common over-the-counter pain reliever is not an NSAID and won't harm the lining of your stomach. (To avoid the risk of liver failure, take no more than 4g per day, and avoid alcohol when you take it.)

○ **Add another protective medication** Some experts recommend the prescription medications sucralfate (Antepsin) and misoprostol (Cytotec) to shield the stomach lining from damage if you must take an NSAID on a daily

Treat an ulcer right

If you're relying on antacids and a bland diet to control ulcer pain, it's time to update your strategy. The only way to prevent dangerous complications such as bleeding and stomach perforation: get tested to confirm a *Helicobacter pylori* infection, which causes most ulcers, then start treatment. A course of antibiotics, usually given along with an acid-reducing proton-pump inhibitor, is the only way to knock out the spiral-shaped germ, which burrows into the protective mucus layer lining the stomach wall, releasing toxins that burn holes in the stomach lining.

basis. However, if you are pregnant or planning to become pregnant, do not take misoprostol, which has been linked to an increased risk of miscarriage and birth defects.

○ **Take care with antidepressants** If you are taking an NSAID along with an SSRI antidepressant such as fluoxetine or citalopram, this will increase the risk of stomach bleeding by a factor of six. If this combination is unavoidable, your doctor may recommend that you take a proton pump inhibitor such as lansoprazole or omeprazole to protect the stomach.

Quit smoking Nicotine in tobacco increases the amount of acid in your stomach and makes it more concentrated. Studies show that smoking raises the ulcer risk seven times higher than normal. Some experts suspect that chemicals in tobacco smoke may somehow work with *H. pylori* to create stomach ulcers.

Cut down on or cut out alcohol Alcohol irritates and erodes your stomach lining and boosts acid production. While it may not cause ulcers on its own, scientists believe that it boosts risk in people with an *H. pylori* infection and those who use NSAIDs regularly. And since half of all adults are infected with this bacterium by the age of 60, holding back on alcohol sounds like a good idea.

Prevention boosters

Start the day with porridge and fresh fruit In a Harvard study of more than 47,000 men, those who ate seven servings of fruit and vegetables a day had a 33 per cent lower risk of developing ulcers than those who had less than three servings daily. Eating plenty of soluble fibre – the type found in pulses, pears and porridge – was found to cut risk by 60 per cent. Experts aren't sure why these foods are protective. One possibility is that soluble fibre becomes a thick gel in your digestive system and may help protect the walls of your upper small intestine from damage by digestive juices.

Eat spinach and beetroot Vegetables such as spinach, lettuce, radishes and beetroot are rich in chemicals that raise levels of nitric oxide in the stomach. Swedish researchers think that higher nitric oxide levels may strengthen the stomach's inner lining so it can better protect itself from digestive acids.

Symptoms to watch for

Burning pain in your abdomen that starts two to three hours after a meal, gets worse at night when your stomach is empty and eases when you eat something. An ulcer may also take away your appetite, cause weight loss, or make you feel nauseated. Get immediate help if you notice blood in your stool or in vomit; a bleeding ulcer can be a medical emergency.

Latest thinking

Three antibiotics are better than two against the ulcer bug. In a review of 10 studies involving more than 2,800 people with ulcers, Italian researchers found that *H. pylori* was eliminated in 93 per cent of the volunteers when they used a 10-day therapy that involved three different antibiotics. Only 77 per cent of those who were given two antibiotics improved.

305

Stress-related disorders

Stress is a normal reaction to things we find challenging. According to scientists, the stress response evolved to prepare primitive human beings to face or run away from danger by triggering physiological changes. But if the challenge persists, the body remains in a state of alert and tension builds up. This can have a negative effect on health, leading to all sorts of mental and physical problems. Here are some stress-relieving strategies to help you stay on an even keel.

39%
The amount by which you could reduce your stress levels by looking forward to something funny.

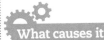

What causes it

The most common stress triggers include: pressure at work, financial worries, family and relationship problems, bereavement, unemployment, moving house, job loss, and changes in sleeping habits.

Take a deep breath

Try this quick and simple exercise if you start to feel stressed.

- Sit or lie in a comfortable position with your arms and legs uncrossed and your back straight.
- Breathing from your abdomen, inhale through your nose, slowly to a count of five.
- Pause and hold your breath for a count of five.
- Exhale through your mouth or nose to a count of five.
- When you have exhaled completely, take two breaths in your normal rhythm and then repeat the second and fourth steps.
- Repeat this sequence for 3 to 5 minutes.

Key prevention strategies

- **Talk it through** Discussing worries with friends, family and colleagues can stop inner tension building up as well as helping to put a different perspective on your problems.
- **Keep active** Regular exercise helps to clear the mind enabling you to deal with problems more calmly. It also releases stress-relieving feel-good endorphins. Aim to do some kind of physical activity that you enjoy for at least 30 minutes on most days.
- **Learn inner calm** Relaxation techniques such as yoga, deep breathing exercises, massage and meditation can help to dissipate stress.
- **Manage your time better** Try to establish a good work/life balance. Make a 'to do' list at the start of every day. Prioritise jobs and do the ones that are most important first. Learn to delegate both work and domestic tasks wherever you can.
- **Watch your lifestyle** Make sure you eat regularly and get plenty of sleep. Avoid drinking more than the safe limits of alcohol – it is all too easy to 'self medicate'. Avoid smoking altogether and don't resort to illegal drugs in the hope that they will make you feel better.
- **Keep a stress diary** Recording thoughts and events can help to identify what triggers your stress – often the first step towards dealing with the problem. Having done this, step back and assess what it is in your life that is making

you stressed. What can you offload or change? How can you establish a better balance between work, social life and family time?

- **Focus on the positive** Change the things you can and accept the things you can't. If you find this hard to do, consider trying cognitive behavioural therapy (CBT), which teaches you how to replace unhelpful patterns of thinking with more positive thoughts.

- **Make space for humour** A US study undertaken in 2008 reported that among the male subjects, levels of three key stress-related hormones, cortisol, adrenaline and dopac, dropped by 39 per cent, 70 per cent and 38 per cent respectively in those who were told they were going to watch a funny film, compared to other members of the group.

- **Doctor, doctor** Your GP may prescribe drugs that can help treat the symptoms of stress such as anxiety, depression, phobias and panic attacks in the short term. In the longer term he or she may recommend counselling such as CBT (above). If your stress is causing additional health problems, your doctor will advise on appropriate treatment alongside measures to help you reduce stress.

Prevention boosters

- **Make 'me' time** Regular leisure activities can help you unwind. Make some time every day for yourself – for example, have a leisurely soak in a hot bath, read a novel, listen to music, go to the cinema – whatever you choose to do make sure you enjoy it.

- **Modify Type A behaviour** If you are a very driven and competitive person, you may also feel under pressure most of the time. You can't necessarily change your character, but building in relaxing leisure activities will help to protect your good health and counteract the ill-effects of stress.

- **Create happy challenges** Setting yourself achievable goals – for example, improving your foreign language skills or taking up a new hobby – boosts confidence, which in turn makes it easier for you to cope with stress in your life.

Visualise it

Visualisation uses the power of the imagination in a directed way to bring about beneficial physical, psychological and emotional changes. Experts believe it can help reduce stress.

Start by conjuring up a mental image of a place you can go to feel calm. It might be a sunken garden with a waterfall, a long sandy beach or the top of a snow-clad mountain. During a stressful day find somewhere quiet where you won't be disturbed, shut your eyes and conjure up an image of you walking into your special place. Breathe slowly and deeply for a couple of minutes as you enjoy being in your haven of calm. As you open your eyes you will feel the tension floating away.

Symptoms to watch for

Disturbed sleep; no longer enjoying the things that you used to; appetite changes; feeling irritable; tiredness and lethargy; inability to concentrate or make decisions; loss of interest in sex; feelings of anxiety and panic attacks; feeling unable to cope.

Latest thinking

In a German study that monitored the brain activity of volunteers while they carried out timed arithmetic puzzles, it was found that the parts of the brain involved in mood, emotion and stress regulation were more active among past and present city dwellers than those who lived in the country. These findings may lead to new stress-reduction strategies.

Stroke

A tiny clot, a rip in a tiny blood vessel – the smallest things can trigger a stroke – a potentially life-altering event that shuts off the flow of blood and oxygen, destroying brain cells. Strokes kill at least five million people worldwide each year and disable millions more, yet most of us put it last on the list of our greatest health fears. The good news is that there's plenty you can do to prevent having a stroke.

up to **40**%
The possible drop in your stroke risk if you lower high blood pressure by just 5 points.

Key prevention strategies

Lower your blood pressure If your blood pressure reading is above 120/80, your risk of suffering a stroke is dramatically higher than that of someone with lower blood pressure. Why? The blood flows through your arteries and veins with greater force, and this increased force poses a triple threat. It damages blood vessels in your brain and in the carotid arteries in your neck that supply brain cells with life-giving oxygen. It can also create fragile 'bulges' in these arteries, which can rupture. And it can make arteries thicken to the point where they squeeze shut. Finally, it can damage the inner lining, allowing plaque to form; pieces of plaque can break off and travel in the bloodstream to the brain. Small wonder, then, that high blood pressure is the number one cause of stroke.

However, if your blood pressure is high, every 5-point drop can cut your stroke risk by up to 40 per cent. This strategy works whether you're 45 or 95. In a UK study of nearly 3,500 people over the age of 80 with high blood pressure, those who used medication to get their reading down to 150/80 cut their risk of stroke by 53 per cent compared to volunteers who received a placebo. That's higher than the healthy target (120/80) mentioned above, but it illustrates the benefits of lowering high blood pressure. Agree your own healthy blood pressure goal with your doctor.

Take TIAs seriously

Before a stroke, 30 to 40 per cent of people get a warning sign: a brief mini-stroke known to doctors as a transient ischaemic attack, or TIA. Symptoms can include loss of strength or sudden numbness in your face, arm or leg; feeling confused or unable to speak; loss of vision; and/or an unusual headache. The symptoms disappear as swiftly as they start, but that doesn't mean the danger has passed. Your risk of having a full-blown stroke in the next two days is 1 in 20, and over the next three months, it's 1 in 10, unless you take action.

Call your doctor immediately and explain what happened. He or she may put you on medications to prevent blood clots, lower cholesterol and reduce blood pressure. In a British study, this combination cut the odds for a major stroke after a TIA by 80 per cent.

You may not even need medication to reach an optimal level. If your blood pressure's top number (systolic) is between 120 and 139, or your bottom number (diastolic) is between 80 and 89, you have what is termed prehypertension – and stand a good chance of reducing your pressure with weight loss, exercise and a healthy, low-salt diet full of fruit, vegetables and low-fat dairy foods. If your reading stays above 140/90 despite lifestyle changes, your doctor may prescribe one or more medications to bring it down.

Reduce 'bad' LDL cholesterol Too much harmful LDL cholesterol in your bloodstream starts the process that leads to the thick streaks of fatty plaque developing inside artery walls, including the carotid arteries supplying your brain. These blood vessels can eventually become so narrowed that the tiniest clot can block blood flow completely.

Reducing LDL with a low-fat diet plus a statin medication shrinks this plaque and protects the brain. In one study of 2,531 men with slightly elevated LDL levels, those who took cholesterol-lowering medication cut their stroke risk by 31 per cent.

Start with a diet low in saturated fat and rich in fruit and vegetables, whole grains, and low-fat dairy foods. Avoid fatty red meat and full-fat dairy foods such as cheese. Lose weight if you need to and stay active. If your LDL levels stay high ask your doctor about taking a statin. (An ideal reading is below 2.5mmol/l if you have other risk factors for cardio-vascular disease; your doctor can advise the safe level for you). If you've already had a stroke, taking a statin can cut your risk of a second stroke by 16 per cent.

Be physically active and snack on nuts Doing both these things can raise levels of HDL cholesterol – the type that removes LDL from the bloodstream. The minimum healthy HDL level is 1.0mmol/l, but higher is better for your brain. In one study, people with the highest HDL cut their risk for the type of strokes caused by fatty plaque build-up by an incredible 80 per cent.

Avoid fatty takeaway foods and alcohol Until recently, experts didn't realise how dangerous triglycerides, another type of blood fat, were for brain health. But in one study, people with the highest levels had triple the stroke risk of those with the healthiest, lowest levels. A healthy triglyceride reading is below 8mmol/l. You can manage high triglycerides by losing weight and cutting down on alcoholic beverages, having grilled or baked fish instead of burgers, and using rapeseed and olive oil instead of butter. Cutting back on refined carbohydrates (found

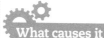

What causes it

Nearly 90 per cent of strokes are the result of a clot breaking off or a bulging area of plaque that cuts off blood flow to part of the brain. The rest happen when a blood vessel in or near the brain ruptures, cutting off the supply of oxygen to surrounding brain cells.

Symptoms to watch for

Classic signs are sudden numbness, weakness or paralysis of the face, arm or leg, usually on one side of the body; sudden difficulty talking or understanding speech; sudden blurred, double or reduced vision; sudden dizziness, imbalance or lack of coordination; sudden severe or unusual headache; confusion. Stroke symptoms that may only affect women include loss of consciousness or fainting; shortness of breath; falls; sudden pain in the face, chest, arms or legs; seizure; sudden hiccups, nausea, tiredness; or sudden pounding or racing heartbeat.

Latest thinking

There's nothing normal about 'high normal' blood pressure. Until recently, experts thought blood pressure readings between 120/80 and 140/90mmHg were perfectly healthy. Now those levels are considered 'prehypertensive' or 'high normal' – and they can raise your risk of dying from heart disease by 58 per cent, making this problem more deadly than smoking.

in white bread, sweets, snack foods and sugary drinks) is also important. Ask your doctor whether fish oil supplements could help (large doses may be needed.)

Stop smoking Smoking just 10 cigarettes a day increases stroke risk by 90 per cent – even if your cholesterol and blood pressure levels are low. Nicotine, carbon monoxide and a cocktail of other chemicals in burning tobacco stiffen arteries, deposit more plaque onto artery walls and make blood stickier and more prone to clotting. Give up now and your stroke risk will begin to fall immediately; within as few as five years your risk falls to that of someone who never smoked.

Fix a fluttering heart Atrial fibrillation (AF) occurs when the upper chambers of the heart quiver instead of beating strongly and steadily, and it quadruples stroke risk. It affects 1 in 25 people over the age of 65 and 1 in 10 over eighty. AF allows blood to pool in the heart and form clots; a strong heartbeat can then send a clot into your brain, resulting in a stroke.

If you're over 65, ask your doctor to assess you. Simply checking your pulse and listening to your heartbeat may be enough, or you may need a test called an electrocardiogram (ECG). The usual treatment for AF involves taking the blood-thinning medication warfarin, which experts say could cut stroke risk by 69 per cent. Yet many people who would benefit from this medication never get it, in part because doctors are cautious about giving it to older people who may bruise or bleed more easily if they have a fall.

Take a daily low-dose aspirin If you've already had a stroke or are a woman at high risk of a stroke, taking a 75mg aspirin tablet daily could protect your brain. In one study, aspirin cut women's stroke risk by 17 per cent (but didn't lower most men's risk). If you're at above-normal risk for stroke – due to high blood pressure, out-of-balance blood fats, atrial fibrillation or a family history of stroke – ask your doctor if low-dose aspirin therapy is appropriate for you.

Prevention boosters

Walk five days a week Taking a brisk hour-long walk five times a week cuts your odds of a stroke almost in half, and half an hour's walk reduces your odds by about 25 per cent. In fact, any vigorous physical activity that burns 1,000 to 3,000kcal per week will cut your risk, including swimming, cycling and most team sports.

Preventive stroke surgery

If the arteries in your neck are blocked by plaque, your stroke risk soars, but surgically clearing them out could cut your odds by 50 to 75 per cent, according to studies. You may be a candidate if you've already had a stroke or mini-stroke or if X-rays using special dyes or other tests reveal that one of the arteries is 75 to 99 per cent blocked. (Warning signs of a blockage include blurred vision, slurred speech or weakness.) The main surgical technique for clearing the arteries supplying the brain—called carotid endarterectomy – involves making an incision in one or both arteries and scraping out the plaque.

Cultivate the fine art of resilience Breathe deeply, sing your favourite song, do yoga or dance. Learning to cope with anxiety and stress, in whatever way works for you, could cut your stroke risk by an extra 24 per cent.

Put fish on the menu Eating grilled or baked oily fish one to four times a week could cut your stroke risk by 27 per cent, possibly because healthy fats in fish can keep blood vessels flexible and discourage plaque. But don't have greasy fish and chips: in a US study from Harvard Medical School, people who ate fried fish just once a week raised their stroke risk by as much as 44 per cent.

Enjoy alcohol in moderation One drink may lower your risk, but having too many raises it, according to Chinese researchers who followed 64,000 men for nine years. Their conclusion was that having one to six units of alcohol per week lowers stroke risk by 8 per cent; having more than 21 units per week raises it by 22 per cent. And don't have all your drinks on one night; experts suggest a maximum of two units on any one day.

Go for whole grains Opt for porridge, wholemeal bread and cereals, and brown rice. Women who ate the most whole grains had a 40 per cent lower risk of stroke than those who ate the fewest, according to a Harvard School of Public Health study.

See also:

Cause 1: Hypertension, page 22
Cause 5: Bad cholesterol balance, page 30
Step 1: Exercise, page 62
Step 3: Quit smoking, page 66
Step 7: Cut back on saturated fat, page 72

Temporomandibular disorder

The joints responsible for your jaw 'popping out' when you open your mouth wide are the temporomandibular joints on each side of your head, and they keep your jaw attached to your skull. They're among the most complicated and commonly used joints in the body, able to move forwards and backwards and from side to side. However, chewing too much, grinding your teeth or having a misalignment in your teeth and/or jaw can all stress the joints or the muscles and ligaments that control them, leading to temporomandibular joint (TMJ) disorder, leading to jaw pain and headaches.

77%
The amount you can reduce jaw pain by doing a daily programme of jaw exercises.

What causes it

Stress, a misaligned jaw, clenching your jaw, grinding your teeth or degenerative joint disease.

Key prevention strategies

Rest your jaw Minimise your chewing and halve the thickness of your sandwiches so you don't have to open your mouth as wide. If you need open your mouth wider than the width of three fingers, your sandwich (or other food) is too thick. It also helps to avoid chewing gum and other chewy foods such as toffees.

See your dentist Our teeth were not meant to grind, so if you grind your teeth (or, if you're not aware of it, your sleeping partner says you do), see your dentist, who can fit you with a mouth guard to wear at night to prevent this major cause of TMJ. You're also more likely to develop TMJ if the teeth in your upper and lower jaws don't come together neatly when you close your mouth. If you have this problem (called malocclusion), ask your dentist to refer you to an orthodontist, who may recommend braces to realign your teeth, improve your bite and reduce your risk of TMJ.

Stop clenching your jaw and grinding your teeth Some people hold tension in their jaws without even realising it, especially when they're under stress. That tension can contribute to or even cause jaw pain to the extent that it becomes painful even to eat. The following tips can help you learn how to relax the muscles that control your jaw.

- **Put a cork in it** Hold a wine bottle cork between your front teeth and relax the muscles around it. Do this whenever you feel yourself clenching or until relaxing those muscles becomes automatic.
- **Try biofeedback** Electromyogram (EMG) biofeedback teaches you to relax your jaw and facial muscles. Sensors that signal when they

detect muscle tension are attached to your forehead, jaw muscles and shoulder muscles. Then you're taught techniques to relax and reduce the tension. After practising for a few weeks, you're able to reduce the tension without the sensors. Ask your doctor or dentist for a referral.

○ **See a cognitive behavioural therapist** This type of therapy can help you realise and change factors, such as your response to stress and anxiety, that contribute to jaw pain. It may provide you with skills to reduce your response to pain and works well for many people when it comes to preventing jaw pain. You don't need many sessions; one study found that pain improved by 50 per cent in people who had just four sessions. Your doctor can help you find a specialist. Combining this type of therapy with biofeedback and a mouth guard works better than any of the three treatments alone.

Prevention boosters

Exercise your jaw Jaw exercises can strengthen and stretch the muscles around the joints. In one study of laser treatment plus exercises and exercises alone, it was the exercises, rather than the laser treatment that produced dramatic reductions in jaw pain. Practise the exercises below several times a day. Try to hold each position for a full 5 seconds and repeat the exercise five times.

○ **Opening** Hold the back of your hand underneath your jaw to create resistance. Open your mouth about 2.5 cm wide while pushing against your hand.

○ **Forward thrust** Hold the back of your hand against the bottom of your jaw to create resistance. Push your jaw forward against the pressure of your hand.

○ **Sideways thrust** Hold the palm of your hand against the side of your jaw that hurts. Push your jaw to that side.

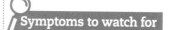
Symptoms to watch for

Jaw pain; neck, back and facial pain; pain in and around the ear; headaches; or ringing in the ear (tinnitus). You may hear a clicking sound when you chew.

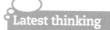
Latest thinking

Injections of botulinum toxin type A (Botox), the same substance used to erase frown lines, into the muscles used to move the jaw have been found to significantly reduce pain in people with TMJ.

See also:

Step 8: *Reduce chronic stress, page 74*

Thrush

85%
The potential reduction for thrush infections if you eat yoghurt containing live *Lactobacillus acidophilus* cultures every day.

The yeast-like fungus *Candida albicans* is naturally present in the body but is kept under control by our complex and delicate ecosystems. However, there are times when this organism can get out of control leading to unpleasant symptoms – a condition commonly known as thrush. Thrush can affect the vagina (where it causes itching, discharge and soreness), the mouth (those who use steroid inhalers for asthma are particularly susceptible), skin folds and, in babies, a particularly 'angry' form of nappy rash. Minimise the risk of candida infection with this advice.

What causes it

Uncontrolled growth of the yeast organisms that live on your skin, in your vagina and in your mouth. The growth occurs in the vagina when the normally acidic environment loses its acidity. Many things can disrupt vaginal harmony, including pregnancy, menstruation, diabetes, oral contraceptives, antibiotics and steroids. Elsewhere, candida overgrowth can be caused by lowered immunity or the presence of a 'yeast-friendly' environment in an area of skin or mucous membrane.

Key prevention strategies

Always opt for cotton underwear To keep vaginal thrush at bay, swap your nylon lingerie for cotton, which allows air to circulate and helps prevent yeast organisms from breeding in the vagina. And always wear briefs under tights.

Keep the area dry After a shower or bath, dry yourself thoroughly, especially the skin folds and genital area, before getting dressed. And change out of a wet swimming costume as soon as possible. Yeast loves damp environments.

Wipe the right way After bowel movements, wipe from front to back, never back to front. One theory about vaginal thrush is that bacteria get into the vagina from the rectum, disrupting the microbial environment that normally keeps this organism in check.

Drugs that prevent disease

Up to 30 per cent of women taking antibiotics are prone to thrush. These medications can kill off beneficial bacteria that keep vaginal flora in balance. If you're taking antibiotics and you're prone to yeast infections, keep some over-the-counter thrush creams or vaginal pessaries (miconazole or clotrimazole) on hand and use them at the first sign of vaginal itching or discharge.

Spoon up some yoghurt Some studies suggest that eating 250g a day of yoghurt that contains live, active bacteria cultures could reduce the risk of recurrent thrush in the vagina and elsewhere in the body.

Check your blood glucose If you've ever made bread, you know that yeast needs sugar to grow. That's why people who have diabetes are much more vulnerable to candida infections, especially vaginal and oral thrush. A recent study has shown that oral thrush is five times more common in people with severe Type 1 (insulin-dependent) diabetes than in the population at large. (See *Diabetes*, starting on page 164 for some prevention tips.)

Avoid oral sex If you're a woman, having your partner perform oral sex five or more times a month can increase your risk of vaginal thrush. Avoid or limit oral sex, if you're susceptible.

Keep your dentures clean Take special care with oral hygiene and keep your dentures clean if you have them. Around 7 in 10 people who wear dentures will develop oral thrush at some stage and this can often be related to inadequate cleaning.

Prevention boosters

Avoid dyes and perfumes Coloured or perfumed toilet paper and scented sanitary pads and tampons can disrupt the normal vaginal environment, so stick to uncoloured and unperfumed products.

Avoid feminine hygiene products There's absolutely no need to use douches, powders or sprays; they can cause irritation and upset the balance of your vaginal flora. Washing the external genital area with water and a mild soap is sufficient for good personal hygiene.

Follow a low-GI diet Just as those with diabetes are more prone to thrush, so too are people with insulin resistance. This condition occurs when cells become resistant to insulin, the hormone that allows glucose into cells, leading to higher than normal blood glucose levels. Foods made with sugar, high-fructose corn syrup and white flour – most shop-bought cakes and pastries as well as biscuits, crackers, crisps and sweetened drinks – all contribute to insulin resistance because they cause rapid rises in blood glucose. White bread and white rice do the same. Instead, eat foods with a low glycaemic index (GI), which have a less marked effect on blood glucose. These include most high-fibre foods such as vegetables, pulses and whole grains; 'good' fats from olives, nuts and avocados; and lean protein foods.

Symptoms to watch for

Vaginal thrush can cause itching and burning in the vagina and the surrounding area (the vulva), as well as vulval swelling; cottage cheese-like vaginal discharge; pain during intercourse. Oral thrush can cause sore, white patches or ulcers in the mouth. In the skin folds or nappy area, thrush infection can cause a bright red and sore rash.

Latest thinking

A tablet designed to help maintain the normal acidity of the vagina could one day be used to prevent recurrent yeast infections. Such a product is currently under investigation.

See also:

Cause 4: *Insulin resistance*, page 28

Tinnitus

Tinnitus – a buzzing, ringing or roaring sound in the ears – affects 1 in 20 people. One theory links it to hearing loss. For some, tinnitus can wreak havoc on their ability to lead normal lives. Whether you've never experienced it or it's just beginning to creep up on you, try to keep the worst at bay with these recommendations.

18%
The percentage of tinnitus sufferers who could have escaped the condition by avoiding excessive noise.

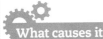

What causes it

Loud noises, noise and age-related hearing loss, excess earwax, infections, heart and blood vessel problems, medications, tumours, allergies, problems related to the jaw and neck.

Symptoms to watch for

A ringing, buzzing, roaring, hissing or whistling noise in your ears, which may be noticeable only when you're in a quiet place.

Key prevention strategies

Turn down the volume One common culprit in tinnitus is noise-related hearing loss, even if the loss isn't severe enough for you to notice. Always protect your ears in noisy environments, such as loud rock concerts or workplaces with noisy machinery, by using sound-excluding earplugs or ear protectors. (See also *Hearing loss*, page 202.) In one 2005 study of tinnitus sufferers, exposure to excessive noise was an associated factor for 18 per cent of cases.

Don't use cotton buds Putting anything in your ears -- including a finger or a cotton bud – can push wax against your eardrum, which can contribute to or worsen tinnitus. A better way to clear the wax is to pour a drop or two of olive oil in one ear and lie on the opposite side for an hour while the oil loosens the wax and brings it to the surface. When you turn over, have a tissue handy to catch the wax and oil.

Cut back on aspirin If you often take aspirin for headaches or other pain, talk to your doctor about alternatives. Overuse can lead to tinnitus. If you're on daily low-dose aspirin therapy, though, don't worry; the amount isn't great enough to cause tinnitus.

Relax your jaw Tinnitus is a common symptom of temporomandibular joint disorder (TMJ), in which the hinge that works the upper and lower jaw and the muscles and ligaments that support the jaw are stressed or misaligned. (See page 312 for prevention tips.)

Watch your medications More than 200 medications have the potential to cause tinnitus as a side effect. If you're hearing ringing or buzzing, ask your doctor if one of your medications could be to blame and whether you can lower the dose or switch to another one. Some of the worst culprits are those that can damage the inner ear, such as quinines (for malaria and rheumatoid arthritis); some diuretics (for high blood pressure); certain antibiotics; and some chemotherapy drugs.

Control your blood pressure
High blood pressure can contribute to tinnitus. You're more likely to hear blood whooshing through blood vessels when the pressure of the flow is strong. Try to control your salt intake and keep your cholesterol in check, since narrowed arteries can cause turbulent – and loud – blood flow. (For further advice, see *High blood pressure*, starting on page 212.)

Already have tinnitus?

Devices that emit soothing sounds can be helpful for those with tinnitus. Neuromonics is a new form of treatment that uses an MP3-like device to deliver specially selected sounds to people with tinnitus as part of an overall treatment approach that includes counselling and support. One study, sponsored by the device's manufacturer, found that, after six months, 86 per cent of people using the device improved at least 40 per cent. The product is not yet marketed in the UK but advice and a range of sound therapy CDs are available from the Tinnitus Society (www. tinnitus.org.uk).

Prevention boosters

Try to stay on top of things Depression, anxiety, stress and tinnitus seem to go hand in hand, although no one's sure which is the chicken and which is the egg. One study found that nearly half of people with disabling tinnitus also had major depression. People with tinnitus who take antidepressants or receive psychotherapy improve more than those who do neither.

Watch what you drink There's some evidence that drinking too much alcohol or too many soft drinks or cups of coffee or tea (caffeine is a likely culprit) can lead to tinnitus.

Check your posture Holding your neck in a hyperextended position, such as when you ride a bicycle, can lead to tinnitus. Look in the mirror and ask yourself: Do I look like a bird pecking for worms? If the answer is yes, your neck is hyperextended. (Read more about proper neck posture in *Neck pain* on page 262.)

Get a blood test Low blood levels of iron or thyroid hormones can sometimes be associated with tinnitus.

Latest thinking

Electrodes implanted in the part of the brain responsible for hearing and then electrically stimulated can suppress the phantom noises of tinnitus. One study of 12 people who underwent the implants showed a 97 per cent reduction in tinnitus.

Urinary tract infections

Women are twice as likely as men to experience urinary tract infections (UTIs). The female urethra is much shorter, giving the bacteria responsible for these painful, often recurrent infections easier access to the bladder. What's more, in women the urethral opening is just a short distance from the anus, making it far easier for bacteria from the bowel to enter. About 6 out of 10 women will have at least one UTI, and about 2 out of 10 will experience them repeatedly.

up to **39**%
The possible reduction in the risk of recurrent urinary tract infections if you drink 250ml of cranberry juice daily.

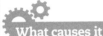

What causes it

Usually infection with bacteria that have originated in the bowel. They spread from the anus to the urethral opening and then to the bladder.

Symptoms to watch for

Burning or pain during urination; feeling that you need to urinate more often than usual; feeling that you need to urinate but are not able to; leaking urine; cloudy, dark, unusually smelly or blood-stained urine.

Key prevention strategies

Practise good hygiene Prevent bacteria from getting in by wiping from front to back after a bowel movement – never from back to front. Use a clean flannel to wash the skin around your rectum (and especially between rectum and vagina) every day when taking a shower or bath.

Drink up The more you drink, the more you urinate and the more bacteria you flush out of your urinary tract. Drinking unsweetened cranberry juice offers the best protection (see *Easy ways to eat more cranberries*, right). Blueberry and other berry juices are also good choices.

Visit the bathroom before and after sex Do two things: urinate to flush any bacteria from the urethra and then wash the area. Although many experts continue to recommend this tactic, research has failed to confirm its effectiveness.

Wear 100 per cent cotton underpants Cotton 'breathes', keeping the area between the legs drier than if you wear underpants made from synthetic fibres, and dry conditions discourage bacteria.

Don't use vaginal douches or other feminine hygiene products Douches and vaginal sprays irritate the urethra and disrupt the natural balance of good and bad bacteria that keeps infections in check.

Prevention boosters

Review your contraceptive method Using a diaphragm and spermicide may increase the risk of UTIs in women with a history of repeated infections. Even condoms with spermicide can raise the risk

Easy ways to eat more cranberries

Cranberry juice for urinary tract infections is one of those folk cures that may really work. An antioxidant compound in cranberries (and blueberries) prevents bacteria from adhering to the cells of the bladder and urinary tract. Most studies on cranberries have been conducted with pure juice (buy unsweetened juice; if it's too tart, dilute with water) or dried cranberry extract pills. Here are five other ways to get this important fruit into your diet.

1. Sprinkle dried cranberries over salads or yoghurt, and mix them into your muesli base instead of raisins.

2. Use fresh cranberries with apples, blueberries, peaches or cherries in pies.

3. Enjoy cranberry relish Combine a bag of fresh cranberries, 225g sugar, the juice of one lemon and a cinnamon stick in a medium saucepan and cook over medium – low heat until the cranberries pop. Cool and serve with pork or chicken.

4. Whip up a cranberry smoothie Blend together a banana, 8ml low-fat mixed berry yoghurt, 8ml cranberry juice and 100g fresh or frozen blueberries.

5. Make cranberry ice cubes Mix equal amounts cranberry juice and water, pour into ice-cube trays, then freeze.

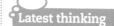

Latest thinking

The bacteria that cause UTIs actually invade bladder cells, taking up residence there more or less permanently and leading to recurrent infections. This may be one reason that prophylactic (preventive) antibiotic therapy works so well. Previously, researchers didn't think the bacteria could get into bladder cells.

of UTIs. Consider changing to a contraceptive method that isn't inserted into the vagina, such as the oral contraceptive pill, or contraceptive injections or implants.

Ask about antibiotics If you're prone to UTIs, ask your doctor about prophylactic antibiotics – antibiotics taken to prevent infection. Whether taken daily, only after sex, or every few weeks, they work to prevent UTIs, according to studies.

Ration the intercourse The more often you have sex, and the more people with whom you have sex in a year, the higher your risk of developing UTIs.

Varicose veins

One-way valves in the leg veins prevent blood flowing backwards, but if the veins expand or the valves weaken – due to an inherited tendency, inactivity, a job that keeps you on your feet, pregnancy or other factors – blood can do just that, causing pooling that leads to twisted, bulging varicose veins and tired, achy, itchy, swollen legs. These steps can protect your legs and keep varicose veins from growing worse if you already have them.

50%
The amount by which you could reduce your risk of varicose veins by drinking a glass of wine most days.

What causes it

Weakened valves in leg veins, which allow blood to pool instead of travelling back to your heart. Age, genetics, lack of exercise, standing for long periods, and extra pressure due to being overweight or pregnant can all make the valves less efficient.

Key prevention strategies

Don't stand when you can sit Standing for long periods every day raises your risk of varicose veins by 60 per cent, say researchers at Finland's Tampere University Hospital. Sitting down instead of standing whenever possible helps by easing pressure on blood vessels. Keep your feet flat on the floor or cross your ankles when you sit; crossing your legs at the knees squeezes veins shut, further blocking blood flow.

Elevate your legs Raising your legs prevents blood from pooling. If you already have varicose veins or simply want to give your leg veins extra help, lie down at home and raise your legs higher than the level of your heart by propping them on pillows or even against a wall so that gravity works to prevent blood pooling in the veins of your legs and feet.

Lose any extra weight you may have put on lately Being overweight puts extra pressure on the veins just below the surface of the skin in your legs. And according to one large Scottish study, being overweight or obese raised the risk of developing varicose veins by as much as 58 per cent. By eating less and getting more aerobic exercise, you'll lose weight and also reduce your risk of developing leg vein problems in the first place.

Rein in vein pain

Horse chestnut seed extract is one remedy for varicose vein discomfort that seems to really work. When Harvard Medical School doctors reviewed 16 well-designed studies of thousands of people with weak valves in their leg veins, they found that those who took the extract had four times less pain than those who got a placebo. Half saw a decrease in swelling, and 70 per cent had less itching. They also reported improvement in feelings of fatigue and heaviness in their legs. UK researchers say this safe botanical may be as effective as compression stockings. Escin, the active ingredient, has strengthened the walls of small blood vessels in lab studies.

The usual dose is 300mg (containing 50 to 75mg of escin per dose) every 12 hours for up to 12 weeks. A supplement is recommended because horse chestnut contains toxins which are removed during processing.

Keep your legs on the move Standing and even sitting still at a desk all day allows blood to pool in your legs. Push it back towards your heart as often as you can. How? If you're sitting, point and flex your feet to boost circulation. If you're on your feet, get the blood moving several times an hour by rising on your toes, shifting your weight from one foot to the other, bending your legs and walking on the spot.

Wear compression stockings These long elastic socks squeeze your legs so blood can't pool as much. They can ease aching and swelling if you have varicose veins and may help prevent them, too. When Japanese researchers measured the legs of 20 people with varicose veins, they found that all grades of compression stockings reduced swelling, but medium and strong-grade stockings worked best. These are labelled '22 mmHg' or '30-40 mmHg'. UK researchers found that the stockings can reduce the amount of blood pooling in leg veins by about 20 per cent.

Wear flat shoes High heels may not cause varicose veins, but wearing them makes your calf muscles less effective at pumping blood back towards your heart when you walk, according to experts at Wake Forest University Baptist Medical Center in the USA.

Prevention boosters

Stop straining Working too hard to have a bowel movement increases pressure on veins in the lower legs. Researchers at Scotland's University of Edinburgh report that this kind of pushing nearly doubled the risk of vein problems in men. To make bowel movements as easy and comfortable as possible, drink plenty of water during the day and increase your fibre intake. (For more tips, read the advice given for *Constipation* on page 146.)

Enjoy a glass of wine Spanish researchers who analysed the health records of 1,778 people found that those who enjoyed a glass of wine every day had a 50 per cent lower risk of varicose veins than those who drank less – or more. Other research suggests that flavonoids and saponins in wine can help keep blood vessels flexible and healthy.

Symptoms to watch for

Enlarged, bulging veins; swelling in your legs and ankles; a 'heavy', painful, or cramp-like feeling in the legs; itching; discoloured skin.

Latest thinking

Exercise your legs even if you wear compression stockings. Scientists in Hong Kong recently discovered a design flaw in the stockings: as study volunteers moved around, their stockings sometimes squeezed more tightly at the widest part of the calves than at the ankles, which could actually promote blood pooling rather than prevent it. The researchers' conclusion was that compression stockings are still worth wearing if you're on your feet all day, but you should also be sure to exercise your calf muscles to help keep blood moving.

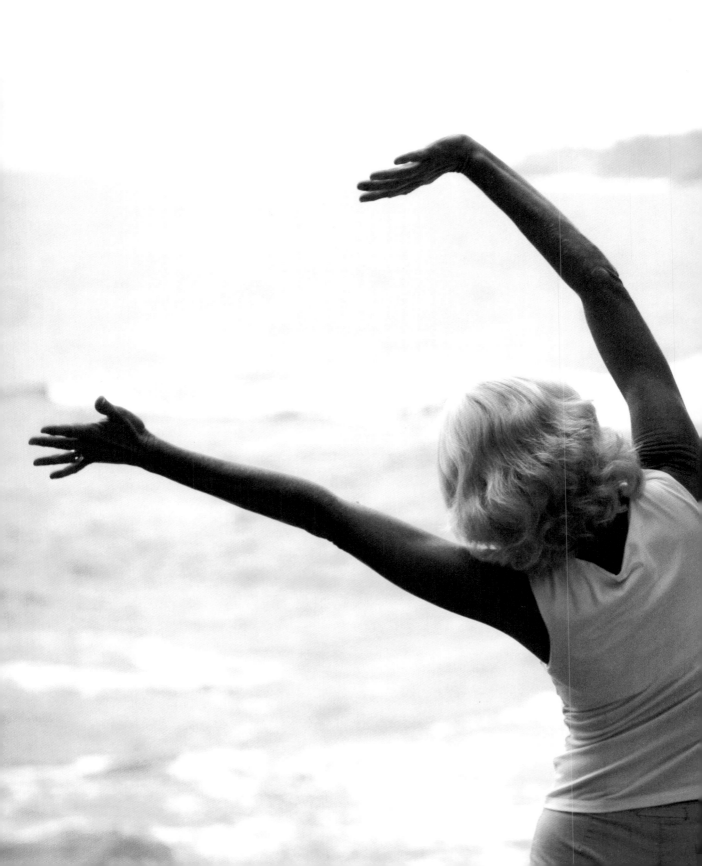

SECTION 3

Exercises

Discover the therapeutic physical exercises that will help you to build strength and relieve a variety of aches and pains throughout your body.

Back strength and flexibility

A strong, supple back is one that's less likely to be injured. Simply doing this series of easy exercises every day can help to protect against back pain and back injury (see page 114). They strengthen and/or lengthen the back muscles, abdominal muscles (which provide support for your back), and even the hamstrings at the back of your legs, which help minimise stress on the lower back. Gradually build up to the number of repetitions suggested.

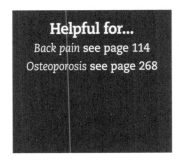

Helpful for...
Back pain see page 114
Osteoporosis see page 268

Hamstring stretch

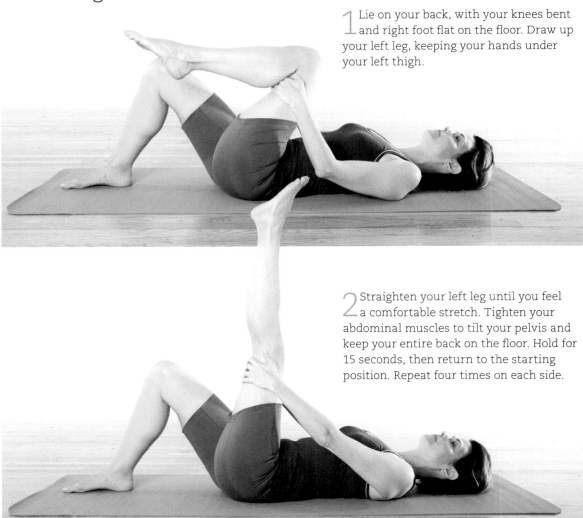

1 Lie on your back, with your knees bent and right foot flat on the floor. Draw up your left leg, keeping your hands under your left thigh.

2 Straighten your left leg until you feel a comfortable stretch. Tighten your abdominal muscles to tilt your pelvis and keep your entire back on the floor. Hold for 15 seconds, then return to the starting position. Repeat four times on each side.

Knee-to-chest stretch

1 Lie on your back, with your knees bent and feet flat on the floor, arms by your sides.

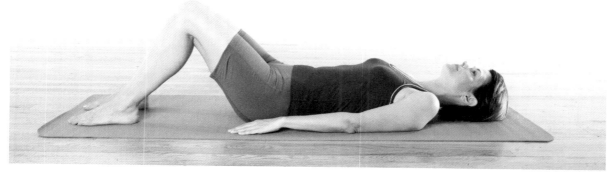

2 Using both hands, pull one knee towards your chest until you feel a comfortable stretch in your lower back. Hold for 15 seconds. Return to the starting position and repeat with the other leg. Repeat four times on each side.

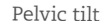

Pelvic tilt

Lie on your back, knees bent and feet flat on the floor. Tighten your abdominal muscles and gently tilt your pelvis backwards to flatten your lower back into the floor. This is a small motion, mostly felt and not seen. Hold for 5 seconds. Repeat ten times.

Back rotation

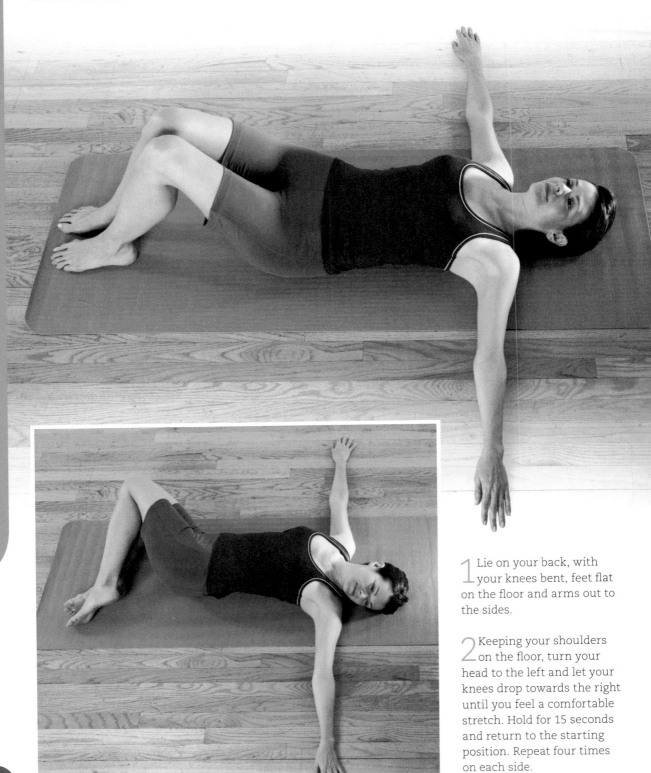

1 Lie on your back, with your knees bent, feet flat on the floor and arms out to the sides.

2 Keeping your shoulders on the floor, turn your head to the left and let your knees drop towards the right until you feel a comfortable stretch. Hold for 15 seconds and return to the starting position. Repeat four times on each side.

Arm and leg lift

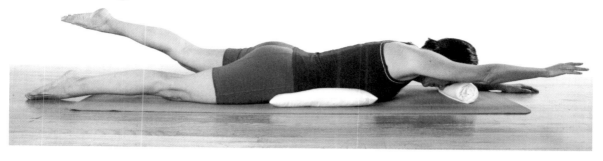

Lie face down with a thin pillow under your stomach and a small rolled towel under your forehead. Tighten your buttocks, then lift your right hand and left leg about 10-20 cm off the floor. Hold for 2 seconds, then lower and repeat on the other side. Continue for 2 minutes. Don't let your back arch excessively while doing this exercise.

Halfway sit-up

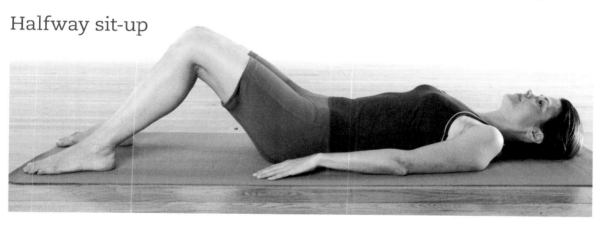

1 Lie on your back with your knees bent and feet flat on the floor.

2 Tucking your chin in towards your chest, stretch your arms out in front of you. Then, using your abdominal muscles, slowly curl your upper body forward, lifting one vertebra off the floor at a time, until your shoulders clear the floor. Keep your chin tucked in. Hold for 3 seconds. Slowly lower yourself to the floor one vertebra at a time. Repeat ten times.

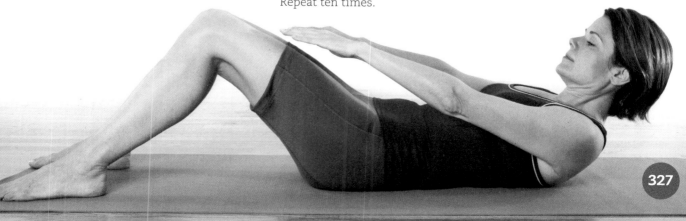

327

Hip bridge and roll down

1 Lie on your back with your knees bent and your legs about hip width apart.

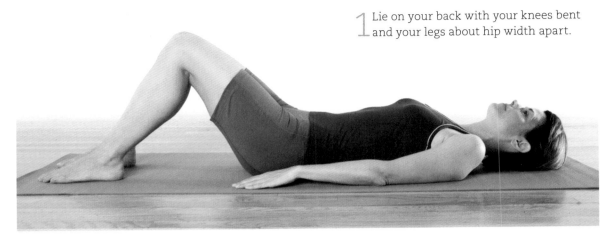

2 Tighten your abdominal muscles, tilt your pelvis backwards and use your buttock muscles to lift your hips until your body forms a straight line from knees to shoulders. Hold for 5 seconds.

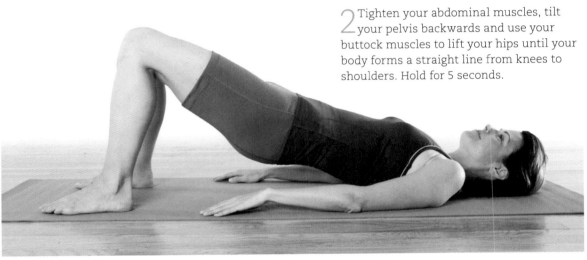

3 Slowly roll your spine back down to the starting position, touching one vertebra at a time to the floor, starting near your shoulder blades and ending with your tailbone. Relax your abdominal muscles. Repeat ten times.

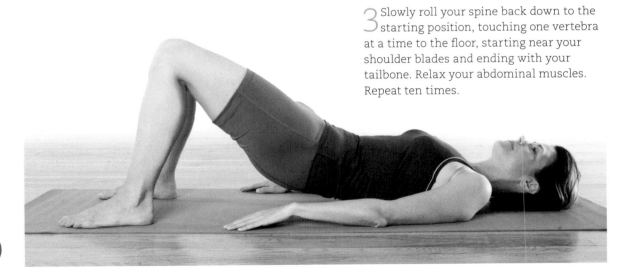

Cat stretch

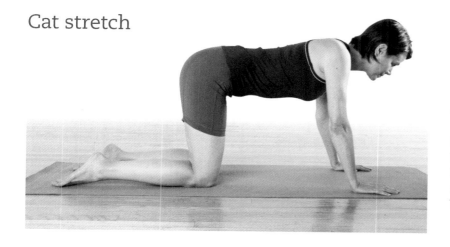

1 Get on your hands and knees on the floor with your knees below your hips, your hands below your shoulders, and your back straight.

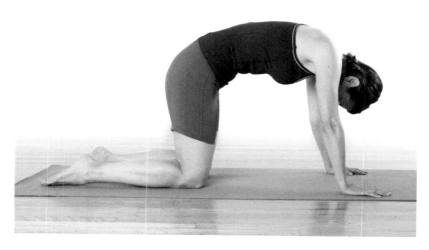

2 Drop your head, tuck your tailbone under and raise the middle of your back. Hold for 5 seconds, then return to the starting position.

3 Raise your head and hips and stick out your buttocks, allowing your back to sag towards the floor. Hold for 5 seconds. Return to the starting position. Repeat ten times.

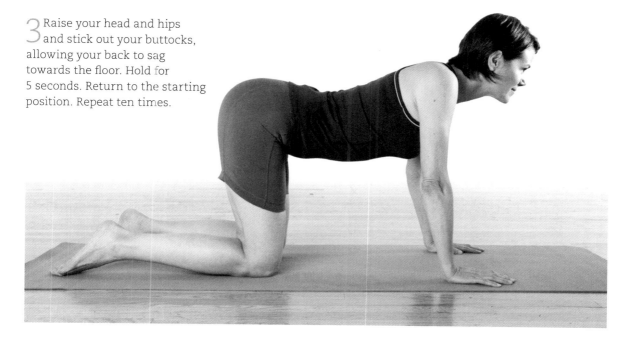

Better balance

Improving your balance and strengthening the muscles in your legs and around your hips helps to prevent falls – and therefore hip and other fractures – a serious risk for osteoporosis sufferers (see page 268) and older people. The following exercises are designed to do just that. Start by holding onto a sturdy chair or table. As you get stronger and your balance improves, hold on more loosely and then with just one finger; finally, don't hold on at all. Keep your abdominal muscles held in during the exercises.

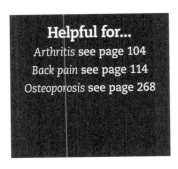

Helpful for...
Arthritis **see page 104**
Back pain **see page 114**
Osteoporosis **see page 268**

Knee bend

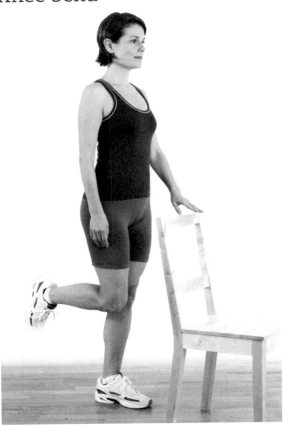

1 Stand straight with one hand on a table or chair back for balance.

2 Bend your right leg at the knee, bringing your foot as far up behind you as possible. Hold for 5 seconds, then lower your foot and repeat with your left leg. Repeat ten times on each side.

Heel raise

1 Stand straight with one hand on a table or chair back for balance.

2 Rise on the balls of your feet as high as possible. Hold for 5 seconds, then lower your heels to the floor. Repeat 15 times. Rest for a minute, then repeat another 15 times.

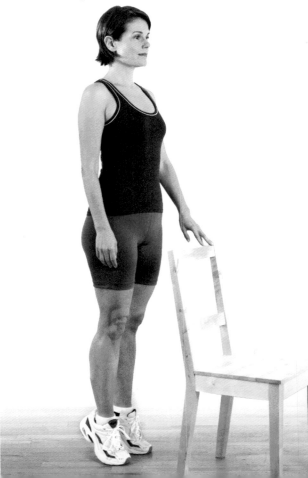

Hip and knee bend

1 Stand straight with one hand on a table or chair back for balance.

2 Slowly raise one knee towards your chest while keeping your waist and hips straight. Hold for 5 seconds, then slowly lower your leg and repeat with the other leg. Repeat ten times on each side.

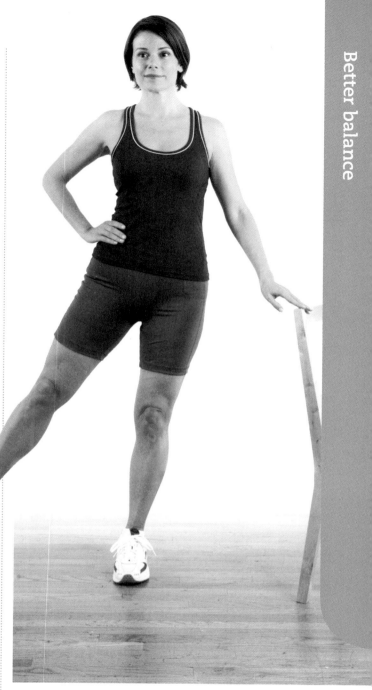

Hip strengthener

1 Stand 30-45cm away from a table or behind a chair. Lean forward and hold onto the support.

2 Slowly lift one leg back and up without bending the knee or letting your back arch. Hold for 5 seconds, then slowly lower your leg and repeat with the other leg. Repeat ten times on both sides.

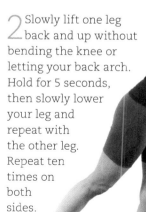

Side leg raise

1 Stand straight and hold onto a table or chair back for support.

2 Keeping your back straight, slowly raise one leg to the side as far as you can. Keep your foot and toes pointing straight ahead. Hold for 5 seconds, then slowly lower your leg and repeat with the other leg. Repeat ten times on each side.

Exercises for hands and wrists

Repetitive wrist and hand motions can lead to repetitive strain injury (RSI) and carpal tunnel syndrome (see page 128). Perform these preventive exercises before you begin work, once an hour while you're doing a repetitive task such as typing and before you go home. Hold each move for 5 seconds. Complete each sequence ten times, then stand with your arms relaxed by your sides for 10 seconds.

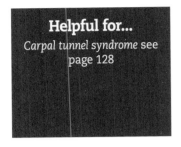

Helpful for...
Carpal tunnel syndrome see page 128

Forearm stretch

1 Press your right hand against a wall, with your fingers open. Firmly press the palm of your hand into the wall.

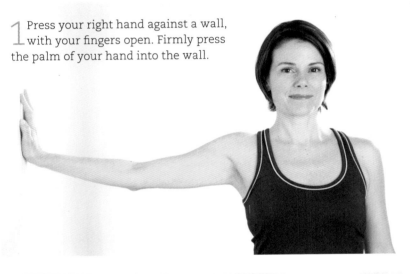

2 Slowly bring the tip of your right shoulder blade forwards, turning your head to the left, until you feel a stretch in your arm.

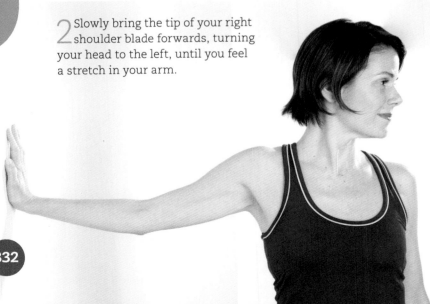

Muscle strengthener

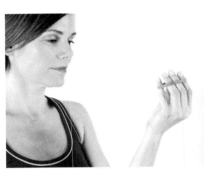

1 Place a thick rubber band around your slightly separated fingertips, near the top.

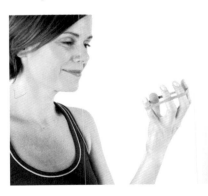

2 Slowly spread your fingers, then close them, keeping a steady resistance against the rubber band.

332

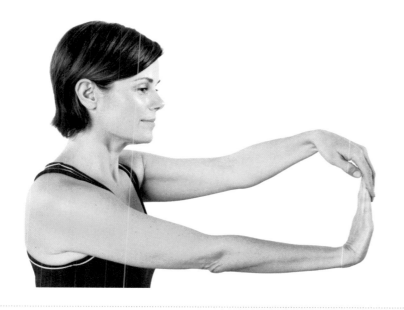

Wrist extender

Hold your right arm out in front of you with your elbow straight. Use your left hand to gently pull back from the base of your fingers until you feel a stretch in the bottom of your forearm. Ultimately your wrist should be bent at a 90-degree angle so your fingers point straight up. Repeat with the left arm.

Fist flex

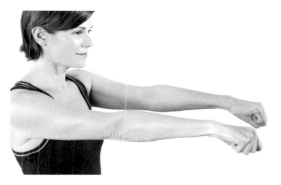

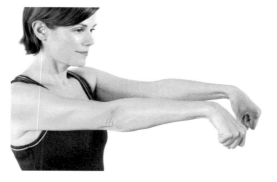

1 Hold your arms straight out in front of you, then make fists with your hands and squeeze as tightly as you can.

2 Keeping your hands in fists, bend your wrists down at a 90-degree angle.

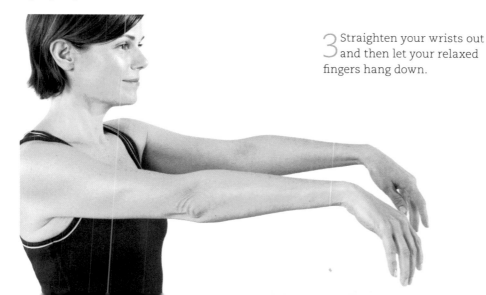

3 Straighten your wrists out and then let your relaxed fingers hang down.

Joint strength

These moves strengthen key muscles that act as shock absorbers for the joints in your legs and arms, helping to protect you against arthritis (page 104) and many types of injury. Ask your doctor if this programme is right for you, then start with 500g weights and an exercise band. Exercise for 10 minutes three times a week. As you become stronger, do more repetitions, increase the weight and switch to an exercise band with greater resistance.

Helpful for...
Arthritis see page 104
Foot problems see page 186
Knee pain see page 246
Osteoporosis see page 268

Calf strengthener

Stand facing a chair back or table with your feet a few centimetres apart and hold on to the chair or table for balance. Rise onto the balls of your feet, then lower. Repeat until your calves feel tired. If this becomes easy after a few weeks, add weight: use a small backpack with a 2kg weight in it (such as a dumbbell). To make it even harder, do the exercise (without the backpack or weight) standing on one leg only.

Foot builder

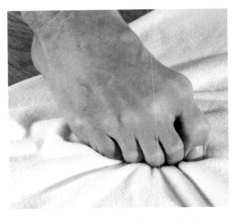

Spread a hand towel in front of a chair. Sit down and put one bare foot near the back edge of the towel. Keeping your heel on the towel, use your toes to gather the fabric and pull it under your foot. Keep going until you've gathered all you can. Repeat with your other foot.

Quadriceps toner

1 Sit on the floor with your left leg straight in front of you and your right leg bent. You can support your back by sitting against a wall or by putting your hands slightly behind you.

2 Keeping your abdominal muscles tight, lift your left leg off the floor. Hold for 3 seconds. Lower and repeat until your leg feels tired. Switch legs and repeat.

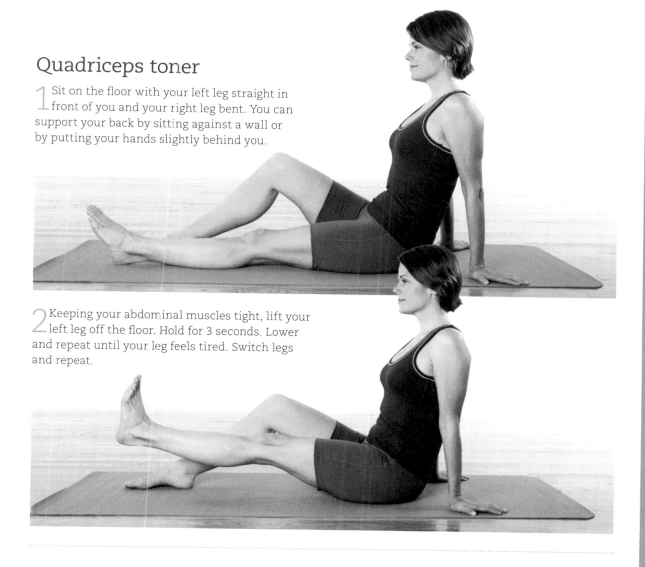

Hip flexor builder

1 Lie on your back on the floor, bend your right knee, keeping your right foot on the floor.

2 Tighten the quadriceps muscle in your left thigh, turn your leg outward slightly and raise it as far as you can (but not above your right knee). Lower and repeat until the muscle feels tired. Switch legs and repeat.

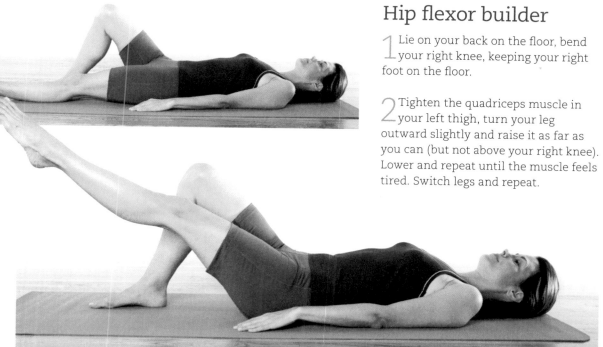

Hamstring builder

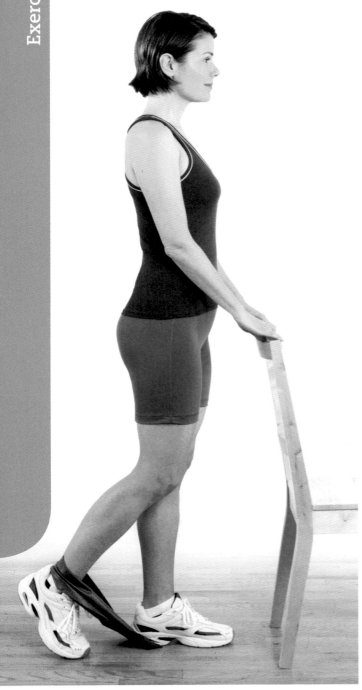
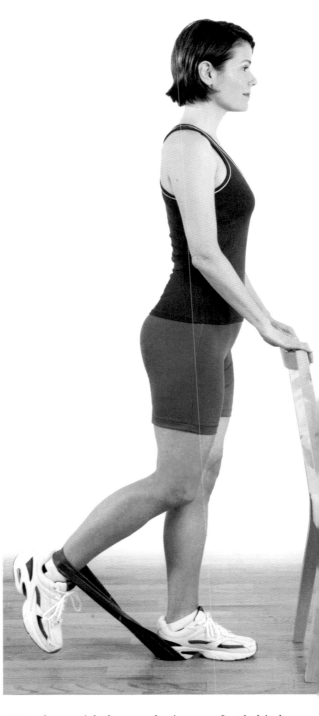

1 Knot an exercise band to make a medium-sized loop. Stand facing a table or sturdy chair that you can use for support. Put one end of the loop under your left foot and the other around your right ankle.

2 Bend your right knee and raise your foot behind you, pulling against the resistance of the band. Keep your abdominal muscles tight and don't let your back arch. Repeat until the back of your thigh feels tired, then switch sides.

Shoulder mobiliser

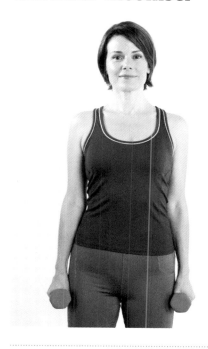

1 Stand and hold a pair of lightweight dumbbells (start with 500g weights) at your sides.

2 Keeping your arms straight, shrug your shoulders upwards, then relax. Repeat 20 times.

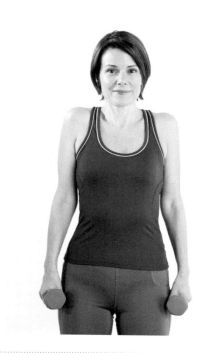

Shoulder strengthener

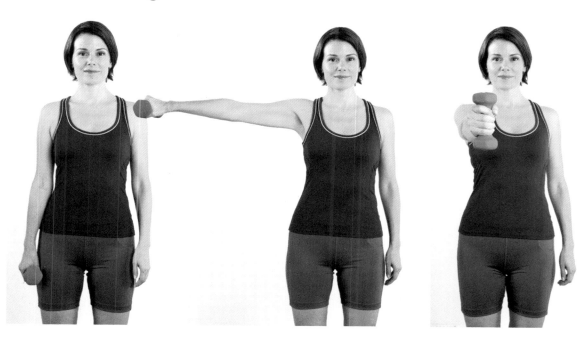

Hold a dumbbell in your right hand, with your arm down at your side. Lift the weight straight out to the side then rotate your elbow joint and swing it slowly out in front of you as far as you comfortably can. Slowly swing your arm back to the side. Repeat five to ten times, then switch hands.

Neck strength and flexibility

Often, pain in the neck area (see page 262) is related to unconsciously tensing your neck, particularly when you're spending hours at the computer or in the car. Next time you're online playing Scrabble, or sitting and knitting for hours at a time, or if you're at your desk feeling stressed (see page 306), remind yourself to do these easy stretching exercises to relieve the tension and to help keep your neck supple. You can strengthen your neck simply by resisting all these motions with your hand.

Helpful for...
Headaches see page 200
Stress-related disorders see page 306

Neck rotation

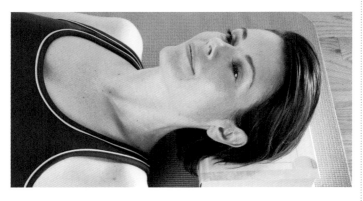

1 Lie on the floor with a large, thick book under your head.

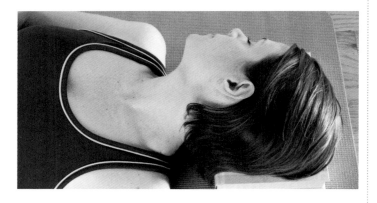

2 Slowly turn your head to one side and hold in that position for 10 to 20 seconds. Repeat on each side three to five times.

Forward tilt

Sit straight. Gently tug your chin down onto your chest and then tilt your head forwards as far as it will go. Hold for 10 seconds, then return to the starting position. Repeat five times.

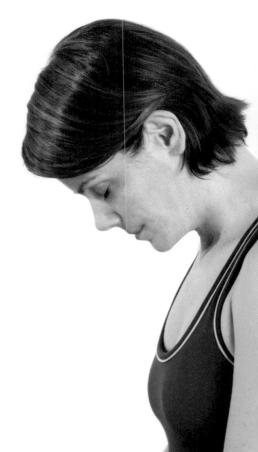

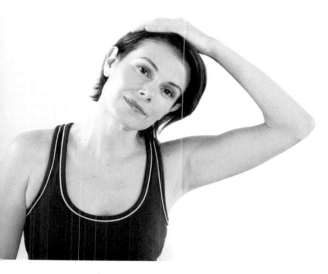

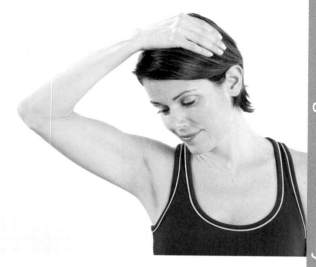

Side stretch

Stand or sit straight and hold the right side of your head with your left hand. Let your right arm hang loosely at your side. Slowly pull your head to the left until you feel a gentle stretch in your neck. Hold for 10 seconds, then repeat on the other side.

Diagonal stretch

Stand or sit straight and hold the left side of the top of your head with your right hand. Let your left arm hang loosely at your side. Slowly pull your head to the right and down, stopping when you feel a gentle stretch on the left side of your neck. Hold for 10 seconds, then repeat on the other side.

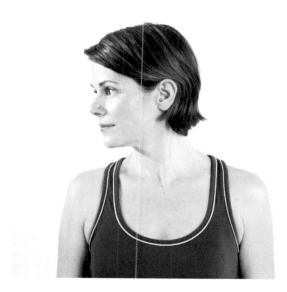

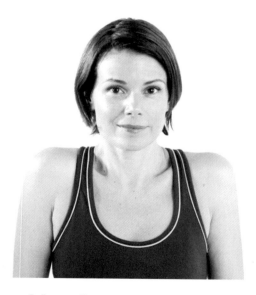

Side tilt

Sit straight and turn your head to the right as far as it will go. Gently tilt your head forwards until you feel the stretch. Hold for 10 seconds, then return to the starting position. Repeat five times on each side.

Shoulder shrug

Stand or sit straight and raise your shoulders up towards your ears until you feel slight tension in your neck and shoulders. Hold for 5 seconds, then roll your shoulders down and relax. Repeat five times.

Index

X, Y, Z

Acknowledgements

Picture credits

Front cover and spine Getty Images/Simon Stanmore, cover design by Conorde Clarke; **2-3** Getty Images/Sam Edwards; **4** Getty Images/Ryan McVay; **5** Getty Images/Dougal Waters; **6** Getty Images/Peter Cade; **7** Getty Images/Rob Melnychuk; **8-9** Getty Images/Dougal Waters; **10** Getty Images/Assembly; **12** Getty Images/James and James; **14** Getty Images/Thomas Schmidt; **16** Getty Images/Floresco Productions; **20** Getty Images/Richard Kolker; **22-33** © Bryan Christie Design; **34** Getty Images/LWA; **60** Getty Images/Sam Edwards; **63** Getty Images/Fuse; **64** iStockphoto.com/Lauri Patterson; **66** iStockphoto.com/Nick Garrad; **68** Getty Images/Fuse; **71** Getty Images/Ian Hooton/SPL; **72** iStockphoto.com/Elena Elisseeva; **75** Getty Images/Paul Grand Image; **77** Getty Images/Moment; **78** Getty Images/Max Oppenheim; **81** ShutterStock, Inc/Tihis; **82** © Reader's Digest; **84** iStockphoto.com/Henrik Larsson; **86** iStockphoto.com/Peter Dazeley; **90-91** Getty Images/Peter Cade; **322-323** Getty Images/Rob Melnychuk; **324-329** © Reader's Digest/Jill Wachter

Disease Free

Published in 2012 in the United Kingdom by Vivat Direct Limited (t/a Reader's Digest), 157 Edgware Road, London W2 2HR.

Disease Free is owned and under licence from
The Reader's Digest Association, Inc.
All rights reserved.

Copyright © 2012 The Reader's Digest Association, Inc.
Copyright © 2012 The Reader's Digest Association Far East Limited
Philippines Copyright © 2012 Reader's Digest Association Far East Limited
Copyright © 2012 Reader's Digest (Australia) Pty Limited
Copyright © 2012 Reader's Digest India Pvt Limited
Copyright © 2012 Reader's Digest Asia Pvt Limited

Adapted from *Disease Free* published by Reader's Digest (Australia) in 2010 and The Reader's Digest Association, Inc. in 2009

Reader's Digest is a trademark owned and under licence from the United States Patent and Trademark Office and in other countries throughout the world.
All rights reserved.

All rights reserved. No part of this book may be reproduced, stored in a retrieval system, or transmitted in any form or by any means, electronic, electrostatic, magnetic tape, mechanical, photocopying, recording or otherwise, without permission in writing from the publishers.

We are committed both to the quality of our products and the service we provide to our customers. We value your comments, so please do contact us on 0871 351 1000 or visit our website at www.readersdigest.co.uk

If you have any comments or suggestions about the content of our books, email us at gbeditorial@readersdigest.co.uk

PROJECT TEAM
Project editor Rachel Warren Chadd
Editor Cathy Meeus
Art editor Hugh Schermuly
Writer Jane Garton
Researcher Angelika Romacker
Proofreader Maureen Kincaid Speller
Indexer Marie Lorimer

FOR VIVAT DIRECT
Editorial director Julian Browne
Art director Anne-Marie Bulat
Managing editor Nina Hathway
Picture resource manager Sarah Stewart-Richardson
Pre-press technical manager Dean Russell
Product production manager Claudette Bramble
Senior production controller Jan Bucil

ISBN 978-1-78020-015-6
Concept code US4927/G
Book code 400-399-UP0000-1

Colour origination by FMG
Printed and bound in China